D1395753

SPORTS MEDICINE
AND ARTHROSCOPY

REVIEW
OF
SPORTS MEDICINE
AND ARTHROSCOPY

MARK D. MILLER, MD

Major, USAF MC
Clinical Assistant Professor of Surgery
Uniformed Services University of the Health Sciences
Bethesda, Maryland
Associate Team Physician
Department of Orthopaedic Surgery
US Air Force Academy Hospital/SGHST
USAF Academy, Colorado

DANIEL E. COOPER, MD

Head Team Physician, Dallas Stars Hockey Club
Assistant Team Physician, Dallas Cowboys Football Club
WB Carroll Memorial Clinic, Associated
Dallas, Texas

JON J.P. WARNER, MD

Assistant Professor of Orthopaedic Surgery
University of Pittsburgh School of Medicine
Orthopaedic and Arthroscopic Surgery
University Orthopaedics, Inc.
Center for Sports Medicine and Rehabilitation
Pittsburgh, Pennsylvania

Suzanne Merrick Edmonds

Medical Illustrator

W.B. SAUNDERS COMPANY

A Division of Harcourt Brace & Company

Philadelphia/London/Toronto/Montreal/Sydney/Tokyo

W.B. SAUNDERS COMPANY
A Division of Harcourt Brace & Company

The Curtis Center
Independence Square West
Philadelphia, Pennsylvania 19106

Library of Congress Cataloging-in-Publication Data
Review of sports medicine and arthroscopy / [edited by] Mark D.
   Miller, Daniel E. Cooper, Jon J.P. Warner ; Suzanne Merrick Edmonds,
   medical illustrator. — 1st ed.

    p.   cm.

    ISBN 0-7216-5281-6

    1. Sports injuries.   2. Arthroscopy.   I. Miller, Mark D.
II. Cooper, Daniel E.   III. Warner, Jon J. P.
    [DNLM: 1. Sports Medicine. 2. Arthroscopy—methods.   QT 260 R454
1995]
    RD97.R49 1995
    617.1'027—dc20

DNLM/DLC   94-22156

Review of Sports Medicine and Arthroscopy   ISBN 0-7216-5281-6

Printed in the United States of America

Last digit is the print number: 9   8   7   6   5   4   3   2   1

To my loving wife, Brenda,
for putting up with yet another "project."

MDM

In loving memory of my special son, Chad Thomas Cooper.
His short life continues to inspire me
and keeps all of this in clear perspective.

DEC

To the women in my life:
my wife, Geraldine;
my grandmother, Dr. Marie;
my mother, Dr. Gloria;
my sister, Lynn;
Elizabeth and Monica;
and my three daughters, Brooke, Lauren, and Christina.

JJPW

Foreword

The combination of increased leisure time and an emphasis on exercise as a means of improving health has led to participation in sports, from gymnastics programs in early childhood to the Senior Olympics. This increased participation has led to an increased incidence of injury.

Although many medical specialties strive to participate in the care of athletes, orthopaedic surgeons have the longest and the most colorful history of participation in sports medicine. Beginning in the 1960s, a few senior orthopaedic surgeons with an interest in sports medicine opened their practices to young orthopaedic surgeons who wished to obtain training in the new subspecialty of sports medicine. These early fellowships were the beginning of orthopaedic sports medicine as a subspecialty. Today, there are over 100 fellowships available for postgraduate training in orthopaedic sports medicine. It is appropriate that Drs. Miller, Cooper, and Warner, all products of these postgraduate fellowship training programs, should produce this excellent review of sports medicine and arthroscopy.

The authors have very carefully produced a concise review of the accepted principles of practice in sports medicine and arthroscopy combined with an excellent up-to-date bibliography of the pertinent sports medicine literature. This text will become "the Bible" for those involved in the medical care of the athlete. Its wide coverage will allow it to be used not only by orthopaedic surgeons but also by all medical and allied health personnel involved in the care of the athlete.

The authors are to be congratulated for producing an excellent book that is easy to read, simple to reference, and detailed in scope. The main purpose of the book is to provide improved care for athletes at all levels of participation. Its simplicity and comprehensiveness permit this with ease.

Jesse C. DeLee, MD
Associate Clinical Professor
  of Orthopaedics
Director, University of
  Texas Health Science
  Center at San Antonio
San Antonio, Texas

Preface

In the tradition of *Review of Orthopaedics,* we have written this book to summarize the state of the art of sports medicine and arthroscopy. Despite the large volume of new textbooks, journals, courses, and special examinations for sports medicine, or perhaps because of it, there appears to be much confusion within the orthopaedic community on even the basic principles of arthroscopy and treatment of sports-related injuries. We have attempted to distill the overwhelming amount of literature from this rapidly evolving subspecialty into a concise, easy-to-follow format. We have drawn extensively from our sports medicine fellowship experiences and from the work of others and we greatly acknowledge our mentors.

Review of Sports Medicine and Arthroscopy is intended for the orthopaedic surgeon with a special interest in sports medicine. We hope that it will serve as both a curriculum guide for sports medicine fellowship programs and a source of information for all orthopaedic surgeons who treat athletes, from the school playground to the professional level. Sports medicine and arthroscopy is a relatively new and exciting subspecialty in orthopaedics. We hope that the reader shares our passion and enthusiasm for our field.

Mark D. Miller, MD
Daniel E. Cooper, MD
Jon J.P. Warner, MD

Contents

I

Lower Extremity

CHAPTER 1

Knee

I. Basic Sciences
  A. Anatomy—Studies of knee kinematics reveal that the knee is much more than a simple hinge type joint, because its motion consists of both rolling and gliding components. A complex array of ligaments, menisci, capsular structures, and musculature must be fully appreciated in order to adequately address pathology of the knee.
   1. Ligaments—Four major ligaments and a number of supporting ligaments and structures make up the knee. The four major ligaments—the anterior cruciate ligament (ACL), posterior cruciate ligament (PCL), medial collateral ligament (MCL), and lateral collateral ligament (LCL)—are addressed in this section, and other ligaments are later addressed on the basis of their location.
    a. Anterior Cruciate Ligament—This ligament has been the subject of intensive research; nevertheless, many differences of opinion regarding the anatomy and function of this ligament remain. The tibial insertion of the ACL is a broad, irregular, diamond-shaped area located directly in front of the intercondylar eminence of the tibia. The femoral attachment of the ligament is a semicircular area on the posteromedial aspect of the lateral femoral condyle (Fig. 1–1). The ACL is approximately 33 mm in length and 11 mm in diameter. Most authorities suggest that the ACL is composed of two "bundles" or portions, but the distinction is based more on function than on anatomy. The anteromedial bundle of the ACL is tight in flexion, and the posterolateral part is tight in extension. The ligament is composed of approximately 90% type I collagen and 10% type III collagen. The ligament's blood supply is primarily from the middle geniculate artery and fat pad (supplied by the inferior medial and lateral geniculate arteries). Mechanoreceptor nerve endings have been identified in the ACL, and they are thought to have a proprioceptive role.
    b. Posterior Cruciate Ligament—Although studies of this ligament lag behind those of the ACL, the PCL has become a popular research subject. The ligament inserts in a sulcus posteriorly, below the articular surface of the tibia, and originates in a broad half-moon or crescent shape anterolaterally on the medial femoral condyle (see Fig. 1–1). The PCL is approximately 38 mm in length and 13 mm in diameter. Like the ACL, the PCL is generally believed to be made up of two components, an anterolateral and a posteromedial portion; some investigators suggest that it has three components. The anterolateral part of the ligament is tight in flexion, and the posteromedial part is tight in extension. Two variable meniscofemoral ligaments may also contribute to the PCL. These ligaments originate from the posterior horn of the lateral meniscus and become intimately associated with the PCL fibers. The anterior meniscofemoral ligament (Humphry) inserts anterior to the PCL, and the posterior meniscofemoral ligament (Wrisberg) inserts posterior to the PCL (Fig. 1–2). Although it has not been studied as extensively as the ACL, the neurovascular supply to the PCL is similar to that of the ACL.
    c. Medial Collateral Ligament—The MCL is a broad, flat ligament composed of separate superficial and deep portions. The superficial MCL (tibial collateral ligament) lies deep to the gracilis and semitendinosus tendons and fascia. This ligament originates at the medial femoral epicondyle and inserts distally into the periosteum of the proximal tibia, with its primary insertion deep to the pes anserinus. Functionally, the superficial MCL appears to have two components. The anterior fibers tighten during the first 90° of motion, whereas the posterior fibers tighten in extension. The deep MCL (middle capsular ligament) is actually a capsular thickening

3

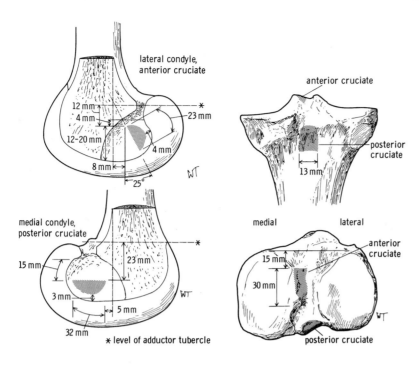

FIGURE 1–1. Origins and insertions of the ACL and PCL. (From Girgis FG, Marxhall JL, Al Monajem ARS. The cruciate ligaments of the knee joint; anatomical, functional and experimental analysis. Clin Orthop 106:216–231, 1975.)

that blends with the superficial fibers at its insertion on the tibia. The deep MCL is often considered to consist of two components based on their proximal-distal relationships: the meniscofemoral ligament (not to be confused with the ligaments of Humphry and Wrisberg) and the meniscotibial (coronary) ligament.

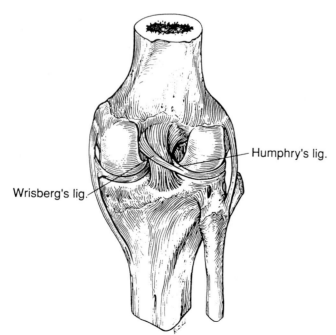

FIGURE 1–2. The relationships between the PCL and the menisco-femoral ligaments (Humphry and Wrisberg). (From Tria AJ, Klein KS. *An Illustrated Guide to the Knee.* New York: Churchill Livingstone, 1992.)

d. Lateral Collateral Ligament—The LCL (fibular collateral ligament) is a cord-like structure that originates on the lateral femoral epicondyle posterior and superior to the popliteus tendon and inserts on the lateral aspect of the fibular head. Because it is located behind the axis of rotation, the LCL is tightest in extension and relaxes in flexion.

e. Ligament Ultrastructure—Like all ligaments, the ligaments of the knee are composed primarily of type I collagen with variable amounts of elastin and reticulin. The "crimp" or sinusoidal pattern collagen that makes up the cruciate ligaments has less amplitude than that of the MCL. Additionally, the width of the MCL collagen bundles is about three times that of the ACL. Electron microscopy studies have confirmed that the MCL has more collagen fibers per unit area than the ACL. Quantitative electron microscopy of the cruciate and meniscofemoral ligaments was recently reported in a study by Marks and colleagues. In this study of young fresh-frozen cadaver ligaments, the mean collagen fibril cross-sectional area was found to vary with location:

CROSS-SECTIONAL AREA (nm^2)

Ligament	Proximal	Central	Distal
ACL	3016	5623	5871
PCL	8546	5382	3690
MCL	10,044	12,437	9181

TRANSAXIAL PLANE JOINT LINE

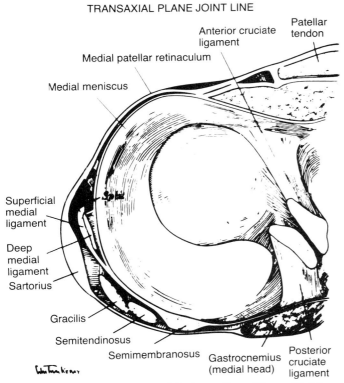

FIGURE 1–3. Medial structures of the knee. (From Warren LF, Marshall JL. The supporting structures and layers of the medial side of the knee. J Bone Joint Surg 61A:56–62, 1979.)

Thus, the ACL enlarges as it courses toward its tibial insertion, and the PCL narrows as it courses toward its tibial insertion.

2. Medial Structures—The medial aspect of the knee is composed of three layers (Fig. 1–3):

Layer	Components
I	Sartorius and sartorial fascia
II	Superficial MCL, posterior oblique ligament, semimembranosus
III	Deep MCL/capsule

The gracilis and semitendinosus tendons as well as the saphenous nerve run between layers I and II. Layers I and II blend anteriorly, and layers II and III blend posteriorly. Dissection between these planes can be limited in these regions.

3. Lateral Structures—The lateral aspect of the knee can also be considered in three layers, although they are less consistent and less well defined than on the medial side (Fig. 1–4):

Layer	Components
I	Lateral fascia, iliotibial tract, biceps tendon
II	Patellar retinaculum, patellofemoral ligament
III	Capsule, LCL, arcuate ligament, fabellofibular ligament

The deep layer may not be discrete in the posterolateral corner of the knee. The arcuate ligament, the LCL, the popliteus, the fabellofibular ligament, the popliteofibular fibers, and the lateral head of the gastrocnemius all contribute to the complex arrangement of the posterolateral corner of the knee. Within layer III, the inferior lateral geniculate artery is deep to the LCL and is vulnerable during aggressive meniscal resection. Posterior structures of the knee are shown in Figure 1–5.

FIGURE 1–4. Lateral structures of the knee. (From Seebacher JR, Inglis AE, Marshall JL, Warren RF. The structure of the posterolateral aspect of the knee. J Bone Joint Surg 64A:536–541, 1982.)

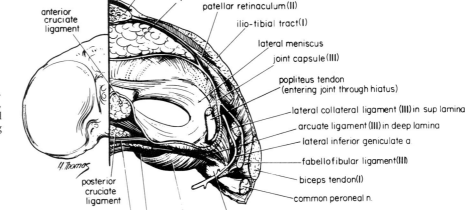

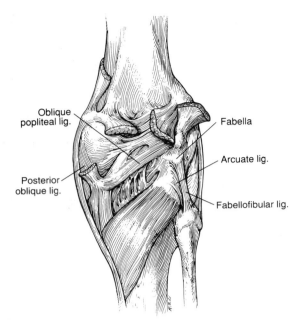

FIGURE 1–5. Relationships of the posterior aspect of the knee. (From Tria AJ, Klein KS. *An Illustrated Guide to the Knee.* New York: Churchill Livingstone, 1992.)

4. Menisci—These crescent-shaped structures are triangular in cross section, tapering to a thin free edge centrally. The menisci are attached peripherally via coronary ligaments, except at the popliteal hiatus (lateral meniscus). Only the peripheral portions of the menisci (20–30% of the medial meniscus and 10–25% of the lateral meniscus) are vascularized, primarily from the medial and lateral genicular arteries. The lateral meniscus is also less vascular in the area of the popliteal hiatus. The medial meniscus is more C shaped, whereas the lateral meniscus forms an incomplete circle or "O" (Fig. 1–6). The transverse (or intermeniscal) ligament connects the menisci anteriorly. The menisci deepen the articular surfaces of the tibial plateau and thus aid in load transmission, reduce stress on articular surfaces, contribute to joint stability, and aid in lubrication and chondral nutrition in the knee.
5. Patellofemoral Joint—The patella, the largest sesamoid bone in the body, articulates with the femoral sulcus and serves as a fulcrum for the quadriceps muscles. The surface of the patella is divided into two large facets—medial and lateral—that are separated by a median ridge. The medial facet varies anatomically and is sometimes divided into a medial facet proper and a small odd facet. This odd facet may develop as a response to functional loads and does not contact the medial femoral condyle except in extreme degrees

of flexion. The variable sizes of the facets have been described by Wiberg, with a type I patella designating medial/lateral facet equality and greater numbers signifying lateral facet predominance. The trochlear surface has also been classified on the basis of the relative sizes of the medial and lateral portions. Because several ossification centers contribute to the patella, failure of fusion (most often involving the superolateral corner [type III] but sometimes involving the inferior [type I] or lateral patella [type II]) can lead to a bipartite patella. The articular cartilage of the patella is the thickest in the body, and the patella is said to be exposed to forces several times body weight. Numerous pathologic entities exist. The term *chondromalacia* is a pathologic description and should not be used as a wastebasket diagnosis for anterior knee pain. Further discussion of these disorders and a guide to subclassification by specific diagnosis follow.

B. Biomechanics—The primary role of the ligaments of the knee is to provide passive restraint to abnormal motion. The ACL is the primary restraint (85%) to anterior translation of the tibia relative to the femur. The PCL serves as the primary restraint (95%) against posterior tibial displacement. Both of these ligaments also serve to regulate the "screw-home" mechanism of the knee (external rotation of the tibia with terminal extension). The MCL, particularly its superficial portion, serves as the primary restraint to valgus angulation. The LCL is then the primary restraint to varus angulation. Both the MCL and the LCL also serve in concert with their

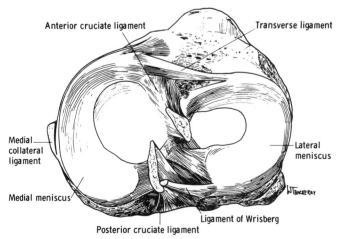

FIGURE 1–6. The shape and relationships of the menisci. (From Warren R, Arnoczky SP, Wickiewicz TL. Anatomy of the knee. In Nicholas JA, Hershman EB [eds]. *The Lower Extremity and Spine in Sports Medicine.* St Louis: CV Mosby, 1986, pp 657–694.)

surrounding posterior structures to control axial rotation of the tibia on the femur.

1. Structural Properties—The tensile strength of a ligament, or the maximum stress that a ligament can sustain before failure, has been characterized for the knee ligaments. In reviewing these studies, however, it is important to consider specimen preparation, age, orientation, and various other factors. The ACL has been reported to have an average tensile strength of 2160 N, and up to 2500 N in young individuals. Although the PCL is generally thought to have a higher tensile strength than the ACL, there is little agreement about the value. The MCL has approximately twice the stiffness and tensile strength of the ACL. The strength of the LCL has not yet been determined. Studies of ACL graft strengths originally reported strengths of approximately 160% of the ACL for a 14-mm patella tendon. A recent study in paired specimens found that the strength of a 10-mm patellar tendon graft averaged 2977 N (approximately 140% of the strength of the ACL). Rotation of the graft 90° increased the tensile strength of the grafts approximately 30%. Animal studies of patella tendon grafts in vivo suggest that the strength of the graft is diminished to 20% of its original value at 6 weeks, and some studies suggest that the graft strength remains <50% at 1 year. However, postmortem analysis of a human graft at 8 months postoperatively demonstrated a tensile strength of 87% of the ACL.

2. Kinematics—The study of knee motion has led to a better understanding of the function of knee ligaments. The four-bar cruciate linkage system has been described to explain the flexion-extension kinematic principles of the knee (Fig. 1–7). This model clarifies the interaction of the ligaments and the central role of the ACL in knee kinematics. As the knee flexes, the instantaneous center of joint rotation (point of intersection of the cruciate ligaments and PCL "links") moves posteriorly during knee flexion, forcing a combination of rolling and gliding to occur between the articulating surfaces. The concept of ligament isometry and its application to the clinical setting remain controversial. Ideally, ligaments (intact and reconstructed) should lie within the flexion axis in all positions of the joint to remain isometric. Ligaments anterior to the flexion axis stretch as the joint flexes, and ligaments posterior to the axis shorten. Various techniques and instruments have been developed in order to achieve

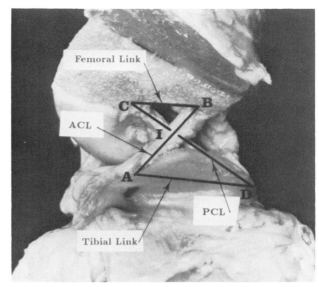

FIGURE 1–7. The four-bar linkage consists of the ACL (AB), the PCL (CD), the femoral link (CB), and the tibial link (AD). (From The geometry of the knee in the sagittal plane. Proc Inst Mech Engin., Vol 20-1989. Part H: J Eng Med, pp. 225–233. Reprinted with permission from the Institution of Mechanical Engineers, London.)

isometry; however, more practical considerations, such as graft impingement and avoiding flexion contracture formation, may be more important.

3. Meniscal Biomechanics—The collagen fibers of the menisci are arranged both radially and circumferentially (Fig. 1–8). The circumferential fibers help dissipate the hoop stress in the menisci, and the combination of fibers allows the meniscus to expand under compressive forces and increase the contact area of the joint. Through full knee flexion/extension, the lateral meniscus has an anteroposterior excursion of approximately 11 mm. That is more than twice the excursion of the

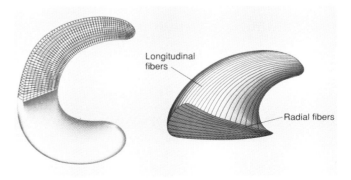

FIGURE 1–8. Longitudinal (circumferential) and radial fibers of the menisci. (From Tria AJ, Klein KS. *An Illustrated Guide to the Knee.* New York: Churchill Livingstone, 1992.)

medial meniscus. The lateral meniscus is also displaced more than the medial meniscus with rotation. Studies have shown that ACL deficiency may result in abnormal meniscal strain, particularly in the posterior horn of the medial meniscus.

II. History and Physical Examination
   A. History—A complete history and clarification of the mechanism of injury set the stage for an accurate diagnosis.
      1. Age-Related Injuries—Certain knee problems and injuries are more common in specific age groups. Adolescent females often complain of anterior knee pain. Younger patients with traumatic injuries often have meniscal tears and ligament injuries, whereas older patients may have degenerative conditions.
      2. Mechanism of Injury—Careful questioning often elucidates the exact cause and position of the knee with an injury. Cutting maneuvers associated with a "pop" with acute onset of swelling are highly associated with ACL tears. Twisting injuries, with moderate swelling, loss of motion, and late mechanical symptoms, are more suggestive of meniscal tears. Dashboard injuries can imply a PCL tear. High-speed accidents are often associated with multiple ligament injuries. Direct trauma to the anterior knee is commonly elicited in patients with patellar injuries. The position of the foot during the injury can be important. A direct blow to the anterior knee with the foot dorsiflexed typically results in patellar injuries; however, a similar force with the foot plantarflexed may result in a PCL injury. Symptoms of "giving way" do not necessarily implicate the ACL, because patients with patellar subluxation or dislocation, as well as individuals with meniscal or chondral flap tears, often have similar complaints. Although somewhat controversial, artificial turf playing surfaces may be associated with a greater number of anterior cruciate ligament injuries, particularly with special teams play in football. A discrete injury often cannot be elicited, and overuse conditions, such as tendinitis, must be considered.
   B. Physical Examination
      1. Observation—Assessment of varus/valgus alignment, leg length discrepancies, and other abnormalities is accomplished first. The feet should be checked for pes planus, because this can be associated with knee symptoms. A careful analysis of gait is also important, but this may not always be possible with acute injuries. A medial or lateral thrust (tibial translation and angular displacement that occurs during the stance phase of gait) may imply chronic posterolateral or posteromedial injury (Fig. 1–9). Pain or inability to squat fully can imply meniscal injury or arthritis. Skin integrity, ecchymoses, erythema, effusion, and patellar positions are also noted.
      2. Range of Motion—Both the injured and the normal knee are checked for motion (normal 0–135° ±5°). Thigh circumference is also measured at a level above the suprapatellar pouch (8–10 cm). Active motion is tested to evaluate the knee for an extensor lag. Range of motion is recorded as extension (hyperextension is recorded with a minus sign) and flexion (e.g., −10 to 135°).
      3. Palpation—An effusion is checked by ballottement of the patella onto the femoral groove or by squeezing the suprapatellar portion of the knee with one hand and attempting to displace fluid across the knee with the other hand. With practice, the amount of fluid can be measured.
      4. Stability Assessment—Straight instability, usually from an isolated injury, is best evidenced by laxity to stress testing in a single plane. Combined injuries demonstrate laxity to stress testing in more than one plane. Demonstration of rotatory instabilities requires special testing. All traumatic knee injuries should be evaluated with a systematic approach to stress the knee in each of its six degrees of freedom (three planes of translation): flexion, extension, varus, valgus, internal,

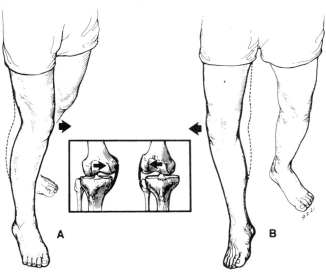

FIGURE 1–9. Medial thrust (*A*) and lateral thrust (*B*) are designated based on the movement of the femur in the coronal plane. (From Tria AJ, Klein KS. *An Illustrated Guide to the Knee.* New York: Churchill Livingstone, 1992.)

and external rotation. A systematic approach, within the limits of a patient's comfort, involves an assessment of active and passive range of motion, varus/valgus testing at 0° and 30° anterior/posterior testing at 30° and 90° (Lachman and drawer tests), and testing for rotatory translation (pivot shift, flexion-rotation drawer, rotation at 30° and 90° of knee flexion).

a. Varus and Valgus Instability—Evaluation of the integrity of the medial and lateral structures is carried out with varus stressing (tests lateral structures) and valgus stressing (tests medial structures) at 0° and 30° extension (Fig. 1–10). Opening at 30° of flexion only (no instability in full extension) is consistent with an isolated collateral ligament injury. As with all ligament injuries, the amount of excursion is determined and is graded on the basis of the following criteria:

Grade	Amount of Opening	Associated Tear
I	0–5 mm	Minimal
II	5–10 mm	Moderate
III	>10 mm	Complete

It is important to note that a difference exists between the "grade" of laxity and the "grade" of ligament injury. Knee position is critical, because isolated collateral ligament injuries are associated with varus/valgus laxity at 30° of knee flexion but with *no* laxity at 0° of flexion. Opening at both 30° and 0° extension is consistent with an injury to both the collateral ligament and other structures. Valgus laxity at 0° implies injury to the posteromedial capsule and an injury to

the PCL and possibly the ACL. Varus laxity (<5° opening) at 0° can be associated with isolated LCL injury; however, greater degrees of laxity are usually associated with combined LCL and posterolateral capsular injuries. Significant varus laxity (>10° opening) at 0° is usually associated with concomitant PCL injury.

b. Anterior Instability—Anterior translation can be evaluated with the knee partially flexed (Lachman) or flexed 90° (drawer). *The Lachman test is the most sensitive examination for assessing the integrity of the ACL, especially in an acute setting.* With the knee flexed approximately 20° to 30°, the examiner's hands are placed on the anterior leg and thigh and the tibia is translated anteriorly (Fig. 1–11). The amount of displacement and the *quality of the endpoint* is recorded. A side-to-side difference of >3 mm is considered pathologic. The *anterior drawer* test is also useful in evaluating the status of the ACL but is less reliable than the Lachman. This test is performed with the knee flexed 90°. The greatest utility of the test is with rotating the position of the foot, allowing assessment of rotatory instability (discussed later).

c. Posterior Instability—As with anterior instability, posterior translation can be evaluated with the knee in various degrees of flexion. *The most sensitive test for detecting isolated PCL injuries is the posterior drawer.* This test, similar to the anterior drawer, is accomplished with the patient supine and the knee flexed 90° (Fig. 1–12). The key to this examination

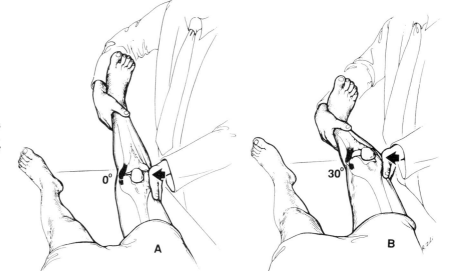

FIGURE 1–10. Varus and valgus stress testing is performed at both 0° (*A*) and 30° (*B*) of flexion. (From Tria AJ, Klein KS. *An Illustrated Guide to the Knee.* New York: Churchill Livingstone, 1992.)

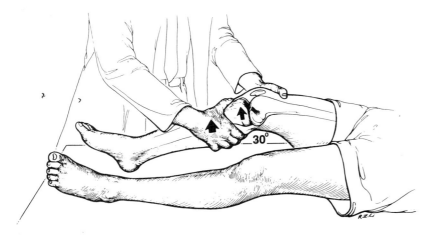

FIGURE 1–11. The Lachman test, which is the most sensitive test for acute ACL injuries, is performed with the knee in 30° of flexion. (From Tria AJ, Klein KS. *An Illustrated Guide to the Knee*. New York: Churchill Livingstone, 1992.)

is accurately assessing the starting point. With a PCL injury, the tibia is posteriorly displaced and the normal "step off" between the medial femoral condyle and the anterior edge of the medial tibial plateau is absent. In fact, some authorities have suggested that the step off should be graded as follows:

Step Off	Instability
+10 mm	0 (normal)
+ 5 mm	1 (mild)
0 mm (flush)	2 (moderate)
− 5 mm or more	3 (severe)

Failure to appreciate this sometimes subtle point may result in a misdiagnosis, one of incorrectly attributing the laxity to an ACL injury. This mistake can be compounded by failing to appreciate the normal ACL "pseudolaxity" during arthroscopic visualization of this ligament in a patient with a PCL injury. Placing an anterior force on the tibia reduces this pseudolaxity and results in a normal-appearing ACL. There is often a decrease in the amount of posterior translation with posterior

drawer testing with the foot in internal rotation because of tightening of the meniscofemoral ligaments (which are often not injured when the PCL is torn). Another test described for detecting PCL and posterolateral corner injury is the *posterior Lachman* (or posterior drawer at 30°) test; in this test, again, the step off is important. Both isolated PCL injury and isolated posterolateral corner injury can result in abnormal posterior translation at 30°.

   d. ACL deficiency—In addition to Lachman and drawer testing, various pivot tests have been described for chronically ACL-deficient knees. All of these tests are based on the fact that in extension or small degrees of flexion, anterior subluxation of the tibia is noted. With further flexion (20–40°), the posterior pull of the iliotibial tract reduces the tibia. The pivot shift has been shown to be due primarily to abnormal anterior translation and is not a rotational phenomenon, as many initially believed. The *pivot shift test* is helpful in assessing chronic ACL injuries and is most accu-

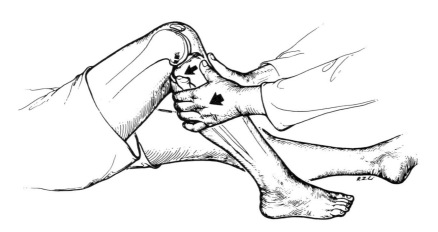

FIGURE 1–12. The posterior drawer test is the most accurate examination for isolated PCL injury. (From Tria AJ, Klein KS. *An Illustrated Guide to the Knee*. New York: Churchill Livingstone, 1992.)

rate with examination under anesthesia. This examination is performed with the patient supine and the leg extended. The foot is held in internal rotation, and a valgus stress is placed on the knee. Gradual flexion results in reduction of the tibia from the subluxed position, resulting in a "clunk" at approximately 20° to 30° of flexion (Fig. 1–13). The *pivot jerk* is a variation of the same test, except that the knee is extended from a flexed position and subluxes from a reduced position at approximately 30° of flexion, resulting in a jerk. The position of hip abduction and external rotation results in accentuation of the pivot phenomenon. Testing with the foot internally rotated, as originally described, is less sensitive but more specific for ACL deficiency. External rotation of the foot allows more sensitivity (good for screening) but is less specific.

e. PCL Deficiency—In addition to posterior drawer/Lachman testing, other tests may supplement the evaluation of the PCL-deficient knee. The *quadriceps active drawer test* involves anterior translation of the tibia with quadriceps contraction and is observed at 70° knee flexion. The *posterior sag sign* demonstrates increased posterior displacement of the tibia (as viewed from the side) with both the hip and knee flexed 90°.

f. Posterolateral Rotatory Instability—Various tests have been described for assessing posterolateral capsular injury. The *posterolateral drawer test* involves increased posterior translation of the tibia with drawer testing with the foot externally rotated. Additionally, with the foot held in neutral, the lateral side of the tibia moves posteriorly on the femur but the medial side of the tibia does not change its position relative to the femur. Some authorities have suggested that a posterior drawer that is more marked at 30° (posterior Lachman) than 90° suggests posterolateral rotatory instability as well. Results of the posterolateral drawer test are highly variable within the physiologic range and are difficult to quantify. The *external rotation recurvatum test* has also been described for detecting posterolateral laxity. This test is performed by simply raising both feet and determining if the knee falls into varus and hyperextension and the tibia rotates externally (Fig. 1–14). The external rotation recurvatum test is specific but very insensitive. Positive results are most marked in cases of combined ACL and posterolateral injury. The *reversed pivot shift test* is similar to the pivot shift test described earlier, except that the leg is held in external rotation and the knee is passively extended. The shift occurs at 20° to 30° of flexion as the posteriorly subluxated lateral side of the tibial plateau abruptly reduces. This test does not have high specificity, however, because an abnormal result can be elicited in otherwise normal knees, particularly during examination under anesthesia, which eliminates the active biceps contraction that can dampen the reversed pivot shift phenomenon. *Increased external rotation* with the knee flexed 30° or 90° has also been associated with posterolateral rotatory instability.

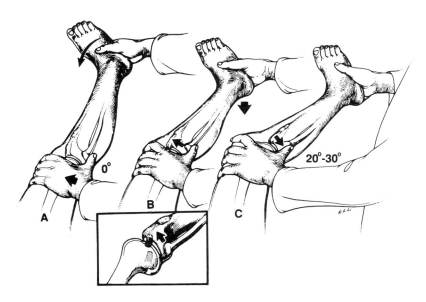

FIGURE 1–13. The pivot shift test is initiated in extension (*A*) and results in extension and reduction of the knee in 20° to 30° flexion (*C*). (From Tria AJ, Klein KS. *An Illustrated Guide to the Knee.* New York: Churchill Livingstone, 1992.)

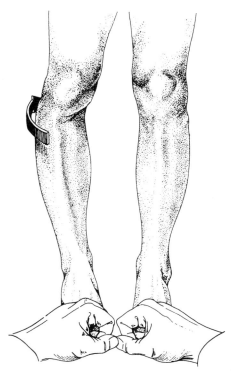

FIGURE 1–14. External rotation recurvatum test. Lifting the feet results in varus angulation, hyperextension, and external rotation of the tibia in patients with posterolateral instability. (From Hughston JC, Norwood LA Jr. The posterolateral drawer test and external rotational recurvatum test for posterolateral rotatory instability of the knee. Clin Orthop 147:85, 1980.)

g. Combined Ligament Injuries—Most cases of combined ligamentous injuries have instability in more than one plane. Combined ACL/PCL injuries have marked anteroposterior (AP) instability, much greater than that of isolated injuries. As implied earlier, a combined collateral ligament and capsular/PCL injury can be detected with varus/valgus instability in full extension.

5. Meniscal Examination—Careful palpation of the joint line may identify tenderness, localized swelling, or a meniscal cyst, all suggestive of meniscal tears. Pain is often exacerbated by hyperflexion. The *squat test*, variously described as asking a patient to squat repetitively or to "duck walk," often elicits symptoms or an inability to perform the test in patients with meniscal tears. The *McMurray* or *flexion-McMurray test* is also helpful in the diagnosis of meniscal tears. This test is performed with a patient supine and the hip and knee flexed (Fig. 1–15). Varus/valgus stress and tibial rotation while extending the knee may result in a palpable pop or click along the joint line in patients with meniscal tears, although complaints of pain with this maneuver can

also be helpful. Various other adjunctive tests such as the *Apley compression test* and the *Steinmann test* (brisk tibial rotation with the knee flexed) have also been described.

6. Patellofemoral Examination—With the patient supine, the patellar alignment and *Q-angle* (angle between the anterior superior iliac spine, patella, and tibial tubercle) are measured. An angle of <15° is generally considered normal. Some examiners prefer to assess the Q-angle with the knee flexed 90° (Fig. 1–16). Angles >8° with this measurement are strongly indicative of an abnormally lateralized distal patella vector. It is important to recognize that if the patella is subluxated, the Q-angle reverts to within the normal range. Patients should also be observed while they are sitting. High and lateral positioning of the patella ("grasshopper eyes"—the patellae appear to be looking up and over the shoulders of the examiner), small patella, patella alta (the patella faces the ceiling rather than straight ahead), dysplasia of the vastus medialis obliquus (proximal medial "hollow" area), and excessive hip anteversion should be noted. The patella is carefully examined with range of motion of the knee to determine if the patella deviates laterally in terminal extension (*J sign*). Palpation of the patella with range of motion may also detect *crepitation,* suggesting a possible chondral injury. Palpation of the patella may elicit pain, and lateral displacement may cause *apprehension* in patients with patellar

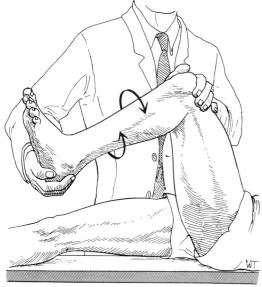

FIGURE 1–15. McMurray test. Note flexion of the hip and knee and rotation of the tibia. Note also the position of the fingers along the joint line. (From Insall JN. Examination of the knee. In Insall JN [ed]. *Surgery of the Knee.* New York: Churchill Livingstone, 1984, pp 55–72.)

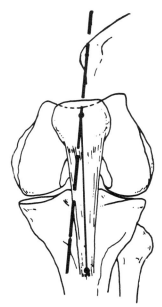

FIGURE 1–16. Quadriceps angle at 90° flexion. Values greater than 8° are consistent with a lateralized distal patella vector. (From Fulkerson JP, Kalenak A, Rosenberg TD, Cox JS. Patellofemoral pain. Instr Course Lect 41:57–71, 1992.)

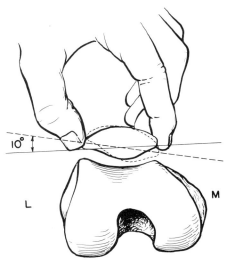

FIGURE 1–18. Patellar tilt is assessed based on a neutral position parallel to the horizontal plane (solid line). A negative tilt is associated with tightness of the lateral restraints. (From Fu FH, Maday MG. Arthroscopic lateral release and the lateral patellar compression syndrome. Orthop Clin North Am 23:601, 1992.)

instability. Measurement of patellar mobility or *glide* is based on the maximum amount of passive displacement (based on a quadrant system) both medially and laterally with the knee flexed 30° (Fig. 1–17). This test evaluates the integrity and tightness of the medial and lateral restraints. *Passive patellar tilt* allows the examiner to determine the tension of the lateral restraints (Fig. 1–18). With the knee fully extended, the patella is manually elevated. A passive tilt of <0° (neutral, i.e., below the horizontal plane) may imply lateral retinacular tightness.

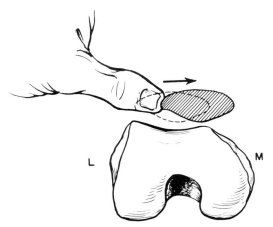

FIGURE 1–17. Patellar glide is measured based on the number of quadrants that the patella can be passively translated over the medial (M) or lateral (L) femoral condyle. (From Fu FH, Maday MG. Arthroscopic lateral release and the lateral patellar compression syndrome. Orthop Clin North Am 23:601, 1992.)

7. Instrumented Knee Laxity Measurement—Although various systems are commercially available, the KT-1000/2000 (MED-metric, San Diego, CA) has been the most widely accepted. The advantage of instrumented measurement of knee laxity is that it yields objective data that can assist the surgeon in quantifying preoperative and postoperative laxity. It is not meant to replace physical examination of the knee. It can be of use in determining partial versus complete ACL tears in an acute setting and is a well-established research tool. Evidence suggests that maximum testing of anterior translation and total posterior-to-anterior translation is probably more accurate with this device when monitoring ligament injuries or reconstructions.

   a. ACL Laxity Measurement—The knee is placed in slight flexion with the use of a thigh support, the foot is supported in 10° to 30° of external rotation, and the KT-1000 device is secured onto the leg with special straps (Fig. 1–19). The 30-pound (134 N) and manual maximum anterior displacements are most commonly reported and are based on the amount of force applied to the device. Side-to-side comparison is recorded, with a difference of >3 mm considered to be significant. Confidence levels of up to 98% can be achieved with experienced examiners. Calculation of the compliance index is also helpful in evaluating acute ACL injuries. Testing is done with 15- and 20-pound loads,

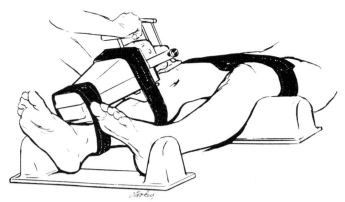

FIGURE 1–19. Instrumented testing of the ACL is accomplished with the knee slightly flexed and the feet in slight external rotation. Variable amounts of force can be applied to the KT-1000 arthrometer. (From Daniel DM, Stone ML. KT-1000 anterior-posterior displacement measurements. In Daniel DM, Akeson WY, O'Connor JJ [eds]. *Knee Ligaments: Structure, Function, Injury, and Repair.* New York: Raven Press, 1990; illustration by Phyllis Stookey.)

and the difference in translation is measured. Differences of >1 mm suggest ACL deficiency.

b. PCL Laxity Measurement—PCL laxity can also be documented with the KT-1000 device, although much less accurately (70% confidence). The key to performing this test is determining the quadriceps-neutral angle for the uninjured knee. This angle is defined as the amount of knee flexion that results in no movement of the tibia with quadriceps

contraction, usually about 70°. The injured knee is then placed at this angle, and the patient is instructed to contract the quadriceps in order to determine the quadriceps-active position. Anterior and posterior measurements can then be determined relative to the quadriceps-active position (Fig. 1–20).

III. Imaging
   A. Plain Radiographs—Standard radiographs of the knee should include a standing AP, standing 45° flexion posteroanterior (PA), lateral, and Merchant or Laurin views. Special views include long cassette lower extremity views, obliques, and stress radiographs.
      1. Standard AP View—The standard AP radiograph should be evaluated for soft tissue abnormalities, the cartilage space, and changes in the subchondral bone. Postmeniscectomy (Fairbank's) changes were described based on this view (Fig. 1–21). Another finding seen on this view includes the presence of a *Segond* fracture, or lateral capsular sign, which represents a capsular avulsion from the lateral tibial metaphysis that is highly associated with ACL disruption. The *Pellegrini-Stieda* lesion is calcification of the MCL, usually near the femoral insertion, resulting from a chronic injury to the ligament.
      2. 45° PA View—The 45° PA flexion weight-bearing view allows better evaluation of cartilage space narrowing than standard AP views. This view is taken with the

INJURED KNEE

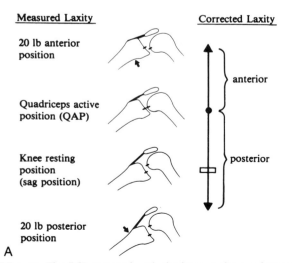

	INJURED KNEE measured laxity	INJURED KNEE corrected laxity	NORMAL KNEE measured laxity	INJURED-NORMAL I-N laxity
20 lb anterior	10	5	4	1
20 lb posterior	3	8	2	6
Quadriceps Active Displacement	+5		0	

A   B

FIGURE 1–20. The PCL is tested with the knee at the quadriceps-neutral angle, and the patient is instructed to contract the quadriceps in order to determine the quadriceps-active position (QAP). Anterior and posterior measurement (*A*) is based on the QAP, and "corrected" laxity values are calculated (*B*). KT evaluation of the PCL is less accurate than that for the ACL. (From Daniel DM, Stone ML. KT-1000 anterior-posterior displacement measurements. In Daniel DM, Akeson WY, O'Connor JJ [eds]. *Knee Ligaments: Structure, Function, Injury, and Repair.* New York: Raven Press, 1990.)

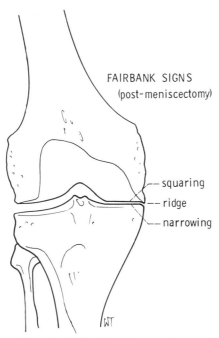

FAIRBANK SIGNS
(post-meniscectomy)

-- squaring
-- ridge
-- narrowing

FIGURE 1–21. Chronic (Fairbank's) changes after meniscectomy include squaring of the condyle, ridging, and narrowing of the cartilage space. (From Insall JN. Examination of the knee. In Insall JN [ed]. *Surgery of the Knee.* New York: Churchill Livingstone, 1984, pp 55–72.)

knees flexed 45° with the anterior aspect of the knees touching the cassette (Fig. 1–22). The beam is oriented parallel to the tibial plateau and centered at the joint line. This view both serves as a notch view and is useful for evaluating osteochondritis dissecans (OCD), osteonecrosis, loose bodies, and osteoarthritis.

3. Lateral View—The lateral radiograph is taken with the patient in a lateral decubitus position and with the knee flexed 30° to 45°. Rotation is controlled to allow the femoral condyles to be superimposed. The condyles can still be discerned, however, because the medial femoral condyle is larger and projects more distally than the lateral condyle, and the lateral femoral condyle has an indentation (sulcus terminalis) at the intersection with the intercondylar line anteriorly. Deepening of the sulcus terminalis of the lateral femoral condyle (lateral femoral condyle notch sign) has been described in patients with chronically ACL-deficient knees. Patella height can be assessed on the basis of three commonly used measurements: the Blumensaat line, the Insall-Salvati index, and the Blackburne and Peel index (Fig. 1–23). Each of these measurements has important qualifiers. Use of the Blumensaat line depends on precise positioning of the knee at 30° flexion. The Insall-Salvati index is affected by patellar spurring and ''inferior patellar nose'' formation. The

Blackburne and Peel index often requires arbitrary determination of the patellar articular surface.

4. Patellar Views—Various views have been proposed to assess the patellofemoral cartilage space and joint congruency. The Merchant view is usually the standard radiograph that is obtained. The technique involves positioning a patient supine with the knee flexed 45° with the cassette placed over the tibia and the beam directed proximal to distal and tangential to the patella. The radiograph is evaluated for articular cartilage loss, tilt, and subluxation of the patella. The Laurin view (20° sunrise) may be more sensitive for patella subluxation/ tilt.

5. Additional Views—These views are ordered only if additional information is needed.
   a. Long Cassette Lower Extremity View— This radiograph, which includes the hip, knee, and ankle, is taken with a patient standing. The anatomic and mechanical axes of the limb can be measured (Fig. 1–24). The difference between the mechanical and anatomic axes is usually 5° ±2°.
   b. Oblique Views—These radiographs

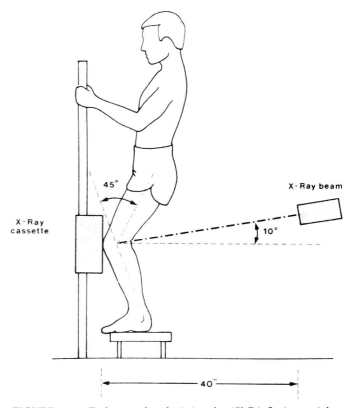

FIGURE 1–22. Technique for obtaining the 45° PA flexion weight-bearing radiograph. (From Rosenberg TD, Paulos LE, Parker RD, et al. The forty-five-degree posteroanterior flexion weight-bearing radiograph of the knee. J Bone Joint Surg 70A:1479–1483, 1988.)

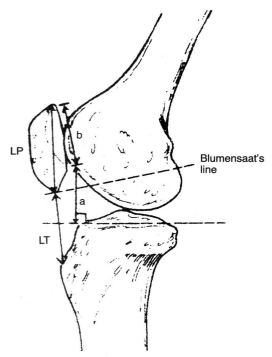

FIGURE 1–23. Composite illustration demonstrating the following three popular methods for evaluating patella alta/baja: (1) Blumensaat line: With the knee flexed 30°, the lower border of the patella should lie on a line extended from the intercondylar notch. (2) Insall-Salvati index: The patella tendon length (LT) to patella length (LP) index should be 1.0. An index >1.2 is considered patella alta, and an index <0.8 patella baja. (3) Blackburne and Peel index: The ratio of the distance from the tibial plateau to the inferior articular surface of the patella (a) to the length of the patella articular surface (b) should be 0.8. An index >1.0 is considered to be patella alta. (From Harner CD, Miller MD, Irrgang JJ. Management of the stiff knee after trauma and ligament reconstruction. In Siliski JM [ed]. *Traumatic Disorders of the Knee.* New York: Springer-Verlag, 1994, pp 357–368.)

may be of use in evaluating subtle fractures about the knee, as well as loose body localization. The views are taken 45° medially and laterally from the AP plane. Oblique views are often useful in evaluating knees with open growth plates.

c. Stress Views—These films are most useful in evaluating occult physeal injuries about the knee. Stress radiographs are also described for evaluation of AP translation with ACL or PCL injuries, although they are rarely used in the United States.

B. Nuclear Imaging—Technetium 99m bone scanning has been very useful in the diagnosis of stress fractures, early arthritis, reflex sympathetic dystrophy (RSD), and other abnormalities about the knee (Fig. 1–25). Imaging of the patella can sometimes be helpful. Scintigraphic patterns associated with a worse prognosis include focal inferior pole uptake and increased trochlear and patellar activity.

Increased uptake can also be seen in the tibial plateau of knees with meniscal tears, as well as in the medial, lateral, and patellofemoral compartments (in that order) with ACL deficiency (probably secondary to meniscal pathology). Fortunately, most of these scans return to a normal appearance after treatment; however, persistence of abnormal findings is highly associated with later development of degenerative changes on plain radiographs. Medial and patellofemoral uptake is also characteristic in patients with chronic PCL deficiency due to increased contact pressures.

C. Magnetic Resonance Imaging (MRI)—MRI has become the imaging modality of choice about the knee. Improved equipment and techniques have revolutionized imaging in the past several years. Imaging of ligament injury, meniscal pathology, and articular cartilage injuries has been well described. Resolution of <1 mm is now possible with three-dimensional acquisition techniques.

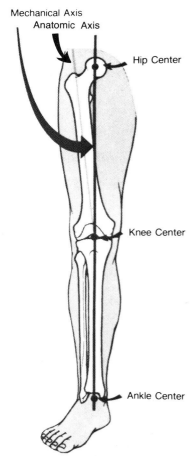

FIGURE 1–24. Knee axes (*arrows*). (From Rohr WL. Primary total knee arthroplasty. In Chapman M [ed]. *Operative Orthopaedics.* 2nd ed. Philadelphia: JB Lippincott, 1993, p 718.)

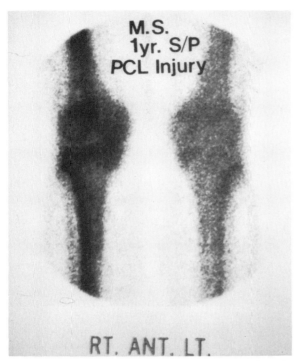

FIGURE 1–25. Technetium bone scan of a patient with a chronic PCL injury. Note the diffuse uptake in the affected right knee. The association of chondral injury with chronic PCL injuries is well documented with bone scan images.

1. Collateral Ligament Injury—The MCL is well visualized with MRI in the coronal plane. Injury to this ligament can be identified by an increase in signal intensity due to hemorrhage and edema, increased thickness, and abnormal configuration and discontinuity of the fibers (Fig. 1–26). Grading of MCL tears is also possible. The LCL can be visualized on coronal images but is often seen better on extreme lateral sagittal images. Discontinuity, displacement, widening, and waviness of the fibers all are consistent with injury to this ligament.

2. Cruciate Ligament Injuries—The ACL is seen well on sagittal views if the knee is placed in 15° to 20° of external rotation. The ACL is usually thinner and brighter than the PCL on MRI (proton-weighted images). The PCL is darker, thicker, and more consistently seen on MRI. Tears of both ligaments can result in nonvisualization, discontinuity of the fibers, and abnormal orientation (Fig. 1–27). Bone bruises or trabecular microfractures are commonly seen on MRI of acute ACL injuries. These lesions are thought to be caused by bony impaction and occur most commonly in the posterolateral tibial plateau and lateral femoral condyle (Fig. 1–28).

3. Meniscal Pathology—Meniscal tears are identified as increased signal intensity within the meniscus that extends to the surface of the meniscus. A grading scale has been developed for characterizing changes within the menisci (Fig. 1–29); however, only lesions that extend to the surface of the meniscus are properly considered meniscal tears. The significance of grades I and II lesions is unknown but likely is related to mucinous degeneration. One study demonstrated that 17% of meniscal lesions reported as grade II were found to be full-thickness tears on arthroscopy. Discoid menisci are well visualized with MRI. Discoid menisci appear thick or elongated (Fig. 1–30). Meniscal cysts are also well visualized on MRI. The cysts are commonly associated with a horizontal tear of the meniscus, which can also be seen on MRI (fluid is evident on T2-weighted images) (Fig. 1–31).

4. Bone Disorders—Osteonecrosis, which occurs most commonly in the medial femoral condyle, can be seen as an area of decreased signal intensity on MRI. Osteochondritis dissecans (OCD) can be well visualized on MRI and can provide information about stability and attachment of fragments that may influence treatment choices. Occult fractures can also be seen on MRI, as can microfractures (discussed earlier).

5. Articular Disorders—Special MRI techniques and sequences (fat suppression, gradient recall, and other images) can provide valuable information about cartilage abnormalities and osteoarthritis. A grading

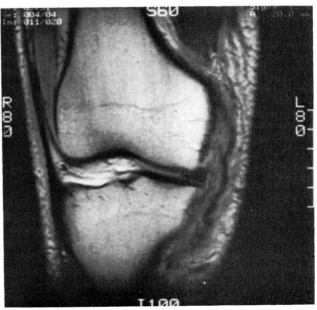

FIGURE 1–26. MRI of an acute MCL injury. Note the waviness and disruption of the fibers of the ligament, as well as diffuse edema.

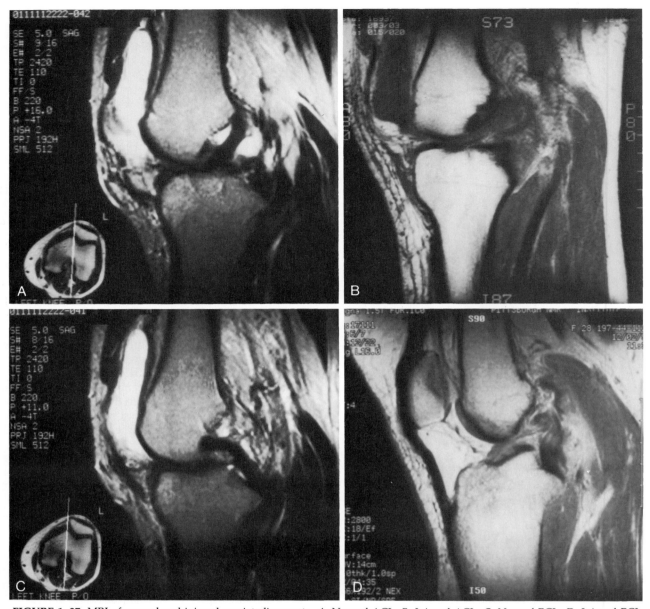

FIGURE 1–27. MRI of normal and injured cruciate ligaments. *A*, Normal ACL. *B*, Injured ACL. *C*, Normal PCL. *D*, Injured PCL.

system for patellar chondromalacia has also been proposed, and preliminary studies suggest that the findings are similar to those seen arthroscopically. Additional information can be obtained by using gadolinium injection for MRI arthrography.

D. Other Imaging
  1. Computed Tomography—Computed tomography (CT) has largely been supplanted by MRI use; however, a few indications for its use remain. CT is useful in evaluating bony lesions, patellar tilt (done at 0° and 20° flexion), and certain fractures. CT arthrography is helpful in evaluating the articular surfaces of the patellofemoral joint.
  2. Arthrography—Arthrography has very few indications in most centers; however, it can still be helpful in remote locations and in evaluating individuals who cannot tolerate MRI. It also has a proven role in evaluating the results of meniscal repair. Meniscal tears are well visualized with arthrography (Fig. 1–32); however, evaluation of lateral meniscal tears is less reliable.
  3. Tomography—Tomography is usually reserved for the evaluation of tibial plateau fractures and is preferred to CT for evaluating this injury.
  4. Thermography—Thermography may be of limited use in evaluating RSD of the knee.
  5. Ultrasonography—Ultrasonography has become an increasingly popular imaging modality for soft tissue lesions of the lower

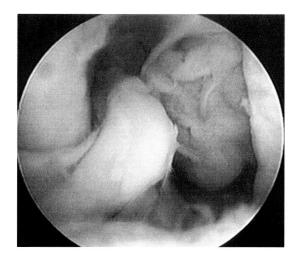

COLOR FIGURE 1. Bucket-handle tear of the medial meniscus displaced into the notch. The tear should be reduced and assessed for reparability.

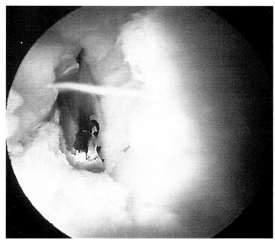

COLOR FIGURE 2. Modified Gillquist (posteromedial) view of a meniscal tear preparation prior to repair. Rasps and shavers can be used to "freshen" both sides of the tear prior to repair.

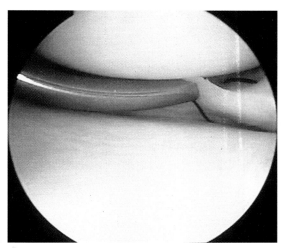

COLOR FIGURE 3. Meniscal repair using the "inside-out" technique. Various horizontal and vertical mattress sutures can be placed, resulting in better coaptation of the meniscus.

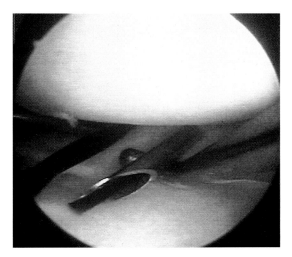

COLOR FIGURE 4. Meniscal repair using the "outside-in" technique. Absorbable (PDS) sutures are introduced through spinal needles placed through separate small longitudinal incisions.

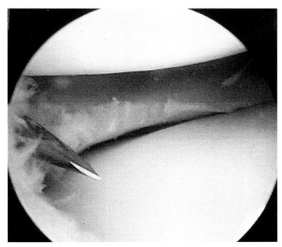

COLOR FIGURE 5. Arthroscopic decompression of a meniscal cyst. A partial meniscectomy has been performed, and the cyst is decompressed through a combination of mechanical decompression through the tear and multiple punctures with a spinal needle, as shown here.

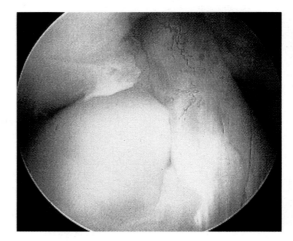

COLOR FIGURE 6. Discoid meniscus seen adjacent to a normal anterior cruciate ligament. Note the thickness of the meniscus.

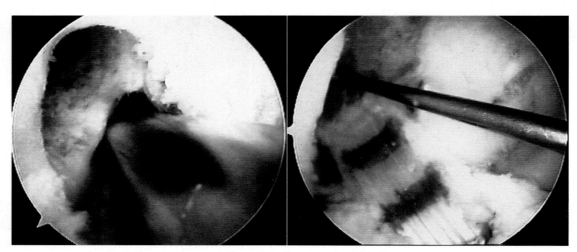

COLOR FIGURE 7. Femoral tunnel placement using endoscopic techniques should leave a posterior cortical rim of approximately 2 mm (*left*). The graft is inserted, and the guide wire is placed anteriorly to facilitate interference screw placement without damage to the graft (*right*).

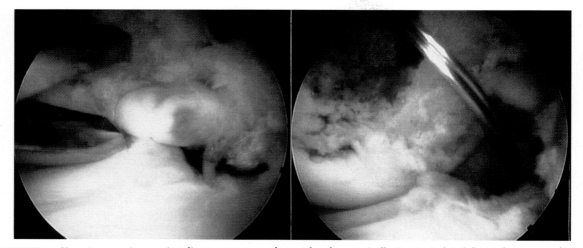

COLOR FIGURE 8. Chronic posterior cruciate ligament tear as observed arthroscopically (posteriorly) (*left*), and passage of 18-gauge wire to facilitate graft placement (*right*).

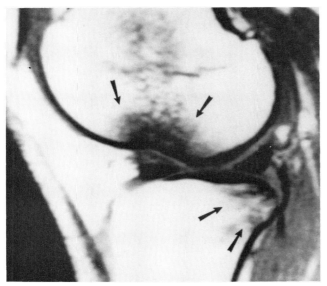

FIGURE 1–28. MRI demonstrating bone bruises or microfractures associated with acute ACL tears. The most common location of these lesions is the posterior tibial plateau and lateral femoral condyle (*arrows*).

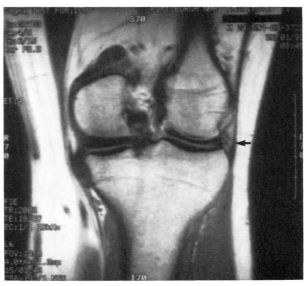

FIGURE 1–30. MRI of discoid meniscus. Note the thickness of the meniscus (*arrow*) compared with the opposite side.

extremity. It is helpful in evaluating patellar tendinitis, hematomas, and various other soft tissue injuries.

IV. Arthroscopy
  A. Principles—The use of the arthroscope in the diagnosis and treatment of disorders about the knee has greatly advanced since the development of the first practical arthroscope by

Watanabe in 1960. Arthroscopic techniques for meniscal, ligamentous, and articular cartilage surgery have been well documented. The benefits of arthroscopic versus open surgical techniques include smaller incisions, less morbidity, improved visualization, and decreased recovery time.
    1. Equipment—Although arthroscopes are available in various sizes and viewing angles, the 4-mm (5.5-mm sheath) 30° arthroscope is most commonly used for knee arthroscopy (Fig. 1–33). A 70° arthroscope is sometimes useful for visualizing

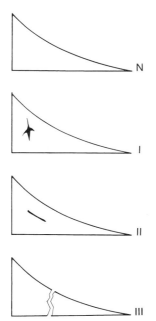

FIGURE 1–29. The classification system used to characterize meniscal tears on MRI. Note that only type III lesions can be demonstrated arthroscopically.

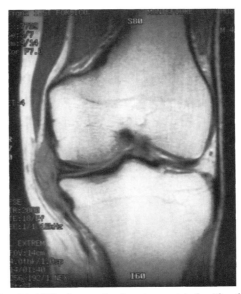

FIGURE 1–31. MRI of a meniscal cyst associated with a horizontal tear of the adjacent meniscus.

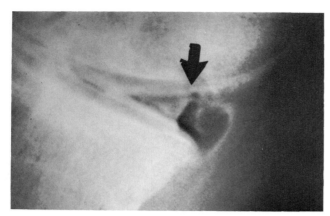

FIGURE 1–32. Arthrogram demonstrating a tear of the medial meniscus (*arrow*).

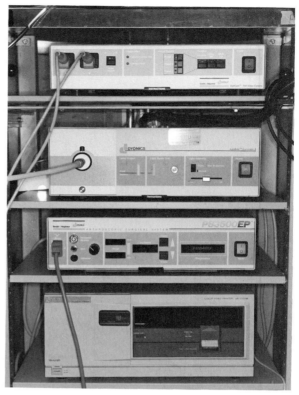

FIGURE 1–34. *Top* to *bottom*, Video, light source, motorized shaver system, and video printer. (From DiGiovine NM, Bradley JP. Arthroscopic equipment and set-up. In Fu FH, Harner CD, Vince KG [eds]. *Knee Surgery*. Baltimore: Williams & Wilkins, 1994.)

the posterior aspect of the knee. A fiberoptic light cord and inflow/outflow tubing are attached to the scope and cannula, respectively. Visualization of the knee joint is accomplished with the use of a video camera, which in addition to a printer can be used to record the procedure (Fig. 1–34). Safe new inflow pumps are now available to improve visibility during operative arthroscopy. Various hand-held instruments have been developed, most designed for performing arthroscopic partial meniscectomies; however, these instruments are also useful for removing loose bodies, for addressing ligament injuries, and for several other purposes (Fig. 1–35). Various blades have been developed for use with motorized shavers (Fig. 1–36). These shavers are effective in removing large amounts of synovium and other tissue and are useful in removing tissue in areas that are difficult to access with hand instruments. Speed and direction of these motorized instruments can be controlled with the use of foot pedals, leaving a surgeon's hands free for arthroscopy. Curved instruments, probes, and shavers are available and can help avoid damage to articular cartilage in "tight" knees. Other instruments that are used in knee arthroscopy include intra-articular cautery, special guides, drills, rasps, and even laser systems.

2. Portals—A number of standard and accessory portals have been described about the knee (Fig. 1–37).

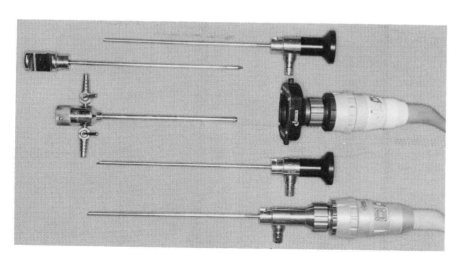

FIGURE 1–33. Arthroscopes, sheath, obturator, and video camera head. (From DiGiovine NM, Bradley JP. Arthroscopic equipment and set-up. In Fu FH, Harner CD, Vince KG [eds]. *Knee Surgery*. Baltimore: Williams & Wilkins, 1994.)

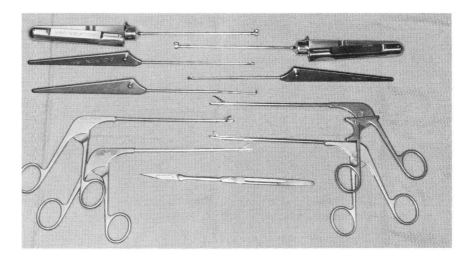

FIGURE 1–35. Arthroscopic hand instruments include baskets, grabbers, probes, and various knives. (From DiGiovine NM, Bradley JP. Arthroscopic equipment and set-up. In Fu FH, Harner CD, Vince KG [eds]. *Knee Surgery*. Baltimore: Williams & Wilkins, 1994.)

a. Standard Portals—Standard arthroscopic portals include a superomedial or superolateral portal used for inflow, an inferolateral portal used for the arthroscope, and an inferomedial instrument portal. The *superior portals* are made with the knee in extension and are placed superior and posterior to the patella. Incisions made parallel to the Langer lines tend to heal with minimal scarring. Care should be taken not to injure the vastus medialis during placement of the superomedial portal. *Inferior portals* are placed with the knee in flexion. Longitudinal incisions placed adjacent to the patella tendon and approximately 1 cm above the joint line (just below the inferior pole of the patella) are usually recommended. Placing these portals too high or too low can damage the articular cartilage or menisci (Fig. 1–38).

b. Accessory Portals—Accessory portals are sometimes necessary for visualization or instrumentation. These are usually established under arthroscopic visualization by first placing a spinal needle into the joint. The *posteromedial portal* is placed 1 cm above the joint line at the posteromedial edge of the medial femoral condyle. The arthroscope is inserted through the notch along the lateral portion of the medial femoral condyle (modified Gillquist view) and into

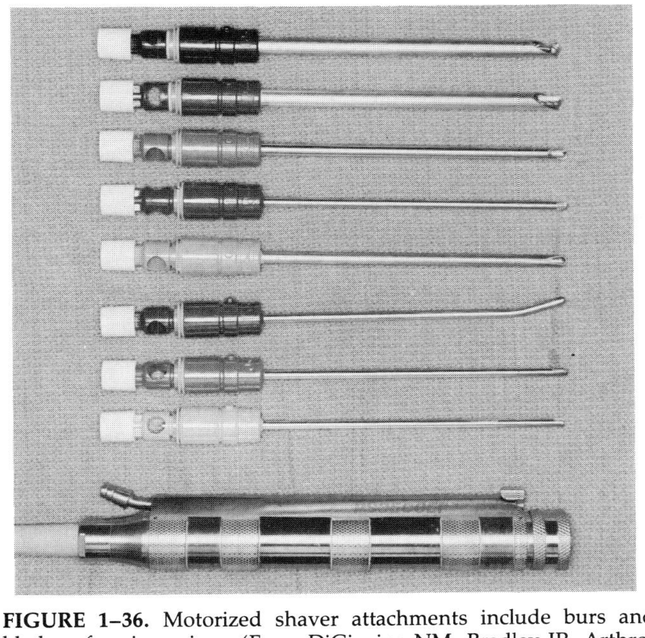

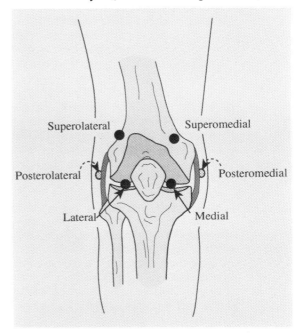

FIGURE 1–36. Motorized shaver attachments include burs and blades of various sizes. (From DiGiovine NM, Bradley JP. Arthroscopic equipment and set-up. In Fu FH, Harner CD, Vince KG [eds]. *Knee Surgery*. Baltimore: Williams & Wilkins, 1994.)

FIGURE 1–37. Commonly used arthroscopic portals. (From Reiman PR, Gardner WG. Septic arthritis. In Fu FH, Harner CD, Vince KG [eds]. *Knee Surgery*, Baltimore: Williams & Wilkins, 1994.)

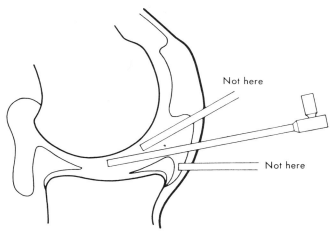

FIGURE 1–38. Anterior inferior portals should allow introduction of the arthroscope just superior to the meniscus and angled parallel to the tibial plateau, to avoid injury to other structures. (From DiGiovine NM, Bradley JP. Arthroscopic equipment and set-up. In Fu FH, Harner CD, Vince KG [eds]. *Knee Surgery*. Baltimore: Williams & Wilkins, 1994.)

the posterior aspect of the knee to visualize the placement of a spinal needle in this portal. The light from the arthroscope illuminates the area around the intended portal, allowing visualization of the saphenous vein (and nerve), which should be avoided when creating this portal. The *posterolateral portal* is located 1 cm above the joint line along the posterolateral edge of the lateral femoral condyle in the interval between the iliotibial band and the biceps tendon. Placement any farther posteriorly can jeopardize the common peroneal nerve. The *transpatellar portal* is located 1 cm distal to the inferior pole of the patella and is angulated to pass above the fat pad. It can be used for central viewing or for grasping. The use of this portal in patients who require autogenous patellar tendon graft harvesting should be undertaken with caution because it may injure the graft. The medial and lateral *midpatella portals* are immediately adjacent to the broadest portion of the patella and can be used for viewing the anterior compartment of the knee. *Far medial and lateral* portals are placed 2 to 3 cm medial and lateral to the anterior inferior portals and may occasionally be helpful for placing accessory instrumentation. The *proximal superomedial portal* is located 4 cm proximal to and in line with the medial edge of the patella. Its use facilitates observation of the patellofemoral joint and the anterior knee.

3. Arthroscopic Technique—Although the sequence is largely a matter of a surgeon's preference, a systematic examination of the

knee should be accomplished before any identified pathology is addressed. The inflow cannula is placed in a superior portal, and the arthroscope is introduced into the inferolateral portal by first inserting a blunt obturator into the notch and then extending the knee, gently directing the obturator under the patella. The obturator is exchanged for the arthroscope, and the inflow cannula is checked. The suprapatellar pouch is examined for adhesions, loose bodies, synovitis, and other pathology, and the arthroscope is then withdrawn slightly and the patellofemoral joint observed. The patella is observed during passive range of motion, and patellar tracking is carefully evaluated. The gutters are carefully evaluated for the presence of plicae, adhesions, or loose bodies, and the arthroscope is then swung into the medial compartment. The medial meniscus is carefully visualized and probed from posterior to anterior (both superior and inferior surfaces), and the articular surfaces of both the tibia and femur are inspected and probed in various degrees of flexion. The intercondylar notch is examined, and the cruciate ligaments visualized and probed. The lateral meniscus and articular cartilage are next evaluated. Finally, if the posteromedial compartment needs further assessment, it is visualized with the modified Gillquist view described earlier. A 70° arthroscope is often helpful to visualize the entire posteromedial compartment. After complete evaluation of the joint, surgical pathology is addressed.

4. Arthroscopic Complications—The most common complication with arthroscopic surgery is iatrogenic articular cartilage damage. The incidence of this complication is probably much higher than reported. Other complications include instrument breakage, extravasation of fluid, hemarthrosis, infection, and neurovascular injury. Complications that are associated with specific procedures are discussed later.

5. Office Arthroscopy—Although use of the arthroscope in the clinic setting is being promoted, relatively few indications for it remain. It should be performed only by surgeons very proficient with the procedure and well trained in arthroscopic techniques, and it should be done for limited diagnostic and/or therapeutic purposes.

V. Menisci
   A. Meniscal Tears
      1. Incidence—Meniscal tears represent approximately 50% of knee injuries that require surgery. The medial meniscus is torn approximately three times more often than

the lateral meniscus. Two types of meniscal tears exist—traumatic and degenerative. Traumatic tears occur in younger patients with sports-related injuries. They may be more peripherally located (and therefore may be amenable to repair) and may be associated with ACL injuries. Degenerative tears usually occur in older patients, are often insidious in onset, and are more commonly complex tears with many different patterns. They usually are not repairable or occur in the age group not well suited for meniscal repair.

2. Classification—Meniscal tears can be classified on the basis of location, orientation, and appearance.
   a. Location—Tears have been classified on the basis of their location in relation to the periphery (and blood supply/healing potential) (Fig. 1–39A). Tears in the extreme periphery are considered to be within the vascular or red zone, and healing is possible. Tears in the central portion of the menisci are located in the avascular zone, and healing is not possible without special techniques. Tears between these two zones, in an indistinct red-white zone, are intermediate in their healing potential. A more specific zone classification of meniscal tears if often useful for documentation purposes (Fig. 1–39B).
   b. Orientation and Appearance—Tears can be classified as longitudinal, radial, horizontal, or oblique based on their orientation. Several terms have been used to describe the appearance of certain meniscal tears, such as bucket-handle (Color Figure 1), parrot-beak, and flap tears (Fig. 1–40). These terms are often combined, and nomenclature can be confusing. Regardless, the length, location, and tear patterns should be documented.

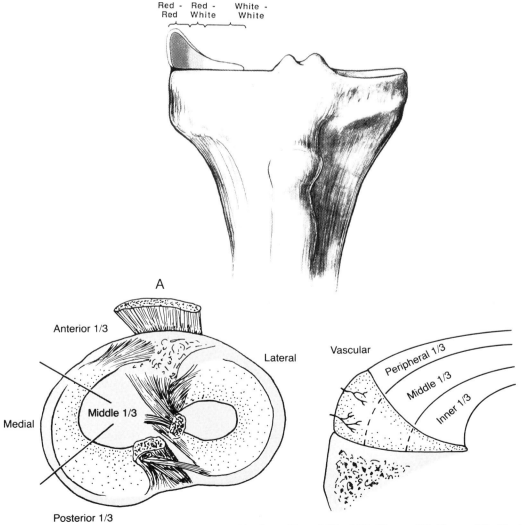

FIGURE 1–39. *A*, Classification of meniscal tears based on potential healing. (From Miller MD, Warner JJP, Harner CD. Meniscal repair. In Fu FH, Harner CD, Vince KG [eds]. *Knee Surgery*. Baltimore, Williams & Wilkins, 1994.) *B*, Classification of meniscal tears based on location (*left*, in relation to circumference; *right*, in relation to radial diameter). (From Browner BD, Jupiter JB, Levine AM, Trafton PG [eds]. *Skeletal Trauma*. Philadelphia: WB Saunders, 1992.)

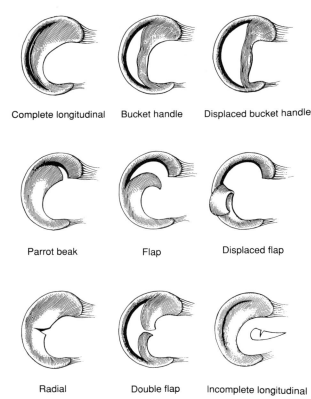

Complete longitudinal   Bucket handle   Displaced bucket handle

Parrot beak   Flap   Displaced flap

Radial   Double flap   Incomplete longitudinal

FIGURE 1–40. Classification of meniscal tears based on appearance and orientation. (From Tria AJ, Klein KS. *An Illustrated Guide to the Knee.* New York: Churchill Livingstone, 1992.)

3. Treatment—Because of the well-known association of meniscectomy with late arthritis, attempts to preserve or repair the meniscus should be the rule rather than the exception. Some small, stable tears may be asymptomatic and do not require treatment. Symptomatic meniscal tears usually need to be surgically addressed, however. Ninety percent or more of athletes with symptomatic tears are unable to return to sports at the same level unless treated. Most surgeons agree that partial-thickness tears, tears that are <5 mm in length, and tears that can be displaced only 1 to 2 mm do not require treatment. Fortunately, total meniscectomy has been largely abandoned as a treatment option. Nevertheless, overly aggressive partial meniscectomies can effectively result in the same outcome. Studies have confirmed increased compartment pressures that are proportional to the amount of meniscus excised. Radiographic Fairbank's changes were present in 50% of patients at 5-year follow-up in one study of arthroscopic partial meniscectomy. Quantification of the amount of partial meniscectomy carried out in each third of the meniscus is important in adequately assessing the long-term effect of partial meniscectomy.

a. Partial Meniscectomy—Various types of surgical equipment and techniques are available for arthroscopic meniscectomy. The meniscus is carefully probed and viewed from different perspectives/portals to determine if the tear is unrepairable. In general, complex, degenerative, and central/radial tears should be treated with partial meniscectomy. Radial and flap tears are simply resected back to a stable rim with an arthroscopic basket forceps (Fig. 1–41). Degenerative tears (Fig. 1–42) are treated similarly. A motorized shaver is often helpful in creating a smooth transition between the tear and the unaffected menisci. Degenerative tears often have horizontal components, and it is essential to ensure that no residual mechanical obstruction remains after resection of these tears. Irreparable or deformed bucket-handle tears (Fig. 1–43 and Color Figure 1) should be reduced and removed by detaching the posterior attachment, partially detaching the anterior attachment, and then avulsing the meniscus from its residual attachment (Fig. 1–44). Partial meniscectomy

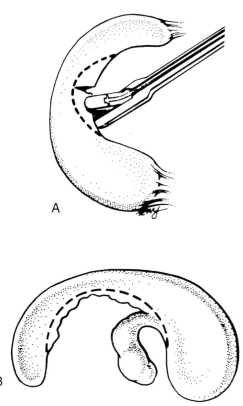

FIGURE 1–41. Outlines of partial meniscectomy necessary for a radial tear (*A*) and a degenerative flap tear (*B*). (From Ciccotti MG, Shields CL, El Attrache N. Meniscectomy. In Fu FH, Harner CD, Vince KG [eds]. *Knee Surgery.* Baltimore: Williams & Wilkins, 1994.)

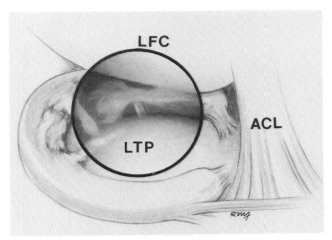

FIGURE 1–42. Degenerative meniscal tear. (LFC = lateral femoral condyle; LTP = lateral tibial plateau; ACL = anterior cruciate ligament.) (From Ciccotti MG, Shields CL, El Attrache N. Meniscectomy. In Fu FH, Harner CD, Vince KG [eds]. *Knee Surgery.* Baltimore: Williams & Wilkins, 1994.)

A   B

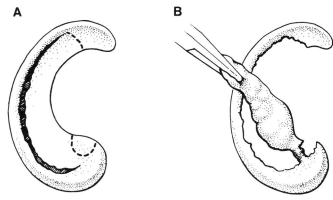

FIGURE 1–44. Technique for excision of a bucket-handle tear includes complete detachment of one edge (*A*) followed by partial detachment of the other attachment and avulsion of the torn meniscal fragment(*B*). (From Ciccotti MG, Shields CL, El Attrache N. Meniscectomy. In Fu FH, Harner CD, Vince KG [eds]. *Knee Surgery.* Baltimore: Williams & Wilkins, 1994.)

using lasers has been proposed. Although still investigational, the neodymium:yttrium-aluminum-garnet (Nd: YAG) contact laser appears to be the most adaptable to arthroscopic applications (Fig. 1–45).

    b. Meniscal Repair–Although meniscal repair was introduced more than a century ago, it has only recently been adapted into routine practice. Four techniques for meniscal repair are currently in general clinical use: (1) open meniscal repair, (2) arthroscopic "inside-out" repair, (3) arthroscopic "outside-in" repair, and (4) arthroscopic "all-inside" repair. Although each of these techniques has advan-

tages and disadvantages, application of individual techniques is largely a matter of a surgeon's preference, experience, and instrument availability.

    (1) Indications—With the exception of open meniscal repair, which is primarily limited to tears in the extreme periphery of the meniscus, the indications for the various techniques of meniscal repair are similar. Histologic studies have demonstrated that the fibrochondrocyte is the cell responsible for healing of meniscal tears. A better understanding of the vascular anatomy and meniscal healing has led several investigators to develop techniques

FIGURE 1–43. Displaced bucket-handle tear of the medial meniscus (MM). (MFC = medial femoral condyle; MTP = medial tibial plateau; ACL = anterior cruciate ligament.) (From Ciccotti MG, Shields CL, El Attrache N. Meniscectomy. In Fu FH, Harner CD, Vince KG [eds]. *Knee Surgery.* Baltimore: Williams & Wilkins, 1994.)

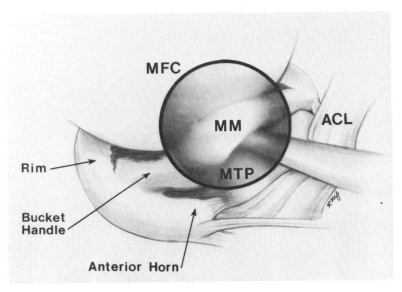

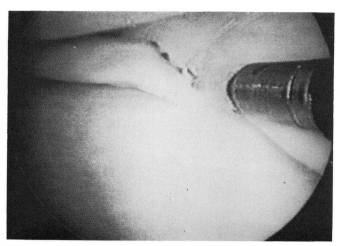

FIGURE 1–45. Arthroscopic view of an Nd:YAG laser partial meniscectomy. (From O'Brien SJ, Fealy S. Laser surgery. In Frymoyer JW [ed]. *Orthopaedic Knowledge Update 4: Home Study Syllabus.* Rosemont, IL: American Academy of Orthopaedic Surgeons, 1993.)

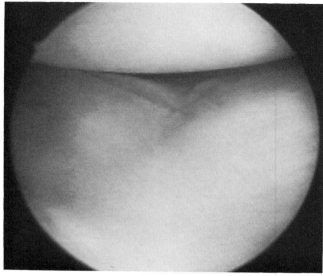

FIGURE 1–46. Arthroscopic view demonstrating a peripheral meniscal tear amenable to repair.

to enhance vascularity in meniscal repair. Animal studies have shown that the use of autogenous clot can significantly enhance meniscal healing in the avascular area of the meniscus. Other investigators have advocated the use of vascular tunnels and vascularized synovial flaps. Clinical reports indicate that meniscal repair failure rate is reduced by using a rasp for parameniscal synovial abrasion or using an autologous blood clot. Several factors must be considered in determining the suitability of a meniscal tear for repair. A patient's age and occupation; the chronicity of the injury; the type, location, and length of the tear; associated ligamentous injuries; and relative urgency to return to sport or activity all are important factors. The ideal candidate for meniscal repair is a young individual with an acute, longitudinal, peripheral meniscal tear that is 1 to 2 cm in length, repaired in conjunction with an ACL reconstruction (Fig. 1–46). There is very little consensus on the relative indications for meniscal repair outside of these ideal parameters. Most surgeons would agree that "red-red" tears should be repaired, and many favor repair of acute "red-white" repairs; however, many of these peripheral tears may be overlooked unless the meniscus is carefully probed. To appreciate meniscal pathology more clearly in the posterior horn, the posteromedial corner is routinely

viewed with a 70° arthroscope via the modified Gillquist approach if there is any question of a tear on routine arthroscopy or preoperative evaluation (Fig. 1–47). Experienced arthroscopists should be prepared to perform a meniscal repair at the time of any knee arthroscopy. It is usually not possible to identify menisci that are repairable preoperatively, but MRI often shows the relative location of tears. Peripheral tears are also more common in association with ACL injuries and should be repaired at the time of ACL reconstruction. Meniscal re-

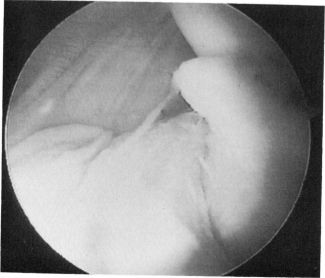

FIGURE 1–47. Arthroscopic view of a posteromedial meniscal tear visualized using the modified Gillquist technique.

pair has been shown to be less successful in ACL-deficient knees. Most authorities recommend concurrent ACL reconstruction at the time of meniscal repair in ACL-deficient knees. The importance of preoperative counseling in this regard cannot be overemphasized.

(2) Techniques—As indicated earlier, there are basically four different approaches to meniscal repair. All of these techniques require the meniscus to be prepared or "freshened" with a rasp or motorized shaver before passing suture (Color Figure 2). The inside-out and outside-in techniques are performed arthroscopically, using mini-incisions to secure sutures to the capsule. The all-inside technique is performed arthroscopically without any additional incisions.

(a) Open Meniscal Repair—Open meniscal repair has a proven record of success, even at 10-year follow-up. The technique basically involves exposure of the capsule through a longitudinal incision, preparation of the meniscal rim and capsular bed, and placement of vertically oriented sutures (strongest and most anatomic repair) at 3- to 4-mm intervals (Fig. 1–48).

(b) Inside-out Meniscal Repair—Inside-out meniscal repair is currently the most popular technique for meniscal repair. It can

be done with a single- or double-barrel cannula. The advantage of the single-cannula technique is that vertically oriented sutures can be placed. Suture placement using the double-barrel cannula system can be accomplished more quickly but gives a surgeon less control over suture placement and can lead to poor coaptation of the repair. The tear is identified and prepared arthroscopically. A small posterior incision is carried down to the capsule, and sutures are placed arthroscopically using specially designed long Keith needles, which are retrieved by an assistant (Fig. 1–49 and Color Figure 3). The assistant is also responsible for retracting the posterior neurovascular structures that are at risk. Care should be taken to stay anterior to the biceps tendon laterally to avoid injury to the peroneal nerve. Medially, an incision in layer I should be made anterior to the sartorius and a retractor placed deep to layer I to protect the saphenous nerve. After placement, the sutures are tied over the capsule, being careful not to entrap small subcutaneous nerve branches.

(c) Outside-in Meniscal Repair—Outside-in meniscal repair uses separate small (1–2 cm) incisions for each pair of sutures. These incisions are made perpendicular to the joint line, and a straight clamp is used to spread the subcutaneous tissue carefully to expose the joint capsule. An 18-gauge spinal needle is placed across the tear from outside to inside, being careful to avoid neurovascular structures in the process. Absorbable 0 PDS suture is passed through the needle into the joint and is secured by a "mulberry" knot tied in the end of the suture (Fig. 1–50 and Color Figure 4). These sutures are tied to adjacent sutures at the end of the procedure. Variations of this technique, which involve retrieving the end of the suture through another needle, can result in placement of horizontal or vertical mattress stitches.

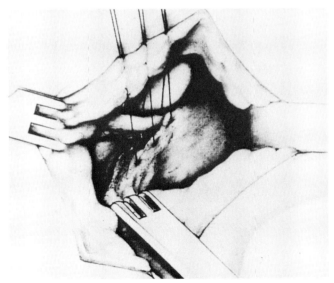

FIGURE 1–48. Open meniscal repair involves reapproximation of the peripheral meniscus to the capsule using vertical mattress sutures. (From DeHaven KE, Black KP, Griffiths HJ. Open meniscus repair. Technique and two to nine year results. Am J Sports Med 17:788–795, 1989.)

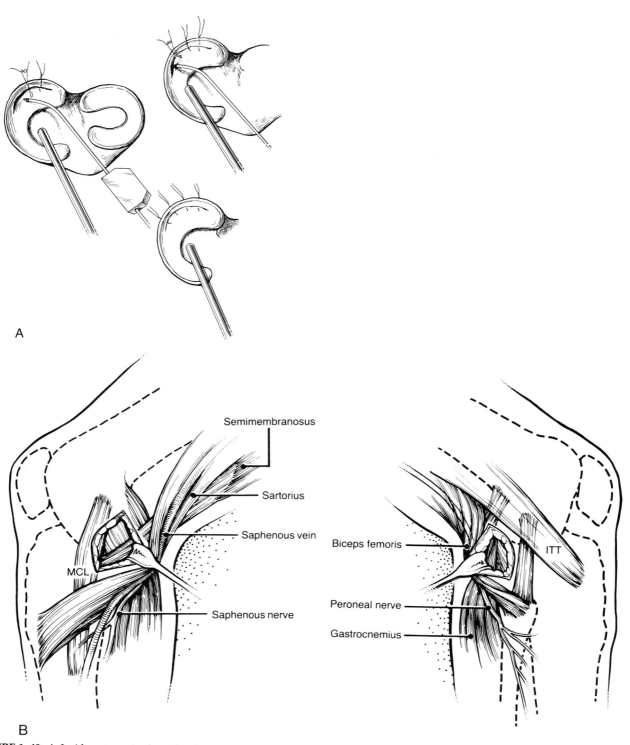

A

B

FIGURE 1–49. *A,* Inside-out meniscal repair using a zone-specific cannula. (From Miller MD, Warner JJP, Harner CD. Meniscal repair. In Fu FH, Harner CD, Vince KG [eds]. *Knee Surgery.* Baltimore: Williams & Wilkins, 1994.) *B,* Incision for retrieval of needles in relation to important structures medially (*left*) and laterally (*right*) (MCL = medial collateral ligament; ITT = iliotibial band.) (From Scott WN [ed]. *Arthroscopy of the Knee.* Philadelphia: WB Saunders, 1990.)

(d) All-inside Meniscal Repair— All-inside meniscal repair is attractive because it does not require additional incisions and at least theoretically avoids any neurovascular risk. After visual- ization and preparation of the tear, a specially designed can- nulated suture hook is used to pierce both sides of the tear, and suture is passed through the lu- men of the hook, across the tear

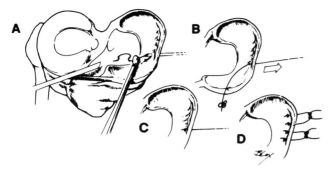

FIGURE 1–50. Outside-in meniscal repair. Note how the knot captures and reduces the meniscal tear. *A*, Suture placed from outside-in through a spinal needle. *B*, ''Mulberry'' knot tied after the suture is retrieved from the anterior portal. *C*, Suture pulled back into the joint adjacent to the meniscus. *D*, Sutures tied together in pairs outside the capsule. (From Hanks GA, Kalenak A. Alternative arthroscopic techniques for meniscal repair: a review. Orthop Rev 19:541–548, 1990.)

(Fig. 1–51). The sutures are secured using a knot pusher that can be introduced arthroscopically.

(3) Results—Several reports have noted an 80% to 90% success rate with meniscal repairs; however, many factors such as the location, chronicity, and type of tear must be distinguished. Although long-term clinical studies are lacking, the use of fibrin clot has been shown to improve healing rates in some clinical studies. Likewise, the use of fibrin

sealant and endothelial cell growth factor has not been studied in humans. Most surgeons agree that meniscal repair is less successful in ACL-deficient knees and advocate combined meniscal repair and ACL reconstruction in this setting. Interestingly, isolated meniscal repair in a stable knee has been reported to be less successful than meniscal repair combined with ACL reconstruction, perhaps owing to the healing response generated by postoperative hemarthrosis.

c. Meniscal Cyst
   (1) Introduction—Much like ganglia in other parts of the body, the cause of meniscal cysts is unknown. These cysts are probably associated with trauma, although others suggest that they are related to synovial implantation or that they represent a myxofibroma. These cysts, which contain a gelatinous fluid similar to synovial fluid, are usually if not always associated with a horizontal meniscal tear (Fig. 1–52). When located on the joint line, they most commonly occur laterally, and they may actually involve some of the meniscus itself.
   (2) Diagnosis—Patients often present with complaints of an insidious onset of discomfort and point to an area of localized swelling. On examination, the cyst can usually be localized, and palpation of the joint line usually elicits tenderness. The cyst is actually more difficult to localize with flexion, and this has been referred to as the *Pisani disappearing sign.*

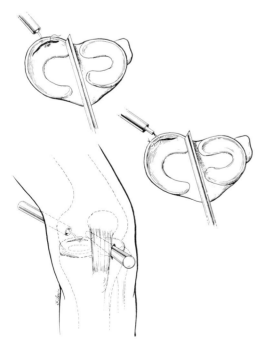

FIGURE 1–51. All-inside meniscal repair. Note positioning of the suture hook. (From Miller MD, Warner JJP, Harner CD. Meniscal repair. In Fu FH, Harner CD, Vince KG [eds]. *Knee Surgery.* Baltimore: Williams & Wilkins, 1994.)

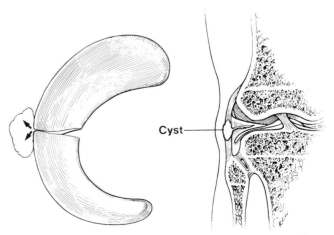

FIGURE 1–52. Meniscal cyst and associated horizontal meniscal tear. (From Tria AJ, Klein KS. *An Illustrated Guide to the Knee.* New York: Churchill Livingstone, 1992.)

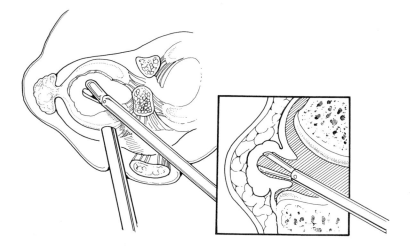

FIGURE 1–53. Partial meniscectomy and decompression of a meniscal cyst through the tear has proven to be effective. (Redrawn from Parisien JS. Arthroscopic treatment of cysts of the menisci. A preliminary report. Clin Orthop 257:154–158, 1990.)

(3) Treatment—The classic form of treatment for meniscal cysts has been partial meniscectomy and en bloc resection. Several articles have reported good success with arthroscopic partial meniscectomy and decompression through the tear (Fig. 1–53). "Needling" of the cyst to allow egress of fluid into the joint is also helpful (Color Figure 5).

(4) Popliteal (Baker) Cyst—This is actually a form of meniscal cyst and is more common than cysts along the joint line. These cysts are usually associated with degenerative medial meniscal lesions. They typically are located in the popliteal fossa between the semimembranosus tendon and the medial head of the gastrocnemius tendon and can extend inferiorly, mimicking a deep venous thrombosis. Treatment can include aspiration or even excision; however, most cysts resolve after partial meniscectomy.

d. Discoid Meniscus
(1) Introduction—Long referred to as the "popping knee syndrome," discoid menisci can be classified as one of three types: (1) incomplete, (2) complete, and (3) Wrisberg variant (also known as lateral meniscal variant with absence of the posterior coronary ligament) (Fig. 1–54). The latter may not be thickened or discoid, but it is commonly included. The cause is largely unknown but is probably not related to an arrest of embryologic meniscal development as was once proposed.
(2) Diagnosis—In addition to mechanical symptoms similar to those associated with meniscal tears, patients

may complain of popping with knee extension. Findings on physical examination are also similar to those in patients with meniscal tears unless the popping can be elicited. Radiographs may be normal, although classic radiographic findings include a widened joint space, squaring of the lateral condyle, cupping of the lateral tibial plateau, and a hypoplastic lateral intercondylar spine. MRI is useful and also helps identify any associated tears in the meniscus.

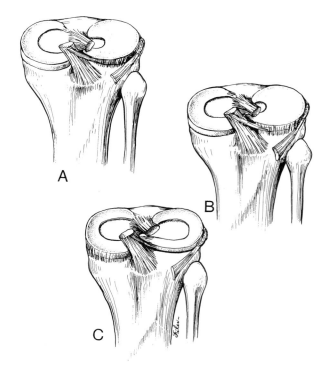

FIGURE 1–54. Three types of discoid menisci. *A*, Partial (incomplete). *B*, Complete. *C*, Wrisberg variant. (From Neuschwander DC. Discoid meniscus. In Fu FH, Harner CD, Vince KG [eds]. *Knee Surgery*. Baltimore: Williams & Wilkins, 1994.)

(3) Treatment—Incomplete and complete discoid menisci found incidentally or not associated with a tear should be left alone (Color Figure 6). Tears in these menisci should be treated with saucerization. A rim of 6 to 8 mm should be preserved. Although some surgeons prefer complete meniscectomy for symptomatic Wrisberg-type menisci, reattachment of these menisci with the same techniques used for meniscal repair has been reported to be successful.

e. Meniscal Transplantation
  (1) Introduction—Although the results in animal models are encouraging, clinical studies of meniscal transplantation are still preliminary. Unfortunately, young patients who have less than total or nearly total meniscectomy, especially lateral meniscectomy, are at significant risk for later development of arthritis. Some patients demonstrate early relentless progressive joint space narrowing. In these patients, meniscal transplantation may be the only treatment option. The ideal surgical candidates are young patients with early chondrosis. The problem is that patients are often asymptomatic and do not seek treatment until they develop advanced chondrosis.
  (2) Meniscal Grafts—Several options are available, including fresh-frozen, freeze-dried, and cryopreserved allografts and various collagen or synthetic scaffolds. Initial experience with freeze-dried (lyophilized) grafts identified a problem with shrinkage and tissue distortion. Cryopreserved grafts (dimethyl sulfoxide used to prepare and stored at −196°C) maintain cell viability and can be stored for prolonged periods but are quite expensive and are not secondarily sterilized. Additionally, it is unclear whether maintenance of cell viability is important, because the grafts are repopulated with host cells during the first 6 weeks after transplantation.
  (3) Techniques—Several techniques have been developed by various investigators. Both open and arthroscopic techniques have been described, using allograft menisci with or without bone plugs. Animal studies of fascia, fat pad, and tendons to replace menisci have been promising; however, early clinical results are less encouraging. Proper graft placement requires an understanding of insertion site anatomy of the meniscal horns (Fig. 1–55):

Meniscus	Horn	Insertion Site
Medial	Posterior	Posterior slope of eminence
Medial	Anterior	Anterior to ACL and eminence
Lateral	Posterior	Just posterior to ACL
Lateral	Anterior	Just anterior to ACL

If performed arthroscopically, the guide should be introduced through the contralateral portal. The arthroscope is placed in the ipsilateral anterior portal, except for the posterior horn of the medial meniscus, which is best viewed through the posteromedial portal. Guide wires are placed under arthroscopic visualization and overdrilled to 5 to 7 mm. The meniscus is introduced, and bone blocks are placed through bony tunnels. The transplanted meniscus is sutured to the periphery, and sutures from the bone blocks are secured over a bony bridge on the tibia (Fig. 1–56).

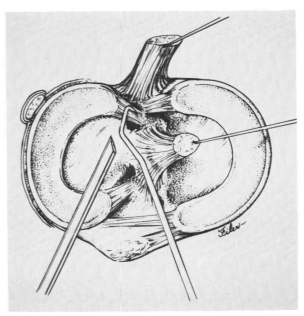

FIGURE 1–55. Arthroscopic guide placement for meniscal transplantation with bone blocks. For the posterior horn of the lateral meniscus (shown here), the guide is placed in the inferomedial portal and the arthroscope is introduced into the inferolateral portal. (Courtesy of Darren L. Johnson, MD.)

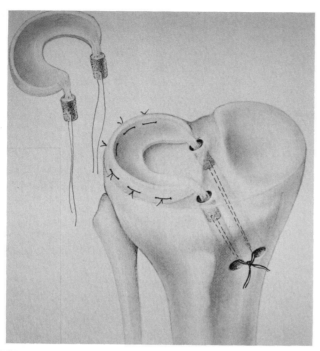

FIGURE 1–56. Meniscal transplantation using the bone block technique. (Courtesy of Christopher D. Harner, MD.)

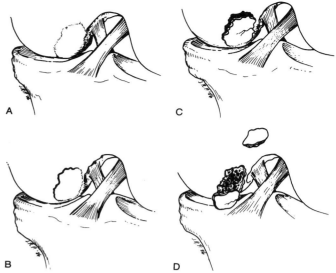

FIGURE 1–57. Classification of osteochondritis dissecans. *A,* In situ lesion. *B,* Early-separation lesion. *C,* Incompletely detached lesion. *D,* Completely detached lesion. (From Rosenberg TD, Paulos LE, Parker RD, Abbott PJ. Arthroscopic surgery of the knee. In Chapman MW [ed]. *Operative Orthopaedics.* 2nd ed. Philadelphia: JB Lippincott, 1993.)

VI. Osteochondral Lesions
   A. Osteochondritis Dissecans (OCD)
     1. Introduction—In OCD, a fragment of subchondral bone and its overlying cartilage are separated from the underlying bone. Although the cause is controversial, OCD is likely a result of trauma. *The lesion is classically located at the lateral aspect of the medial femoral condyle.* Lateral lesions are more likely to be located centrally on the condyle. Various classification schemes have been proposed, based on location of the lesion, age of the patient (*children with open growth plates usually fare well regardless of treatment*), and description of the lesion. Classification based on a description of the fragment and amount of separation are helpful in planning treatment (Fig. 1–57):

Category	Description
I. In situ	Softened area covered by intact cartilage
II. Early separation	Articular cartilage defect, stable flap
III. Incompletely detached	Flap of cartilage attached by hinge
IV. Completely detached	Full-thickness injury with one or more loose bodies: A. Loose within bed B. Displaced

     2. Diagnosis—Patients usually present with vague, poorly localized complaints and oc-casionally with mechanical symptoms. Findings on physical examination depend on the stage of the disease but may include an effusion or localized tenderness. Some patients may have a Wilson sign (pain with internal rotation and extension of the knee that is relieved with external rotation). Radiographs, particularly the notch or flexion weight-bearing view, are helpful in localizing the lesion (Fig. 1–58). Nuclear imaging can be helpful in identifying subtle lesions and may have a role in evaluating progression of the process. Larger lesions are more likely to be loose. MRI can be helpful in evaluating the status of the overlying carti-

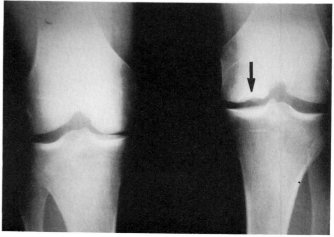

FIGURE 1–58. Radiograph demonstrating advanced osteochondritis dissecans of the medial femoral condyle (*arrow*).

lage; however, arthroscopy is usually required, particularly in older symptomatic patients.

3. Treatment—OCD in younger patients with open physes (juvenile OCD) may not require treatment (except activity modification) unless significant symptoms and effusions develop. Boys younger than 14 to 15 years and girls younger than 12 to 13 years have a favorable prognosis. OCD in adults usually is symptomatic and almost invariably leads to late-onset osteoarthritis unless treated. Even with treatment, however, the prognosis may be guarded. The treatment of in situ lesions may include retrograde drilling (with or without supplemental bone grafting). Lesions that are in the early separation stage may need to be secured with K-wires, special screws, or absorbable K-wires. Incompletely detached lesions usually resolve well with removal of underlying fibrous tissue, some form of chondroplasty, and then reduction and fixation of the flap (Fig. 1–59). Treatment of completely detached lesions usually necessitates removal of loose bodies (often too damaged for replacement), some form of abrasion chondroplasty, and consideration for osteochondral allograft replacement for larger lesions.

B. Cartilage Injury—Although the distinction between articular cartilage injury and OCD is not always clear, the distinction is sometimes important. These lesions are usually related to rotational forces in direct trauma. Most cases are located in the weight-bearing area of the medial compartment (usually the medial femoral condyle). Diagnosis is difficult because patients present with symptoms similar to meniscal injury (including an effusion), and because these injuries involve only cartilage, radiographic findings are normal. These lesions can be classified on the basis of their arthroscopic appearance and frequently are

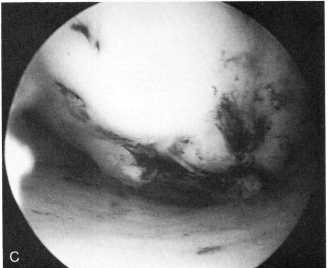

FIGURE 1–59. Treatment of an osteochondral flap tear. *A,* Flap tear of the medial femoral condyle. *B,* The flap is lifted back, and a series of small punctures or microfractures are made in the subchondral bone. *C,* The flap is replaced and secured with bioabsorbable pins.

delaminating injuries (Fig. 1–60). Studies have suggested that poor function and progressive chondral injury are more likely in chronically ACL-deficient knees after partial meniscectomy than in stable knees after meniscectomy. The most appropriate treatment for chondral injuries is still evolving; however, most surgeons recommend debridement of partial-thickness cartilage tears and some type of chondroplasty for cartilage lesions extending to bone. Drilling of the bed and contouring of the sides of the lesion or use of the microfracture technique has been successful at least in the short term. Treatment of the degrading-type injuries, which are probably best attributed to arthritic changes, is more controversial. Large lesions and mirror lesions on both articular surfaces are less likely to be successfully treated with arthroscopic techniques. Although shown to be efficacious in animal studies, continuous passive motion is expensive, and better clinical data are needed to confirm that this expense is justified.

C. Osteochondral Injuries—Osteochondral injuries are easier to diagnose than purely cartilaginous injuries because the bony component of the injury can be seen radiographically. These injuries are most often a result of a patellar dislocation and can involve the patella (usually the medial facet of the patella or the lateral femoral condyle). Treatment should consist of excision of small fragments and replacement of large thick pieces when possible (Fig. 1–61). General guidelines include replacement of fragments composing more than 25% of the joint surface area. Fixation options include Herbert screws, biodegradable pins, and fibrin adhesive. Cartilage transplantation with autografts and allografts is becoming more popular but can be associated with several problems. Several techniques have been described, but results are preliminary. The use of fibrin clot to fill smaller defects has been successful in animal studies, and the possibility of future clinical application is encouraging.

VII. Synovial Lesions
  A. Pigmented Villonodular Synovitis (PVNS)—Although PVNS can occur in both diffuse and localized forms, it most commonly affects the knee joint. Patients may present with pain and swelling and may have a palpable mass. Imaging studies may demonstrate bony erosion, and MRI clearly demonstrates the soft tissue lesions. Treatment includes synovectomy, which can be performed arthroscopically if multiple portals and careful techniques are used. Histology, which is similar to that of giant cell tumor of tendon sheath, is notable for foam cells (histiocytes), fibrous tissue, giant cells, and hemosiderin deposition. More extensive surgical procedures and local chemotherapy may be necessary in refractory cases.
  B. Synovial Chondromatosis—This proliferative disease of the synovium can be associated

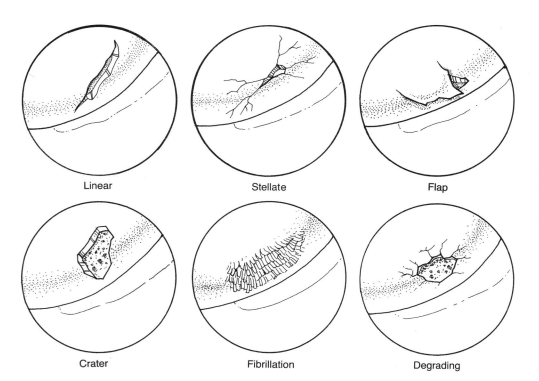

Linear   Stellate   Flap

Crater   Fibrillation   Degrading

FIGURE 1–60. Classification of chondral lesions of the femoral condyles. (Redrawn from Bauer M, Jackson RW. Chondral lesions of the femoral condyles: a system of arthroscopic classification. Arthroscopy 4:97–102, 1988.)

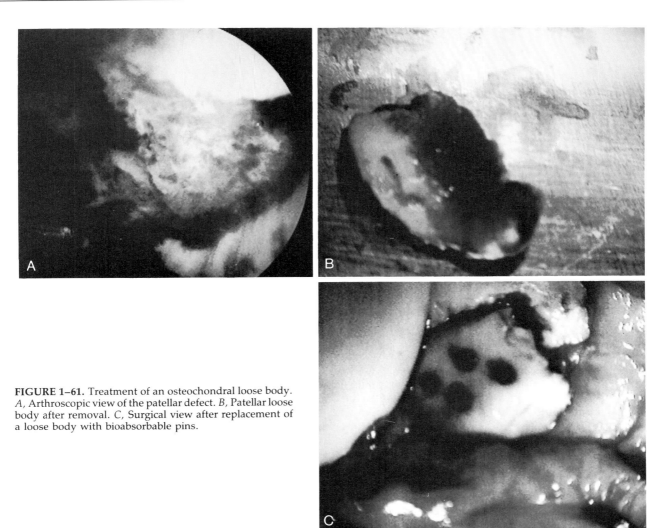

FIGURE 1–61. Treatment of an osteochondral loose body. *A,* Arthroscopic view of the patellar defect. *B,* Patellar loose body after removal. *C,* Surgical view after replacement of a loose body with bioabsorbable pins.

with cartilaginous or osteocartilaginous metaplasia resulting in loose bodies in the joint. The disease presents in three phases:

Phase	Description	Characteristics
1	Early	Chondrometaplasia, no loose bodies
2	Transitional	Active synovial disease, loose bodies
3	Late	Loose bodies, no synovial disease

Late in the course of the disease or in recurrent cases, the loose bodies can coalesce. Treatment consists of loose body removal with or without synovectomy. Some believe that the procedure can be performed arthroscopically with the use of posterior portals.

C. Arthroscopic Synovectomy—This can be carried out for the previously described proliferative diseases or for various other conditions including pauciarticular juvenile rheumatoid arthritis and hemophilia. The technique is accomplished with six portals: (1) superomedial,

(2) superolateral, (3) inferomedial, (4) inferolateral, (5) posteromedial, and (6) posterolateral (Fig. 1–62). Synovial resection should be carried out systematically, beginning posteriorly under direct visualization using a modified Gillquist approach. The suprapatellar pouch and gutters are next addressed through the superolateral and superomedial portals. The portals are then switched, and the inferior portions of the joint are resected using the inferior portals while using the superior portals for visualization. While viewing through the contralateral inferior portal, the perimeniscal synovium is resected through the ipsilateral inferior portal.

D. Synovial Plicae—These represent synovial folds that are embryologic remnants of partitions originally separating what begins as three synovial compartments of the knee. Four plicae have been described: suprapatellar, infrapatellar, medial, and lateral, based on their relation to the patella. The incidence of symptomatic or pathologic plicae is the subject of controversy, and a regional influence

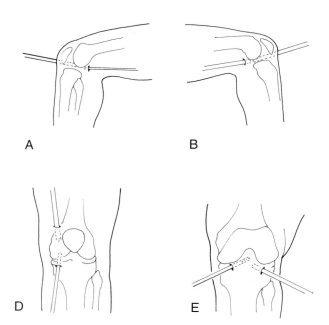

A   B

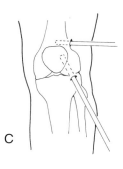

C

D   E

F

FIGURE 1–62. Technique of arthroscopic synovectomy with a six-portal technique. *A,* Posterolateral compartment. *B,* Posteromedial compartment. *C,* Suprapatellar pouch. *D,* Gutters. *E,* Anterior intercondylar area. *F,* Perimeniscal area. (Redrawn from Rosenberg TD, Tearse DS, Kolowich PA. Synovectomy of the knee. In McGinty JB [ed]. *Operative Arthroscopy.* New York: Raven Press, 1991, p 377.)

is noted. The most commonly described plica of clinical significance is the medial patellar plica. This plica, which originates just superior to the patella and passes over the medial femoral condyle and inserts into the fat pad, can become irritated and thickened from trauma or inflammation. This can occasionally cause abrasion of the medial femoral condyle at approximately 30° to 40° of flexion (Fig. 1–63). Some surgeons believe that the diagnosis may be made clinically by noting tenderness and occasional popping over the condyle. Conservative treatment is the rule; however, arthroscopic resection is occasionally necessary. The medial plica is best viewed from the suprapatellar lateral portal and divided/excised using a curved basket introduced through the anterolateral portal. A shaver, introduced through the anteromedial portal, can be helpful in removing any residual tissue. The amount of resection that is necessary is a matter of opinion, and there is considerable controversy about when resection is necessary. One report noted that symptom relief was better if there were clear pathologic changes and if a "kissing lesion" was present on the medial femoral condyle. An otherwise normal and incidentally detected plica should not be surgically resected.

VIII. Ligamentous Injuries
  A. Anterior Cruciate Ligament (ACL)
    1. Introduction—Although injury and treatment of ACL tears have become a major focus in orthopaedics, considerable controversy still surrounds the natural history of this injury. Many authorities have suggested that ACL deficiency produces abnormal kinematics and may result in late

degenerative changes in the knee. However, associated meniscal pathology may have even more of an effect on the development of late osteoarthritis. Studies have suggested that chronic ACL deficiency is associated with a higher incidence of complex meniscal tears not amenable to repair. Nevertheless, Daniels and colleagues noted a disturbing finding, that ACL reconstruction may be more closely tied to the development of arthrosis than ACL deficiency. However, this study was not

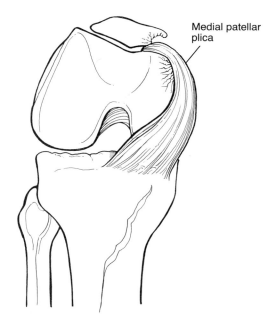

Medial patellar plica

FIGURE 1–63. Medial patellar plica (shelf) with associated chondromalacia of the patella and medial femoral condyle.

without limitations. Long-term European studies have found worse progression of degenerative joint disease (DJD) in knees with ACL and meniscectomy versus meniscectomy alone. Nevertheless, considerable controversy remains about the ideal treatment of this injury. Treatment decisions must be individualized on the basis of patient's age, activity level, degree of instability, associated injuries, and other factors (Fig. 1–64). Most surgeons recommend ACL reconstruction for patients who actively participate in sports, because of the risk of recurrent reinjury, in particular meniscal tear.

2. History and Physical Examination—ACL injuries are often a result of low-velocity, deceleration, rotational injuries and frequently are noncontact injuries. A certain subgroup of patients appear to have stenotic intercondylar notches and are more susceptible to ACL injury including bilateral ACL rupture. The notch-to-width index has been described, with an average value of 0.23 for males and 0.21 for females. One report showed an extremely high ACL injury rate in women who participate in intercollegiate basketball; however, it is unclear if notch stenosis or other factors (ligament size or tensile strength) were responsible for this phenomenon. Valgus/external rotation or hyperextension forces are most common. Most patients relate hearing or feeling a "pop" at the time of injury, and most patients are unable to return to sports immediately after injury. Instability or giving way is a common complaint. Acute hemarthrosis is also typical. Associated injuries are common. MRI studies of acute ACL injuries suggest that bone contusions or bruises commonly occur in conjunction with ACL injury and may be related to the mechanism of injury,

suggesting that a subluxation or near-dislocation occurs with ACL injury (see Fig. 1–28). Meniscal tears are also common, occurring in about 60% to 75% of knees with ACL injuries (not all tears require treatment, however). Combined ligamentous injuries are also relatively frequent, more so with contact injuries. The classic triad as described by O'Donoghue (ACL-MCL-medial meniscus) is actually less common than the ACL-MCL-*lateral* meniscus triad. *The Lachman test* (described in the physical examination section) *is the most sensitive test for ACL injury* (particularly with a "soft" endpoint). The pivot shift/jerk is also very helpful in evaluating an ACL-deficient knee, especially with examination under anesthesia. Instrumented laxity measurement, most commonly with the KT-1000 or KT-2000 (Med-metric, San Diego, CA) has been commonly accepted for reporting results of ACL treatment and, with the use of the compliance index, may have some practical application in evaluating an acutely injured knee. Plain radiographs should be an integral part of the evaluation, and if a knee dislocation is a possibility, then arthrography should also be carried out. MRI has become a helpful adjunct to examination, especially in equivocal situations, but it should not be a routine study for an acutely injured knee.

3. Treatment—The various options for ACL reconstruction range from nonoperative to endoscopic reconstruction.

   a. Nonoperative Treatment—Nonsteroidal medications and physical therapy are initiated early to reduce the amount of effusion and regain motion. *This is recommended for all patients, including operative candidates before surgical reconstruction to reduce the incidence of knee stiffness.* For patients electing to pur-

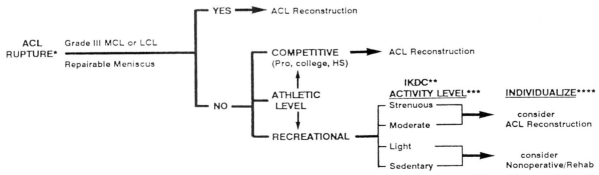

FIGURE 1–64. Algorithm for the treatment of ACL ruptures. (*midsubstance tears; **IKDC = International Knee Documentation Committee; ***activity level: strenuous = jumping/pivoting sports; moderate = heavy manual work, skiing; light = light manual work, running; sedentary = activities of daily living; ****based on age, arthritis, occupation, activity modification, other medical conditions, etc.) (From Spindler KP, Walker RN. General approach to ligament surgery. In Fu FH, Harner CD, Vince KG [eds]. *Knee Surgery*. Baltimore: Williams & Wilkins, 1994.)

sue continued nonoperative management, muscle rehabilitation and gradual return to sports are advocated. Temporary bracing may be appropriate for a patient's comfort. Emphasis is on closed-chain quadriceps rehabilitation. Open-chain quadriceps resisted extension with knee flexion of 120° to 60° and full arc activities such as cycling are recommended. On occasion, an ACL tear may heal enough to restore stability; however, this is certainly the exception to the rule. Patients should avoid provocative positions/maneuvers and may not be able to return to their preinjury activity level. The use of functional knee braces has been shown to be of limited value in sports. Although they may limit knee movement in certain positions, they also reduce proprioception. Knee braces only function to decrease anterior translation at low loads and rates of load application.

b. Primary Repair—Most surgeons agree that primary repair alone is no longer a viable option for an intrasubstance tear, because the ACL does not heal well. Primary repair with augmentation has been reported to be more successful, but the prolonged postoperative protection that is required may result in muscle atrophy and knee stiffness. Additionally, primary repair requires early surgical intervention, which has been shown to be a factor in the development of postoperative stiffness. Repair of bony avulsion injuries may be reasonable if the ligament is still viable and has not stretched excessively with the injury.

c. Extra-articular Repair—Several procedures have been developed to address the lateral aspect of the ACL-deficient knee, including the Macintosh, Ellison, and Losee procedures. These procedures, which basically involve a tenodesis of the iliotibial tract, may reduce or eliminate the pivot shift but do not reliably diminish anterior translation. One long-term study of the Ellison procedure noted increasing laxity and poor results over time. Many authorities later advocated these repairs in conjunction with intra-articular reconstructions; however, more recent reports have noted that they do not have any added benefit over intra-articular ACL reconstruction alone.

d. Intra-articular Reconstruction—This has become the gold standard for active patients with an ACL injury. Several graft sources have been advocated, and two different techniques have been developed.

(1) Graft Selection—Three general categories of grafts are available for ACL reconstruction: autografts (most commonly bone-patella tendon-bone [BPTB] followed by hamstrings), allografts (BPTB or Achilles tendon), and prostheses (complete replacement [e.g., Gore-Tex]). Additionally, grafts can be combined with a ligament augmentation device. The BPTB autograft is the most popular graft and in numerous studies has been shown to be an excellent choice. Nevertheless, some morbidity is associated with graft harvesting, including the risk of patellar fracture and the development of late patellofemoral pain. It should be noted that 20% to 25% of patients with chronic ACL deficiency have patellofemoral pain. The incidence of patellofemoral symptoms after BPTB reconstruction was reported to be approximately 30% when older rehabilitation methods were used. Hamstring grafts have become popular in some centers and are said to be associated with less morbidity. Although the hamstring graft is not as mechanically strong as BPTB grafts, some surgeons advocate double-, triple-, or quadruple-thickness grafts that may exceed the mechanical strength of BPTB grafts. One potential drawback to the use of hamstring grafts is that fixation must be performed with soft tissue techniques or with sutures tied over a post. Both of these methods have been shown to be mechanically inferior to bone-bone fixation with interference screws. Reports comparing hamstring and BPTB autografts demonstrated greater laxity in the hamstring group in patients with chronic ACL deficiency. Allografts have the advantage of no donor site morbidity, and procedures can be carried out through smaller incisions. Potential risks include transmission of human immunodeficiency virus (<1:1 million with optimal screening methods, including donor autopsy). Additionally, grafts that are irradiated with >2.5 millirad (centigray) lose mechanical strength. A few reports have described widening of osseous tunnels with allografts. An additional

issue is the possibility of an immune reaction with the use of allograft tissue. Although this has not clinically been a problem, more research needs to address this area. Allografts have also been demonstrated to have a delayed graft incorporation time in animal studies when compared with autografts, and initial reports suggest that stability may not be as reliable as with autogenous tissue. Therefore, the full implications of these findings and modifications for postoperative rehabilitation have yet to be determined. Finally, the use of prosthetic ligaments cannot be recommended. Numerous reports in the literature describe the high failure rate of Gore-Tex and Dacron grafts. These grafts have also been associated with atraumatic effusions and osteolysis (Fig. 1–65). The use of the ligament augmentation device has also fallen out of favor. Several studies have demonstrated that reconstructions carried out with this device are no better than reconstructions without the device. The device has also been implicated in some cases of graft failure because of stress shielding. However, some evidence suggests that it may be of use to augment a smaller, weaker graft.

(2) Surgical Principles—ACL reconstruction can be accomplished with a two-incision arthroscopically assisted (or miniarthrotomy) tech-

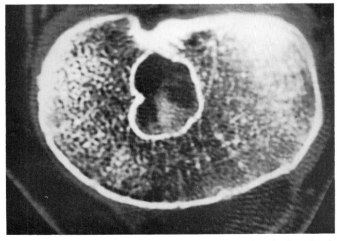

FIGURE 1–65. Proximal tibial osteolysis associated with chronic effects of Gore-Tex prosthetic graft placement. (From Sledge SL, Steadman JR, Silliman JS, et al. Five year results with the Gore-Tex anterior cruciate ligament prosthesis. Am J Knee Surg 5:65–70, 1992.)

nique (Fig. 1–66) or a one-incision endoscopic technique (Fig. 1–67). The main difference between the techniques is in the preparation of the femoral tunnel—outside in (two incision) or inside out (endoscopic). For both techniques, diagnostic arthroscopy is carried out and meniscal pathology addressed (sutures are placed for meniscal repair but not tied until the ACL reconstruction is completed). BPTB graft harvesting should include minimal trauma to the patella with careful technique, as well as incisions in the patella tendon that parallel the fibers and do not violate the underlying fat pad. Semitendinosus and gracilis tendon harvesting should be performed with the knee flexed and the saphenous nerve (which crosses the gracilis) protected. A notchplasty is completed (the inferolateral corner and roof are common sites of impingement), leaving 3 mm of clearance for the graft in all positions of knee flexion. Tunnels are prepared, and the edges are smoothed to avoid graft impingement. A subtle but important difference in the two techniques is the orientation of the graft at the intra-articular edge of the femoral tunnel. With the two-incision technique, the graft is fixed at the lateral cortex, and the ligamentous portion of the graft enters the notch in the anterior portion of the tunnel. With the endoscopic technique, the tendinous portion of the graft occupies the most posterior portion of the tunnel, with the bony portion of the graft anterior. This has implications for tibial tunnel placement: The tunnel must be more posterior for endoscopic techniques and should be more anterior for two-incision techniques. For the endoscopic technique, the tibial tunnel is started at a point midway between the tibial tubercle and the posteromedial edge of the tibia (Fig. 1–68). For the endoscopic technique, the femoral tunnel should be placed posteriorly, leaving only a 1- to 2-mm posterior cortical rim (Color Figure 7). The ideal femoral placement is slightly more posterior when using a two-incision technique, because the graft lies in the anterior part of the tunnel as it enters the knee. A small

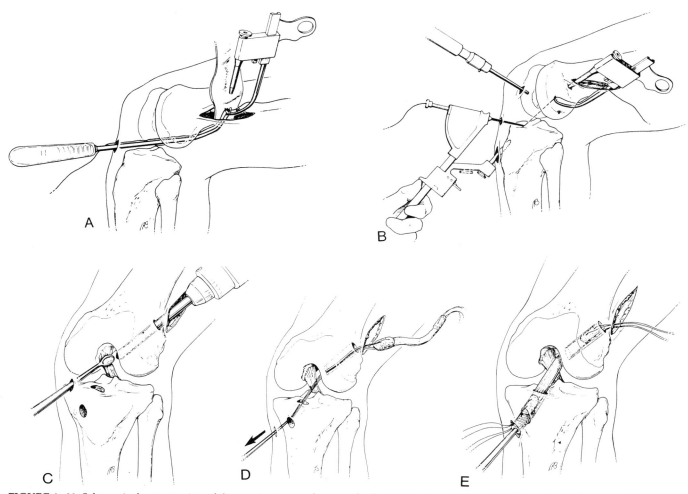

FIGURE 1–66. Schematic demonstration of the two-incision technique of ACL reconstruction. *A,* Femoral guide placed in the "over the top" position with the graft. *B,* Femoral and tibial guides fixed. *C,* Femoral tunnel drilled over K-wire. *D,* Passage of the patella tendon graft. *E,* Graft fixation. (From Diment MT, Sebastianelli WJ, DeHaven KE: Arthroscopically assisted anterior cruciate ligament reconstruction using a central third patellar tendon autograft and two incisions. Op Tech Sports Med 1:45–49, 1993.)

amount of posterior cortical rim is reamed, also. Anterior graft placement, a common error, can lead to graft impingement. It is best avoided by completely clearing and visualizing the posterior cortex of the lateral femoral condyle before placing the femoral tunnel. Ideally, both ends of the graft are secured with interference screws. The graft length occasionally precludes fixation of the tibial side in this manner. This situation, which is more common with the endoscopic technique, can be remedied by securing the bony portion of the graft into a trough on the anteromedial tibia and using a combination of bone staples or sutures tied over a screw and washer for fixation. Before fixation, the knee is extended and the graft is tensioned. Graft tensioning should be performed with the knee near full extension.

(3) Postoperative Rehabilitation—Rehabilitation principles have evolved and have accelerated for ACL reconstruction. Although the concept is controversial, most surgeons advocate early motion and progressive weight bearing. Because of concern of excessive graft tension, some surgeons have advocated avoiding quadriceps loading from 45° of flexion to full extension for 2 to 3 months postoperatively. Return to full activities as early as 6 months postoperatively is possible with more aggressive rehabilitation programs. Of course, the risk of graft damage may be increased with overly aggressive programs. Closed-chain kinetic exercises have been developed and

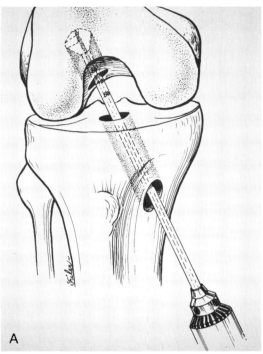

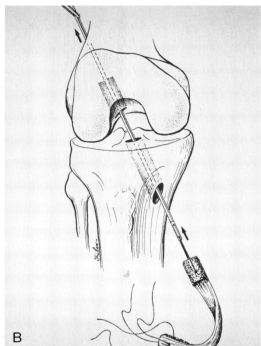

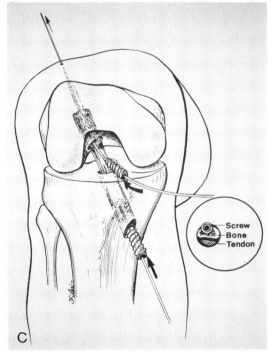

FIGURE 1–67. Single-incision (endoscopic) technique for ACL reconstruction. *A,* Transtibial drilling of femoral tunnel after K-wire is placed 6–8 mm anterior to the posterior cortex of the lateral femoral condyle. *B,* Graft passage from the tibia to the femur. *C,* Graft fixation with interference screws. (From Miller MD, Fu FH. Arthroscopic allograft ACL reconstruction. Op Tech Sports Med (in press).

promoted to minimize anterior tibial translation with active terminal extension.

(4) Complications—Complications in ACL surgery are often a result of technique. These include patella fracture, aberrant tunnel placement, graft rupture from impingement, failure of fixation, and other problems. Loss of motion after ACL reconstruction can also be a difficult problem. Knee stiffness most often is a result of operating in the acute setting, and it is best to wait until full motion is regained and the effusion has resolved (usually 3–4 weeks) before ACL reconstruction. Immediate postoperative motion is also important in avoiding this complication. Failure to achieve early

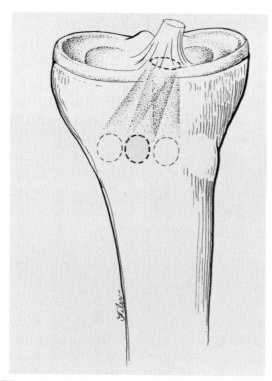

FIGURE 1–68. Ideal tibial tunnel location for graft placement should be midway between the tibial tubercle and the posteromedial edge of the tibia (*shaded area*). (Courtesy of Eric Olson, MD.)

extension can lead to development of a cyclops lesion (Fig. 1–69), infrapatellar contraction syndrome, or more generalized arthrofibrosis. A flexion contracture can result in quadriceps weakness and patellofemoral pain because of increased contact forces. Achieving complete knee extension early postoperatively should be a priority.

e. Treatment of Partial ACL Tears—The natural history or even the existence of partial ACL tears remains controversial. Even the definition of partial ACL tears is not agreed on. Some authorities have suggested that the diagnosis be made arthroscopically and only in patients with a normal pivot shift (an abnormal pivot shift connotes a functionally complete ACL tear). Noyes and colleagues suggest that with 50% disruption of the ACL on arthroscopy, patients have a 50% chance of progressive instability in high-demand activities and a 75% chance of knee reinjury. These investigators also suggested that AP translation of 5 mm or more versus the opposite side was associated with a poor prognosis.

f. ACL Deficiency in Arthritic Knees— Treatment of combined DJD and ACL

deficiency should be individualized. In patients with both significant ACL instability and varus knees from isolated medial compartment DJD, combined ACL reconstruction and upper tibial osteotomy may be an option (Fig. 1–70). The osteotomy is first accomplished, and then the ACL is reconstructed using endoscopic techniques. Patients should not be expected to fare as well as younger patients undergoing ACL reconstruction alone. Long-term results are unknown, because this is best considered a salvage procedure. ACL reconstruction alone may be successful in selected young patients with combined ACL deficiency and osteoarthritis ("knee abusers"). However, once again, the long-term results of these procedures are unknown.

g. Treatment of ACL Injuries in Adolescents—Patients with ACL injuries and open physes present a difficult problem to a reconstructive surgeon. Because of the risk of physeal injury with standard techniques, some surgeons recommend extra-articular procedures only for younger patients with symptomatic ACL-deficient knees. Special techniques that do not violate the tibial physis (tunnel is placed proximal to the

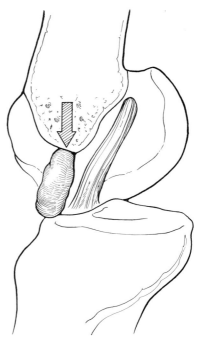

FIGURE 1–69. A cyclops lesion resulting from residual tissue anterior to an ACL graft can block full extension. (Redrawn from Schaefer RK, Jackson DW. Arthroscopic management of the cruciate ligaments. In McGinty JB [ed]. *Operative Arthroscopy.* New York: Raven Press, 1991, p 415.)

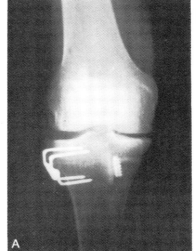
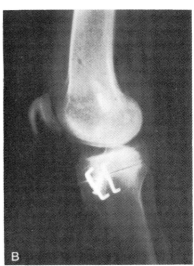

FIGURE 1–70. AP (A) and lateral (B) radiographs after combined upper tibial osteotomy and ACL reconstruction. (From Miller MD, Fu FH. The role of osteotomy in the anterior cruciate ligament deficient knee. Clin Sports Med 12:705, 1993.)

physis), with hamstring graft placement in the over-the-top position, have had some success in these patients and are preferred to extra-articular procedures.

  B. Posterior Cruciate Ligament (PCL)
    1. Introduction—PCL injuries are more common than once believed and may cause chronic morbidity. The PCL serves two major functions: (1) It serves as the primary restraint against posterior tibial displacement, and (2) in conjunction with the ACL, it regulates the screw-home mechanism of the knee (external rotation in terminal extension). The PCL is also a secondary restraint to varus/valgus and rotatory instability. Injury to the PCL can affect these important functions, causing abnormal knee kinematics. Although PCL has not been the subject of as much laboratory and clinical investigation as ACL, it is becoming a focus of research.
    2. History and Physical Examination—Several mechanisms can result in PCL injury (Fig. 1–71).

MECHANISMS OF PCL INJURY

1) Direct anterior blow to the proximal tibia with the knee flexed
2) Hyperflexion, with or without #1
3) Hyperextension (after the ACL tears)
4) Varus or valgus (after the respective collateral ligament tears)
5) Combinations of #1 through #4

Most injuries occur in young males involved in motor vehicle–related accidents (the so-called dashboard injury) and contact sports (especially football [anterior blow to tibia with foot plantar flexed]). Acutely, patients may have a mild effusion, evidence of anterior tibial contusions, or popliteal ecchymoses. Many patients

with isolated PCL injuries may not initially have recognized the significance of their injury but present late with complaints of medial or patellofemoral aching pain. Patients may occasionally complain of instability, but physical examination is often more helpful in these cases. Physical examination for PCL injuries was described earlier; the most sensitive test for PCL injury is the posterior drawer at 90° (Fig. 1–71D). Posterolateral instability, which can be associated with PCL injuries, involves injury to the posterolateral corner (arcuate ligament, lateral collateral ligament, popliteus, popliteofibular ligament, and lateral head of the gastrocnemius). Testing for integrity of the posterolateral corner was described earlier. Patients with chronic PCL/posterolateral corner injuries may ambulate with a varus thrust. Thorough evaluation of *all* knee ligaments is essential in order to identify knees with combined ligament injuries. The role of instrumented testing for posterior laxity in the knee has not been well defined in the current literature. The use of devices that have been devised for measurement of anterior laxity may not be applicable to posterior laxity measurement. In contrast to ACL injury, associated meniscal pathology in PCL-deficient knees is unusual. Radiographs should be carefully reviewed for any evidence of avulsion fractures of the PCL. This is important, because these fractures should be fixed acutely, even if they are only minimally displaced, to avoid long-term morbidity. In cases of posterolateral instability, avulsion fracture of the fibular head or the Gerdy tubercle and the presence of a nondisplaced fracture of the medial tibial plateau should be ruled out. The medial femoral

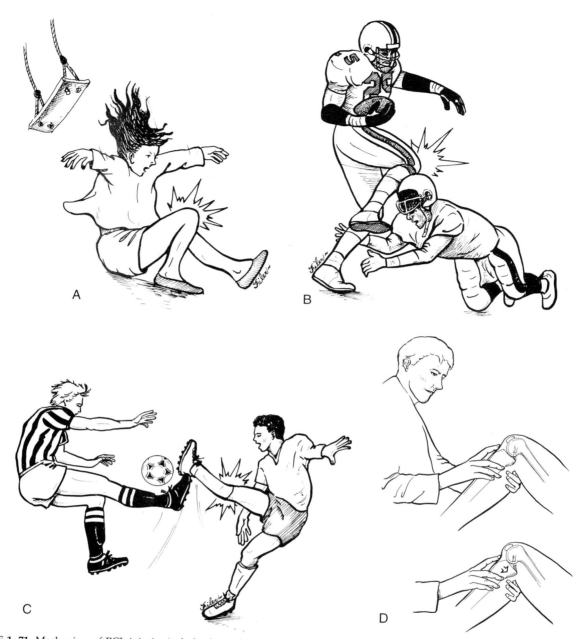

FIGURE 1–71. Mechanism of PCL injuries includes hyperflexion with a downward force (*A*), hyperflexion with an anterior tibial force (*B*), and hyperextension (*C*). *D*, Palpating the anteromedial tibia for the normal step off is important in diagnosing PCL injury. (From Miller MD, Harner CD, Koshiwaguchi S. Acute posterior cruciate ligament injuries. In Fu FH, Harner CD, Vince KG [eds]. *Knee Surgery*. Baltimore: Williams & Wilkins, 1994.)

condyle and patellofemoral joint should be carefully evaluated because of the reported association of arthralgia with PCL injuries, particularly with chronic injuries. Nuclear imaging can be a helpful adjunct to assess early articular cartilage damage. MRI can also be useful, especially in determining the location of the tear and in identifying other associated soft tissue injuries (see Fig. 1–27). In one study, MRI had 100% sensitivity and specificity in identifying complete tears of the PCL. MRI in acutely injured knees can sometimes be helpful, because clinical examination is obscured by swelling and a patient's guarding. How-

ever, one must be careful not to rely solely on MRI findings. All MRI findings must be confirmed by clinical examination. Examination under anesthesia is still the most important determining factor in our surgical approach to knee ligament injuries.

3. Treatment—At present, most authorities recommend nonoperative treatment for acute isolated PCL injuries and reserve surgical reconstruction for symptomatic chronic PCL injuries, acute bony avulsions, and acute combined injuries.
   a. Nonoperative Treatment—Acutely, isolated PCL injuries should be managed by splinting the knee in extension until

the pain subsides, followed by early motion. It is essential that rehabilitation of PCL injuries emphasize open-chain quadriceps strengthening. Functional knee braces have not been shown to be effective in nonoperative management of PCL injured knees. Long-term follow-up studies have expressed little agreement about the natural history of the PCL-deficient knee. Although many have reported satisfactory results with nonoperative treatment of isolated PCL injuries, others have reported good subjective but only fair objective results. A follow-up study of nonoperatively treated isolated PCL injuries suggests that significant activity-related pain and degenerative changes (especially in the medial compartment) are common with this form of treatment. PCL injury results in a poor clinical outcome when associated with rotatory laxity, quadriceps weakness, meniscectomy, patellar chondrosis, and gross laxity. Of most concern is the reported increase in degenerative arthritis associated with chronic PCL instability. This has led some surgeons to adapt a more aggressive approach to acute PCL injuries; however, this is still a matter of considerable controversy. It has been well documented that nonoperative treatment of combined ligament injuries involving the PCL is less successful than in isolated PCL injuries. At this time, most surgeons recommend surgical reconstruction for *combined* ligament injuries, acute or chronic (Fig. 1–72).

  b. Primary Repair—It has long been established that acute repair of bony PCL avulsion fractures is appropriate and avoids the morbidity associated with nonunion of this fracture. These fractures are best approached posteriorly and are ideally secured with screw fixation for larger fragments or primary repair with sutures through small drill holes for smaller fragments (Fig. 1–73). Follow-up studies of such repairs have reported consistently good results. Unfortunately, as with the ACL, primary repair of interstitial tears of the PCL has been largely unsuccessful.

  c. Reconstruction—Various surgical techniques have been reported for PCL reconstruction, with highly variable results. Procedures such as transfer of the medial head of the gastrocnemius or hamstring tendons have been advocated and performed, with mixed results. Hughston reported good subjective but discouraging objective results using the medial head of the gastrocnemius. Insall transferred the medial head of the gastrocnemius with a bone block but reported a failure in two of eight patients. Kennedy believed that recurvatum and posterior drawer signs are not markedly improved by this procedure because the transfer functions dynamically, and explains that when the tibia is forced posteriorly, the contraction of the medial head of the gastrocnemius tends to reduce the upper tibia anteriorly. Other authorities disagree and do not recommend this procedure. Other dynamic transfers, such as the popliteus tendon, double tendon (gracilis and semitendinosus), and semimembranosus, are not successful and are mentioned for historical purposes. If surgical reconstruction is to be performed, attempted re-creation of the normal anatomy yields the best possible clinical result. A current technique, developed in conjunction with intensive laboratory research, is based on attempting to reproduce the normal anatomy. With current graft availability and surgical technique, it is possible to reproduce only one of the two components of the PCL. Because it is anatomically and biomechanically a more

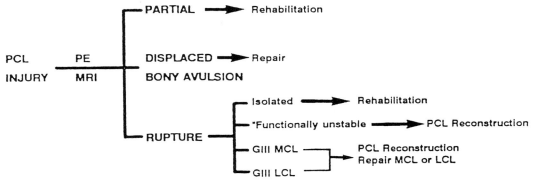

FIGURE 1–72. Algorithm for treatment of PCL injuries. (From Spindler KP, Walker RN. General approach to ligament surgery. In Fu FH, Harner CD, Vince KG [eds]. *Knee Surgery*. Baltimore: Williams & Wilkins, 1994.)

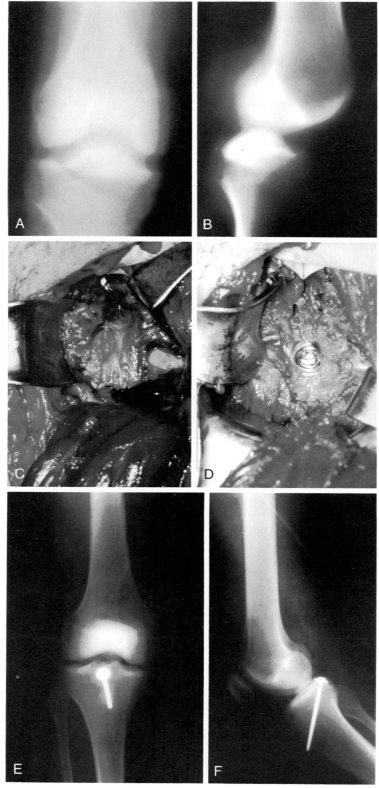

FIGURE 1–73. Primary repair of a PCL avulsion. *A* and *B*, Preoperative tomograms demonstrating a displaced avulsion fracture of the PCL. *C* and *D*, Operative reduction and fixation of the avulsed fracture. *E* and *F*, Postoperative AP and lateral radiograph demonstrating anatomic reduction and fixation of the fracture fragment. (From Miller MD, Harner CD, Koshiwaguchi S. Acute posterior cruciate ligament injuries. In Fu FH, Harner CD, Vince KG [eds]. *Knee Surgery.* Baltimore: Williams & Wilkins, 1994.)

substantial structure, it is preferable to reconstruct the anterolateral portion of the PCL. One surgical technique, which uses fresh-frozen Achilles tendon allograft but is adaptable for use with other grafts, is summarized in Figure 1–74 (see also Color Figure 8). Autologous and allograft patellar tendon and allograft Achilles tendon are currently acceptable grafts for PCL reconstruction.

d. Postoperative Rehabilitation—Postoperatively, the knee is placed in a hinged knee brace that is initially locked in extension. Placing the knee in full extension allows the anterolateral component of the PCL to be under the least amount of tension and minimizes gravitational forces. Quadriceps exercises such as straight leg raising and quadriceps sets are initiated early in the rehabilitation period. Passive range of motion is begun 2 to 4 weeks postoperatively, depending on the extent of the reconstruction. Patients ambulate with crutch assistance initially and are allowed to bear weight as tolerated with the brace locked in full extension, unless collateral reconstruction was performed as well. In the early rehabilitation period, emphasis is placed on avoiding posterior tibial translation, and therapists have an active role in controlling the tibia while performing passive range of motion exercises. Patients are allowed to return to normal activities when functional testing demonstrates similar results at the contralateral knee, usually 8 to 12 months postoperatively.

e. Chronic PCL Injury—Chronic injuries may present a significant challenge to a reconstructive surgeon. Associated medial compartment arthritis may be best addressed with a valgus osteotomy. The most challenging problem involves the chronic PCL and posterolateral corner injury. If a patient has a varus thrust on the injured side, a valgus osteotomy is indicated. Subsequent reconstructive surgery can be performed after a 3- to 6-month recovery period. If a patient does not have a varus thrust, then a posterolateral corner reconstruction can be performed concurrently with PCL reconstruction. Numerous different techniques have been described for posterolateral instability, including arcuate complex advancement popliteus tendon recession, popliteal bypass, and biceps tenodesis. A current approach to this problem is to anatomically reconstruct the lateral collateral ligament and reinforce the posterolateral corner (arcuate ligament complex) using local tissue, autologous BPTB autograft, or allograft. The popliteal bypass procedure as described by Muller has not proven to be successful in the long term. Further study is needed to clarify the proper role of these procedures.

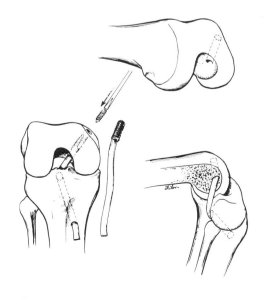

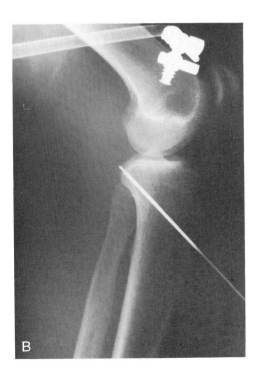

FIGURE 1–74. A, Composite drawing of PCL reconstruction technique. B, Intraoperative lateral radiograph demonstrating the proper location for a tibial guide wire before overdrilling the tunnel. (From Miller MD, Harner CD, Koshiwaguchi S. Acute posterior cruciate ligament injuries. In Fu FH, Harner CD, Vince KG [eds]. *Knee Surgery.* Baltimore: Williams & Wilkins, 1994.)

A

B

f. Complications—Complications associated with PCL reconstruction can be considered in two categories: (1) immediate and (2) delayed. Immediate complications are primarily related to neurovascular injury, infection, or technical errors. The popliteal vessels are at significant risk during tibial tunnel preparation. It is important to visualize the guide pin and drill, to retract the capsule, and to finish the tunnel by hand. Injury to these vessels necessitates immediate repair by a vascular surgeon. Compressive neuropathies can be avoided by paying special attention to positioning of all extremities and adequately padding any vulnerable areas. This is especially important for combined ligament injuries because of the length of the procedure. Peroneal nerve injury can accompany PCL injury, especially in knees with combined injuries involving the posterolateral corner. Careful neurologic examination preoperatively is essential in all cases of suspected PCL injury. Most neurapraxias resolve with conservative management (up to 18 months). Primary neurorrhaphy of complete injuries should be considered. Unfortunately, recovery after these severe palsies is associated with a decidedly poor regenerative potential. Imprecise tunnel placement, graft tensioning, and insecure fixation can result in early postoperative laxity. Delayed complications include loss of motion, avascular necrosis, and recurrent or persistent laxity. Loss of motion after PCL reconstruction differs from motion loss after ACL reconstruction. PCL reconstructed knees often require extra time to regain flexion. Approximately two thirds of patients regain full flexion within 3 to 6 months postoperatively; however, about one third of patients take 9 months to a year to achieve full flexion. This problem can be exacerbated by technical errors in graft placement or overtensioning the graft. The problem of avascular necrosis following PCL reconstruction bears special consideration. Several cases of avascular necrosis of the medial femoral condyle following PCL reconstruction have been reported. The cause of this phenomenon is unclear; however, tunnel location and size with respect to the medial femoral condyle merit further research. Placing more than one tunnel in the medial femoral condyle may increase the risk of avascular necrosis in the setting of multiple ligament reconstruction. Recurrent laxity after PCL reconstruction is common. Almost all PCL reconstructions develop some mild laxity. For this reason, surgery is generally recommended only for moderate to severe posterior instability. Persistent laxity is more common with improper tensioning, divergent tunnel placement, or combined ligament injuries that are not adequately addressed at the time of surgery.

C. Collateral Ligaments
1. MCL injuries—These injuries most commonly occur as a result of valgus stress to the knee, although forced external rotation is less commonly a contributing factor. Pain and instability with valgus stress testing at 30° and no instability at 0° confirm the diagnosis of an isolated MCL injury. Any valgus instability at 0° or moderate instability at 30° suggests a combined ligament injury. Current treatment recommendations for isolated MCL injuries include bracing and early motion. *Nonoperative treatment is advocated for all isolated MCL injuries* (Fig. 1–75). Prophylactic bracing at certain positions may be efficacious when used in football players. Treatment of combined MCL and ACL injuries is more controversial. Surgical treatment of the MCL at the time of ACL reconstruction can result in loss of motion. Because this is more of a problem with MCL injuries that are proximal to the joint line, the physical examination can help guide the decision about the timing of surgery. Reconstruction of the ACL and nonoperative management of associated MCL injuries have been shown to be successful. For chronic injuries that do not respond to nonoperative management, various procedures have been developed to repair the medial structures. These techniques are usually necessary only for reconstruction of combined chronic instability patterns. Most of these procedures consist of proximal advancement of the MCL and reinforcement of the semimembranosus and posteromedial structures (the semitendinosus tendon may be used for this) (Fig. 1–76).
2. LCL Injuries—These injuries are less common than MCL injuries. Varus stress at 0° and 30° of knee flexion is used to evaluate the LCL. Isolated injury to the LCL is less common than combined injury with the posterolateral corner or cruciate ligaments. In contrast to isolated MCL injury, isolated LCL grade III tears yield a small amount of angulation (varus) laxity (up to 4°) in full extension. It is difficult to appreciate the degree of posterolateral disruption in the acute injury. Because of excellent results

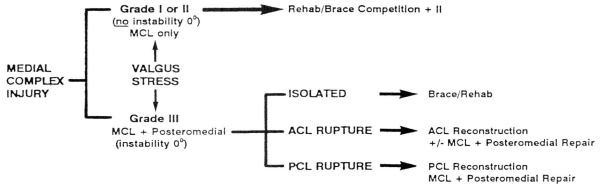

FIGURE 1–75. Algorithm for treatment of MCL injuries. (From Spindler KP, Walker RN. General approach to ligament surgery. In Fu FH, Harner CD, Vince KG [eds]. *Knee Surgery*. Baltimore: Williams & Wilkins, 1994.)

of early primary repair in acute injuries and fair to poor results of reconstructive procedures in chronic posterolateral instability, an aggressive approach to lateral knee ligament injuries is indicated. Examination under anesthesia is a vital step in this process. If laxity is mild (≤3° of increased varus and <10° of increased external rotation), then nonoperative treatment can be successful. For these injuries, it is far preferable to err in favor of surgical exploration and primary repair than to underdiagnose or fail to repair more significant lateral or posterolateral injuries. Combined injuries may necessitate LCL repair in conjunction with other reconstruction (Fig. 1–77). Posterolateral corner injuries should also be addressed in conjunction with LCL repair. Early anatomic repair of the posterolateral corner appears to be most successful. Numerous procedures have been proposed

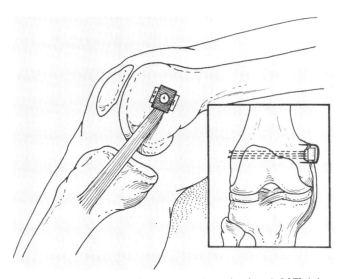

FIGURE 1–76. Technique for reconstruction of a chronic MCL injury. (From Paulos L, Drawbert JP, Rosenberg TD. Knee; soft tissue injuries. In Fitzgerald RH Jr [ed]. *Orthopaedic Knowledge Update 2.* Park Ridge, IL: American Academy of Orthopaedic Surgeons, 1987, p 416.)

for reconstruction of chronic injuries, including posterolateral corner advancement (Muller), biceps tenodesis (Clancy), and various bypass procedures (Muller) (Fig. 1–78).
D. Multiple Ligaments
   1. Introduction—Injuries to multiple ligaments, especially combined ACL/PCL injury, raise the possibility of an unrecognized knee dislocation. When knee dislocation occurs acutely, it is essential that closed reduction and a careful neurovascular examination be performed immediately, with regular follow-up neurovascular assessment. The risk of vascular injury with knee dislocation is high, so liberal use of arteriography is indicated (Fig. 1–79). Vascular injury must be corrected within 6 to 8 hours to decrease the need for amputation. Peroneal nerve injury is also common with knee dislocations, occurring in as many as 40% of cases. Approximately half of these nerve injuries are permanent.
   2. Classification—Knee dislocations are classified on the basis of the direction that the tibia is displaced (Fig. 1–80). Most dislocations are anterior or posterior. Anterior dislocations are usually a result of hyperextension, generally resulting in posterior capsule, ACL, and PCL injury. Posterior dislocations are usually a result of a high-energy anterior force on the tibia and most often result in PCL and ACL injury. Although possible, it is unusual for one of the cruciate ligaments to remain intact after a complete dislocation. Lateral dislocations may occur with valgus force, and medial dislocations with a varus force. Rotatory dislocations are unusual but are produced by a twisting force. The irreducible posterolateral dislocation is the most frequent rotatory dislocation, caused by combined valgus and rotatory forces on the flexed knee. The knee is irreducible by closed

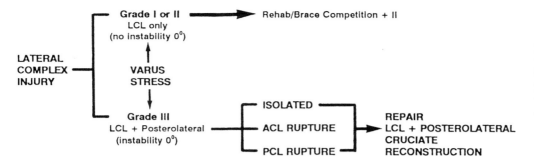

FIGURE 1–77. Algorithm for treatment of LCL injuries. (From Spindler KP, Walker RN. General approach to ligament surgery. In Fu FH, Harner CD, Vince KG [eds]. *Knee Surgery.* Baltimore: Williams & Wilkins, 1994.)

means because of invagination of the medial capsule/MCL. The medial femoral condyle buttonholes through the medial capsule. Open reduction should be performed early to avoid skin necrosis. Occult dislocations may be present in a patient with a spontaneously reduced knee. A high index of suspicion is appropriate in patients with marked or combined instability that is not attributable to a single ligamentous injury.

3. Treatment—Emergent surgical indications include (1) popliteal artery injury, (2) open dislocation, and (3) irreducible dislocations. Even with these circumstances, repair and reconstruction can be delayed, unless substantial dissection is necessary (usually with irreducible dislocations). Early treatment for all other injuries includes closed reduction and immobilization in approximately 20° to 30° of flexion. Substantial controversy surrounds the need for operative repair. Meyers and Harvey reported better functional results in patients treated operatively; however, the opposite conclusion was reached by Taylor and colleagues. Sisto and Warren noted a slight decrease in range of motion but improved stability with surgical repair.

Other reports also confirm generally better results with operative repair/reconstruction. Most surgeons recommend delaying the surgery for 5 to 7 days to ensure that there is no vascular injury. Surgical techniques are also controversial, with most surgeons favoring open repair/reconstruction. Fractures are reduced and rigidly fixed before performing soft tissue procedures. Capsular injuries are repaired from deep to superficial. Cruciate avulsions can be repaired to bone. Interstitial injuries to the cruciates must be reconstructed (Fig.

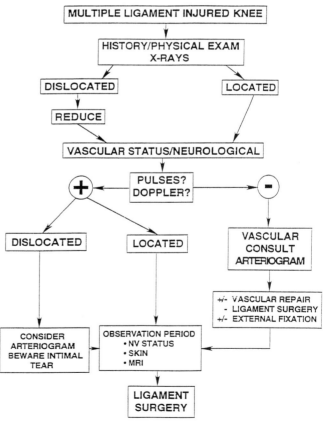

FIGURE 1–79. Algorithm for treatment of multiple knee ligament injuries. (From Marks PH, Harner CD. The anterior cruciate ligament in the multiple ligament-injured knee. Clin Sports Med 12(4):825–838, 1993.)

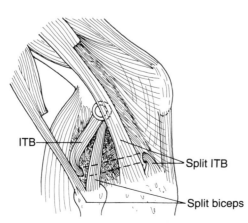

FIGURE 1–78. Technique for chronic posterolateral corner reconstruction. (ITB = Iliotibial band.) (From McMahon MS, Bolard AL. Collateral ligament injuries. In Siliski JM [ed]. *Traumatic Disorders of the Knee.* New York: Springer-Verlag, 1994, pp 301–313.)

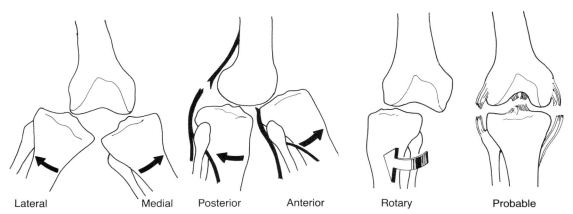

FIGURE 1–80. Classification of knee dislocations. (Redrawn from Bloom MH. Traumatic knee dislocation. In Chapman MW [ed]. *Operative Orthopaedics*. Philadelphia: JB Lippincott, 1988, pp 1633–1640.)

Lateral   Medial   Posterior   Anterior   Rotary   Probable

1–81). Priority should be given to early restoration of the PCL and collateral ligament stability. Early motion is paramount to avoid a high incidence of stiff knee after these combined procedures.

IX. Anterior Knee Pain
 A. Introduction—No longer grouped into the broad and ambiguous category of *chondromalacia*, patellofemoral pain has been classified into various different conditions owing to better understanding (Table 1–1). This classification scheme makes a clear distinction between trauma in an otherwise normal knee and conditions that are related to abnormalities listed as patellofemoral dysplasia. It has been recognized that patellar instability rarely occurs in a "normal" knee and that preexisting abnormalities in the patellofemoral joint (e.g., patella alta or a shallow intercondylar sulcus) or extensor mechanism (e.g., vastus medialis obliquus deficiency or abnormal Q-angle) are usually a predisposing factor. Chondromalacia patellae is a pathologic diagnosis; if the cause of this condition is known, the condition should be classified as such. Occasionally, the cause cannot be determined, and the term *idiopathic chondromalacia* is reserved for these cases. OCD and plicae were discussed in preceding sections and are not reiterated in this section.
 B. Trauma
  1. Introduction—A complete discussion of trauma about the knee is beyond the scope of this text. Nevertheless, the effect of occult trauma on the later development of patellar disorders is probably underappreciated. Patella dislocations are rare in normal knees. Treatment of acute traumatic patella dislocation usually requires operative intervention only in cases of osteochondral fractures. Fractures most commonly involve the lateral condyle or medial patellar facet (Fig. 1–82). With traumatic

avulsion of the vastus medialis obliquus in a previously normal knee, surgical repair and early motion may be most efficacious. Tendon ruptures and overuse injuries are addressed separately.
  2. Tendon Ruptures
   a. Quadriceps Tendon Rupture—These injuries typically occur in patients older than 40 years and occur three times more frequently than patellar tendon ruptures. The mechanism of injury typically is indirect trauma. For both quadriceps and patellar tendon midsubstance ruptures, underlying conditions such as arthritis, fatty degeneration, infection, gout, metabolic disease, calcific tendinitis, and other conditions may be predisposing factors. Patients may present with acute onset of knee pain and marked loss of function. A palpable defect may be present, and active extension is limited. An extension lag is usually present. Anatomic repair should be accomplished if the rupture is diagnosed acutely. Delayed repair may best be managed with the Scuderi technique (Fig. 1–83), using a triangular flap of quadriceps tendon to repair the defect. Chronic repairs may also be repaired using a Marti technique (Fig. 1–84). It may occasionally be necessary to supplement the repair with exogenous tissue (e.g., using hamstring tendons). Overall, results after quadriceps tendon repair are superior to those of patellar tendon repair.
   b. Patellar Tendon Rupture—In contrast to quadriceps tendon rupture, patellar tendon ruptures usually occur in younger patients and are most often caused by direct trauma. Although still unusual, bilateral ruptures are more common for patellar tendon ruptures than quadriceps tendon ruptures. On

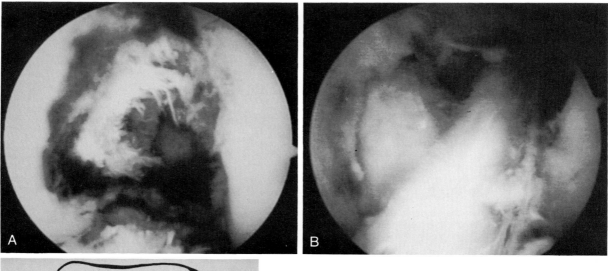

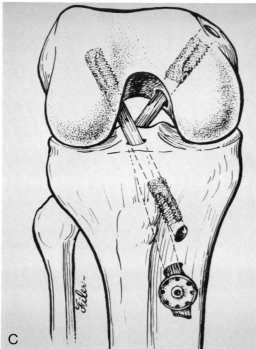

FIGURE 1–81. Arthroscopic view of combined ACL and PCL injury. Before (*A*) and after (*B*) reconstruction with allograft tissue. *C*, Illustration of technique for combined reconstruction.

examination, a defect may be found and the patella is often displaced cephalad. Acute tears should be repaired primarily. Temporary stabilization with wire or nonabsorbable suture (McLaughlin technique) is appropriate (Fig. 1–85). However, care should be taken to avoid overtightening, resulting in patella infera. Intraoperative lateral radiographs can be taken and compared with the uninjured knee.

3. Overuse Injuries
   a. Patellar Tendinitis (Jumper's Knee)— This is a common cause of knee pain in jumping athletes (especially basketball and volleyball participants). Patients present with anterior knee pain and tenderness in the patellar tendon near its origin on the patella. *It is important to note that the tenderness is often more significant when the knee is in extension rather than flexion.* Treatment is first directed at rest, strengthening, stretching, and therapeutic modalities. Cross training with avoidance of high loading impact activities is often an effective technique. Orthoses such as a patellar tendon strap may be of some benefit.

TABLE 1–1. CLASSIFICATION OF PATELLOFEMORAL DISORDERS

I. Trauma (conditions caused by trauma in the otherwise normal knee)
  A. Acute trauma
    1. Contusion (924.11)
    2. Fracture
      a. Patella (822)
      b. Femoral trochlea (821.2)
      c. Proximal tibial epiphysis (tuberlce) (823.0)
    3. Dislocation (rare in the normal knee) (836.3)
    4. Rupture
      a. Quadriceps tendon (843.8)
      b. Patellar tendon (844.8)
  B. Repetitive trauma (overuse syndromes)
    1. Patellar tendinitis ("jumper's knee") (726.64)
    2. Quadriceps tendinitis (726.69)
    3. Peripatellar tendinitis (e.g., anterior knee pain of the adolescent due to hamstring contracture) (726.699)
    4. Prepatellar bursitis ("housemaid's knee") (726.65)
    5. Apophysitis
      a. Osgood-Schlatter disease (732.43)
      b. Sinding-Larsen-Johansson disease (732.42)
  C. Late effects of trauma (905)
    1. Posttraumatic chondromalacia patellae
    2. Posttraumatic patellofemoral arthritis
    3. Anterior fat pad syndrome (posttraumatic fibrosis)
    4. Reflex sympathetic dystrophy of the patella
    5. Patellar osseous dystrophy
    6. Acquired patella infera (718.366)
    7. Acquired quadriceps fibrosis
II. Patellofemoral dysplasia
  A. Lateral patellar compression syndrome (LPCS) (718.365)
    1. Secondary chondromalacia patellae (717.7)
    2. Secondary patellofemoral arthritis (715.289)
  B. Chronic subluxation of the patella (CSP) (718.364)
    1. Secondary chondromalacia patellae (717.7)
    2. Secondary patellofemoral arthritis (715.289)
  C. Recurrent dislocation of the patella (RDP) (718.361)
    1. Associated fractures (822)
      a. Osteochondral (intra-articular)
      b. Avulsion (extra-articular)
    2. Secondary chondromalacia patellae (717.7)
    3. Secondary patellofemoral arthritis (715.289)
  D. Chronic dislocation of the patella (718.362)
    1. Congenital
    2. Acquired
III. Idiopathic chondromalacia patellae (717.7)
IV. Osteochondritis dissecans
  A. Patella (732.704)
  B. Femoral trochlea (732.703)
V. Synovial plicae (727.8916) (anatomic variant made symptomatic by acute or repetitive trauma)
  A. Medial patellar ("shelf") (727.89161)
  B. Suprapatellar (727.89163)
  C. Lateral patellar (727.89165)

Orthopaedic ICD-9-CM Expanded Diagnostic Codes in parentheses. (From Merchant AC: Classification of patellofemoral disorders. Arthroscopy **4**:235, 1988.)

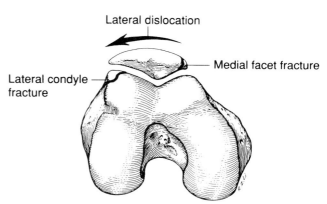

FIGURE 1–82. Patellar dislocation can be associated with osteochondral fractures of the lateral femoral condyle or medial facet of the patella. (From Tria AJ, Klein KS. *An Illustrated Guide to the Knee.* New York: Churchill Livingstone, 1992.)

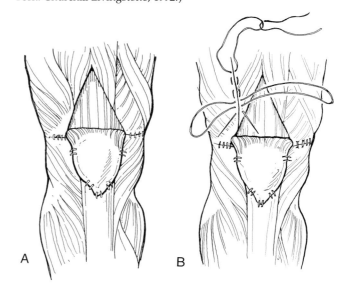
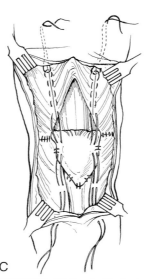

FIGURE 1–83. Scuderi technique for repair of quadriceps tendon ruptures. *A*, A partial-thickness triangular flap of quadriceps tendon is turned down to reinforce the surgical repair. *B*, Bunnell pullout sutures/wires are placed on the medial and lateral portions of the tendon. *C*, Sutures/wires are pulled down and tied over padded buttons.

Isokinetic and plyometric exercises should be avoided, because these may exacerbate the condition. Nonoperative management is usually effective; however, operative excision of the painful, degenerated tendon fibers may occasionally be necessary (Fig. 1–86).
  b. Quadriceps Tendinitis—Although not as common as patellar tendinitis, this

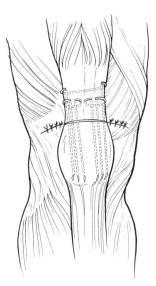

FIGURE 1–84. Marti technique for quadriceps tendon repair. Sutures are passed through vertical drill holes in the patella and are tied at the inferior pole. The retinaculum is repaired directly.

condition, which is also related to overuse, can be just as debilitating. Patients may complain of painful clicking and may report a history of trauma (forced contraction of the quadriceps). Treatment includes quadriceps rehabilitation and modalities to include ultrasound. Operative intervention is occasionally necessary. Arthroscopic debridement of the undersurface of the quadriceps tendon may be possible in selected cases.

c. Peripatellar Tendinitis—This ill-defined condition may be related to hamstring tightness in adolescents and usually responds to hamstring stretching exercises.

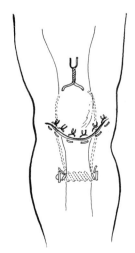

FIGURE 1–85. McLaughlin technique for temporary wire augmentation of patellar tendon repairs. Nonabsorbable suture can also be used for this purpose. McLaughlin recommended removing the hardware at 8 weeks; other surgeons recommend delaying removal until 10 to 12 weeks postoperatively.

d. Prepatellar Bursitis (Housemaid's Knee)—The prepatellar bursa is the most common form of bursitis about the knee (Fig. 1–87). Prepatellar bursitis is often associated with a history of prolonged kneeling. Thickening of the skin over the anterior patella and swelling in the bursa are common. Abrasions must be carefully inspected to rule out any possibility of infection. Surgical excision of the bursa may occasionally be necessary.

e. Iliotibial Band Friction Syndrome—This condition is caused by excessive friction between the iliotibial band and the lateral femoral condyle. Although this condition is more common in runners, it has been noted with increasing frequency in other athletes, particularly cyclists. Findings include localized tenderness over the lateral epicondyle, reproduced by local pressure during flexion and extension of the knee (maximum at 30° knee flexion). Nonoperative management is usually effective. It may occasionally be necessary to excise a small portion of the posterior aspect of the iliotibial band (Fig. 1–88).

f. Semimembranous Tendinitis—This condition occurs most commonly in male athletes in their early 30s and is characterized by pain and inflammation at the insertion of the direct head of the semimembranosus tendon at the posterior tubercle of the tibia. Nuclear imaging can help in diagnosis. Treatment is conservative.

4. Late Effects of Trauma
   a. Patellofemoral Arthritis—Injury to the articular cartilage may be exacerbated by patellar malalignment. This may further erode cartilage, causing pain and crepitation. Lateral release may be beneficial in the early stages; however, once advanced cartilage injury is present, other procedures may be necessary. Options include patellectomy, anterior transfer of the tibial tubercle (Maquet), and anteromedial transfer of the tibial tubercle. The first two options have been associated with excessive morbidity, including reduction of the quadriceps efficiency by up to 30% with patellectomy and skin necrosis, nonunion, and anterior compartment syndrome with the Maquet procedure. Anteromedial transfer of the tibial tubercle, as described by Fulkerson, combines a lateral release with anterior and medial transfer of the tibial tubercle. Bone graft is added to elevate the tibial tubercle further in cases with advanced patello-

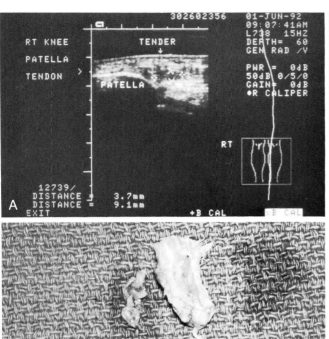

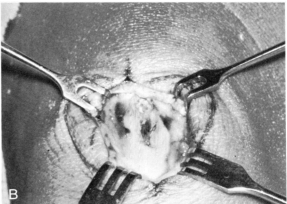

FIGURE 1–86. Example of surgical excision of degenerative patellar tendon after prolonged nonoperative treatment. *A*, Ultrasonography demonstrates the area of the damaged tendon. *B*, Surgical incision. *C*, Removal of damaged tendon fibers.

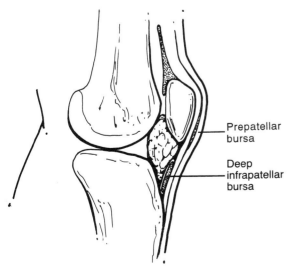

femoral arthrosis (Fig. 1–89). Patellofemoral joint arthroplasty currently has no role for isolated patellofemoral arthritis. Patellar or trochlear osteotomies have had limited success in European studies; however, they have not been popular in the United States. The value

of abrasion, spongialization, and drilling of the patella is unproven.
  b. Anterior Fat Pad Syndrome (Hoffa Disease)—Trauma to the anterior fat pad can lead to fibrous changes and pinching of the fat pad between the femoral condyles and tibial plateau with knee

FIGURE 1–87. Bursae around the knee include the prepatellar bursa and the infrapatellar bursa. (From Walsh WM. Patellofemoral joint. In DeLee JC, Drez D Jr. *Orthopaedic Sports Medicine: Principles and Practice.* Philadelphia: WB Saunders, 1994, pp 1163–1248.)

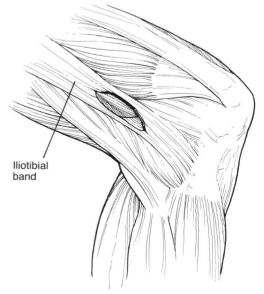

FIGURE 1–88. Treatment of iliotibial band friction syndrome includes excision of a posterior portion of the iliotibial band.

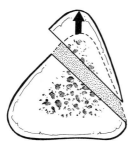

FIGURE 1–89. Anteromedial transfer of the tibial tubercle with the addition of a bone graft, as described by Fulkerson, can allow elevation of the tubercle without many of the risks associated with the Macquet operation.

extension. The condition, which occurs more commonly in patients with genu recurvatum, usually resolves with time. Initial treatment includes activity modification, ice, and padding of the knee. Surgical excision may occasionally be necessary to reduce pain and increase motion. Fat pad fibrosis with painful extension loss as a sequela of knee ligament (ACL) surgery is a separate entity and is a form of arthrofibrosis.

c. Other Effects—Other sequelae of trauma include other forms of fibrosis and RSD of the patella. RSD is characterized by pain out of proportion to the injury sustained. Abnormal vasomotor, thermoregulatory, neurotrophic, sympathetic, and parasympathetic activities typify this exaggerated response to injury. Three stages of RSD are recognized:

Phase	Length	Characteristics
I	3 months	Swelling, edema, increased temperature hyperhidrosis, allodynia
II	6 months	Brawny edema, loss of motion, trophic changes
III	Indefinite	Pale, cool, dry skin; glossy appearance, stiff knee

The stages of RSD are less well defined in the knee than in the upper extremity, and the symptoms are more varied, with disproportionate pain being the hallmark. RSD may be associated with marked osteopenia of the patella as visualized on the lateral or Merchant view (Fig. 1–90). Patients with RSD may present with a "flamingo gait," walking on crutches with only one leg and the other in a flexed position. Although loss of motion is common, as many as 50% of patients have normal motion. Early recognition and treatment are the most important factors leading to resolution and good results. Rehabilitation (transcutaneous electric nerve stimulation, range of motion, hot-cold soaks), nonsteroidal anti-inflammatory drugs, counseling, and occasionally lumbar sympathetic or epidural blocks may be necessary. Although diagnostic arthroscopy or patellar surgery should be avoided to avert exacerbation of the syndrome, surgery may be indicated in some patients to eliminate the triggering pathology. This should be considered only after a series of blocks have controlled the symptoms of RSD.

5. Patellofemoral Dysplasia
   a. Lateral Patellar Compression Syndrome/Excessive Lateral Pressure Syndrome—*Lateral patellar compression syndrome* and *excessive lateral pressure syndrome* are synonymous terms related to *patellar malalignment without associated instability.* The condition is diagnosed clinically (tight lateral retinaculum, normal mobility and normal Q-angle) and radiographically (abnormal patellar tilt

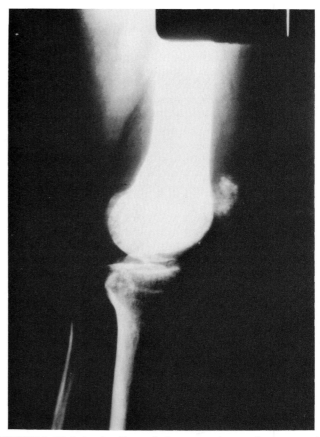

FIGURE 1–90. Lateral radiograph demonstrating patchy osteopenia of the affected patella in reflex sympathetic dystrophy.

without subluxation) (Fig. 1–91). Tilt and compression can lead to patellofemoral pain from lateral retinacular strain and articular cartilage injury. Treatment includes activity modification, nonsteroidal anti-inflammatory drugs, and rehabilitation. Arthroscopy and lateral release may occasionally be required. Arthroscopic confirmation of the diagnosis includes observation that the patella does not articulate medially by 40° of knee flexion, and no evidence of lateral subluxation is found with range of motion. The lateral release can be performed arthroscopically or open and should extend from the lateral joint line to the superior pole of the patella. *It is essential to ensure that adequate hemostasis is achieved after a lateral release.* After the procedure, the patella should be able to be passively tilted 80° (Fig. 1–92). Surgeons should exercise prudence in the diagnosis and surgical treatment of this entity, because most patients do not require surgery.

b. Patellar Instability—Recurrent subluxation or dislocation of the patella is associated with *excessive patellar mobility on examination and radiographic evidence of patellar subluxation/dislocation.* Besides lateral displacement of the patella on radiographs, a shallow intercondylar sulcus or patellar incongruence may be seen. Chronic dislocation of the patella is the most severe form of instability, because the patella never returns to the trochlea throughout the range of motion. This condition may be exacerbated in adolescents with the so-called miserable malalignment syndrome. Femoral anteversion, genu valgum, and pronated feet may contribute to symptoms associated with patellar instability. As for most patellar disorders, the initial treatment is nonoperative. Realignment procedures can be based proximally, distally, or both. Bony procedures are contraindicated in a skeletally immature knee. Most proximal procedures include a lateral release with medial reefing (Fig. 1–93). The Roux-Elmslie-Trillat procedure consists of lateral release, medial capsular reefing, and anteromedial transfer of the tibial tuberosity on a periosteal hinge. This procedure is indicated in patients with recurrent subluxation/dislocation and an increased Q-angle (>15°). Another distal realignment procedure, described by Fulkerson, involves anteromedial transfer of the tibial tubercle by taking advantage of the geometry of the proximal tibia (Fig. 1–94). The logic of medial reefing has recently come into question, because it has been shown that it increases patellofemoral contact forces.

6. Chondromalacia—Although this term has

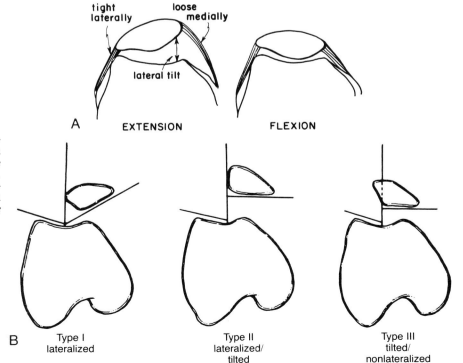

FIGURE 1–91. *A,* Tight lateral retinaculum associated with increased strain with flexion. (From Fu FH, Maday MG. Arthroscopic lateral release and the lateral patellar compression syndrome. Orthop Clin North Am 23:601, 1992.) *B,* Excessive patellar tilt can be characterized on plain films and CT (From Scott WN. *Arthroscopy of the Knee.* Philadelphia: WB Saunders, 1990, p 162.)

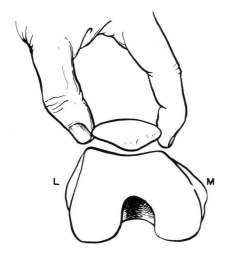
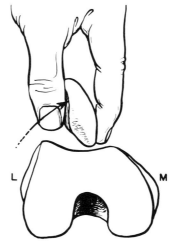

FIGURE 1–92. The patella should be able to be passively tilted 80° after lateral release (L = lateral; M = medial). (From Fu FH, Maday MG. Arthroscopic lateral release and the lateral patellar compression syndrome. Orthop Clin North Am 23:601, 1992.)

fallen into disrepute, articular cartilage degeneration occurs frequently in the patella. This can occur secondary to malalignment or may occasionally be idiopathic. The classification scheme developed by Outerbridge is still in common use today (Fig. 1–95). Treatment is best directed at avoidance; however, arthroscopic drilling may be appropriate for established lesions.

7. Abnormalities of Patellar Height—Both patella alta (high-riding patella) and patella baja/infera (low-lying patella) are judged on the basis of lateral radiographs using various techniques (see Fig. 1–23). Certain factors such as patellar deformity, tibial tubercle deformities, spurring, and the position of the knee can lead to various degrees of error in these measurements. The Insall-Salvati ratio and the Blackburne-Peel ratio are the most reliable. The latter is prefera-

ble in cases of deformity of the tubercle or patella. These conditions can be acquired or congenital and may contribute to other patellofemoral disorders. Patella alta is related to patellar instability, because the patella is abnormally high and is not constrained within the femoral sulcus. Patella baja is often a result of retinacular, fat pad, and patellar tendon fibrosis with contracture.

X. Childhood and Adolescent Knee Disorders
   A. Physeal Injuries—The distal femoral physis, which contributes 70% of femoral growth, is more commonly injured than the proximal tibial physis. The most common type of injury to this physis is a Salter-Harris type II fracture (Fig. 1–96). Patients may present with pain and swelling and often are unable to ambulate. Special oblique views or stress radio-

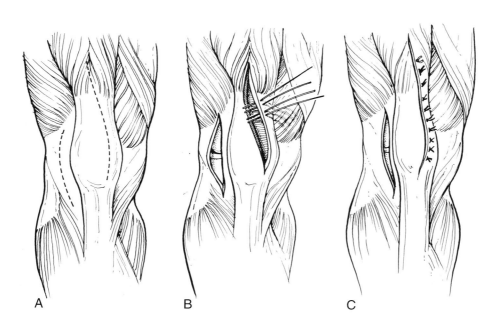

FIGURE 1–93. Proximal patellar realignment includes both lateral release and medial reefing. *A,* Planned incision. *B,* Procedure. *C,* Final result.

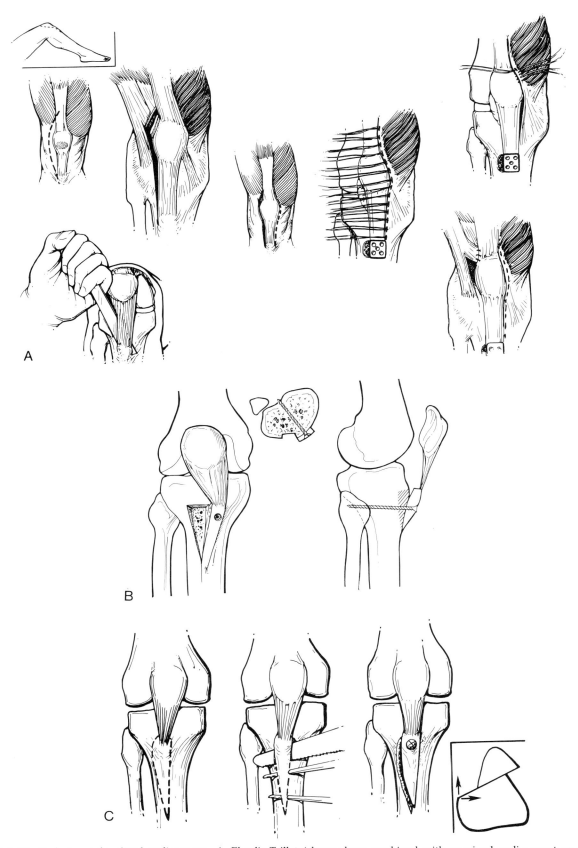

FIGURE 1–94. Techniques for distal realignment. *A,* Elmslie-Trillat (shown here combined with proximal realignment as described by Hughston). (From Walsh WM. Patellofemoral joint. In DeLee JC, Drez D Jr. *Orthopaedic Sports Medicine: Principles and Practice.* Philadelphia: WB Saunders, 1994, pp 1163–1248.) *B,* Bone block transfer (as described by Miller and LaRochelle). (Redrawn from Miller BJ, LaRochelle PJ. The treatment of patellofemoral pain by combined rotation and elevation of the tibial tubercle. J Bone Joint Surg 68A:419–423, 1986.) *C,* Anteromedial transfer (without added bone graft) as described by Fulkerson. (From Walsh WM. Patellofemoral joint. In DeLee JC, Drez D Jr. *Orthopaedic Sports Medicine: Principles and Practice.* Philadelphia: WB Saunders, 1994, pp 1163–1248.)

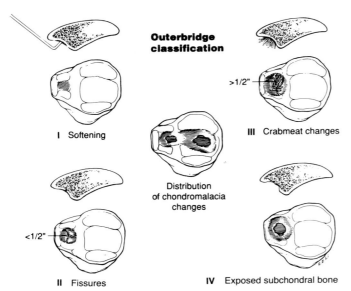

Outerbridge classification

I Softening

II Fissures

III Crabmeat changes

IV Exposed subchondral bone

Distribution of chondromalacia changes

>1/2"

<1/2"

FIGURE 1–95. Outerbridge classification of chondromalacia. (From Tria AJ, Klein KS. *An Illustrated Guide to the Knee.* New York: Churchill Livingstone, 1992.)

graphs may be necessary to identify nondisplaced fractures. MRI may also be helpful in diagnosing subtle fractures that may occur in the sagittal or coronal plane. Closed reduction and immobilization usually results in satisfactory results; however, the incidence of late leg length discrepancy and thigh atrophy is high after fractures of the distal femoral growth

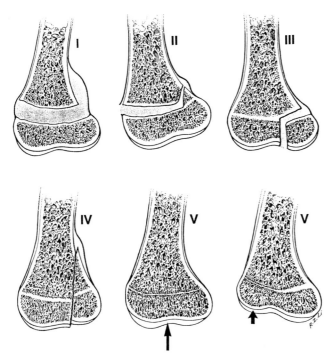

FIGURE 1–96. Salter-Harris classification of distal femoral fractures. (From Tria AJ, Klein KS. *An Illustrated Guide to the Knee.* New York: Churchill Livingstone, 1992.)

plate. Open reduction is indicated for Salter-Harris III and IV fractures or if an unsatisfactory reduction is obtained with a Salter-Harris I or II fracture.

B. Ligament Injuries—Injuries to the MCL are relatively common in children. Closed treatment, as in injuries in adults, usually results in successful results. Midsubstance injuries to the ACL have been noted to be more frequent in recent years. Treatment of these injuries remains controversial. Most surgeons favor a trial of nonoperative management initially. In patients with residual pain, swelling, and giving way or in those patients with an unstable but repairable meniscal tear, surgical treatment may be the only option. Because of the concern over growth disturbance, many procedures have been developed to reconstruct the ACL without violating the growth plate. Unfortunately, none of these procedures are as successful as an intra-articular reconstruction with standard tibial and femoral drill holes. Most authorities recommend delaying these procedures until <1 cm of growth remains in the distal femoral physis. Cutting sports should be avoided during that time. ACL avulsion fracture of the intercondylar eminence of the tibia is relatively common, especially with bicycle accidents in children 8 to 15 years old. Treatment involves closed reduction or, failing this, arthroscopic reduction and fixation of the fragment. The knee is then immobilized in 20° to 30° flexion or the position that results in the most anatomic reduction. Surgical treatment is favored for types II and III fractures that cannot be reduced with closed methods (Fig. 1–97).

C. Extensor Mechanism Disorders
1. Acute Injuries to the Extensor Mechanism—Patellar dislocation is more common in adolescents than adults. Treatment includes immobilization for 3 weeks, followed by quadriceps rehabilitation.

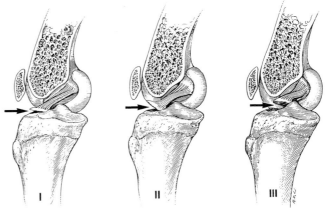

I   II   III

FIGURE 1–97. Classification of tibial eminence fractures. (From Tria AJ, Klein KS. *An Illustrated Guide to the Knee.* New York: Churchill Livingstone, 1992.)

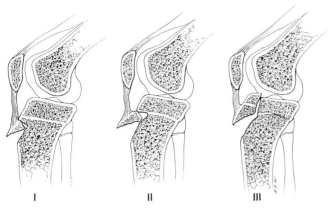

FIGURE 1–98. Classification of tibial tubercle physeal fractures. (From Tria AJ, Klein KS. *An Illustrated Guide to the Knee.* New York: Churchill Livingstone, 1992.)

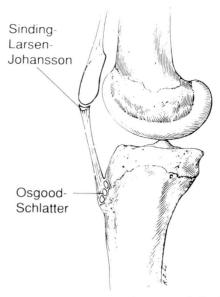

FIGURE 1–99. Osgood-Schlatter disease and Sinding-Larsen-Johansson disease are types of traction apophysitis affecting the knees of adolescents.

Arthroscopic evaluation may be appropriate for acute high-energy trauma with a suspected chondral or osteochondral injury. Fractures of the tibial tuberosity can also occur in adolescents (Fig. 1–98). Treatment of this minimally displaced fracture in patients who can fully extend their knee is closed. Open reduction and internal fixation is recommended for all other fractures.

2. Overuse Injuries
   a. Bipartite Patellae—Most commonly an incidental finding, bipartite patellae can occasionally cause anterior knee pain aggravated by squatting, kneeling, or jumping. The most common location for bipartite patellae is superolateral, although inferior and lateral or multipartite patellae can also occur. Treatment includes activity modification. Rarely, excision of the symptomatic fragment and quadriceps retinacular repair may be required.
   b. Traction Apophysitis (Fig. 1–99)
      (1) Osgood-Schlatter Disease—This is a common condition in adolescent athletes. Patients (usually boys) may complain of activity-related discomfort and swelling and tenderness of the tibial tubercle. The condition is bilateral 20% to 30% of the time. It is thought to be caused by repetitive stress on the immature patellar tendon–tibial tubercle–tibial junction. Activity modification and occasionally immobilization are usually successful. Surgical excision of symptomatic ossicles may occasionally relieve prolonged symptoms.
      (2) Sinding-Larsen-Johansson Disease— This condition is caused by repetitive traction on the immature, inferior pole of the patella and is usually encountered earlier than Osgood-Schlatter disease (age 11 versus 13 years). Treatment is also nonoperative. Surgical treatment for jumper's knee is occasionally required for older children.

Selected References

Basic Sciences

Amiel D, Frank CB, Harwood FL, et al. Tendons and ligaments: a morphological and biochemical comparison. J Orthop Res 1:257–265, 1984.

Arnoczky SP, Warren RF. Microvasculature of the human meniscus. Am J Sports Med 10:90–95, 1982.

Arnoczky SP. Anatomy of the anterior cruciate ligament. Clin Orthop 172:19–25, 1983.

Butler DL. Anterior cruciate ligament: its normal response in relacement. J Orthop Res 7:910–921, 1989.

Cooper DE, Deng XH, Burnstein AL, Warren RF. The strength of the central third patellar tendon graft. A biomechanical study. Am J Sports Med 21:818–824, 1993.

Daniel DM, Akeson WH, O'Connor JJ (eds). *Knee Ligaments: Structure, Function, Injury, and Repair.* New York: Raven Press, 1990.

DeLee JC, Riley MB, Rockwood CA Jr. Acute posterolateral rotary instability of the knee. Am J Sports Med 11:199–206, 1983.

Fu FH, Harner CD, Johnson DL, et al. Biomechanics of knee ligaments: basic concepts and clinical application. J Bone Joint Surg 75A:1716–1725, 1993.

Furman W, Marshall JL, Girgis FG. The anterior cruciate ligament: a functional analysis based on postmortem studies. J Bone Joint Surg 58A:179–185, 1976.

Girgis FG, Marshall JL, Al Monajem ARS. The cruciate ligaments of the knee joint: anatomical, functional and experimental analysis. Clin Orthop 106:216–231, 1975.

Heller L, Langmen J. The menisco-femoral ligaments of the human knee. J Bone Joint Surg 46B:307–313, 1964.

Hughston JC, Eilers AF. The role of the posterior oblique ligament in repairs of acute medial (collateral) ligament tears of the knee. J Bone Joint Surg 55A:923–940, 1973.

Jackson DW, Grood ES, Goldstein JD, et al. A comparison of patellar tendon autograft and allograft used for anterior cruciate ligament reconstruction in the goat model. Am J Sports Med 21:176–185, 1993.

Marks PH, Harner CD, Livesay GA, Koshiwaguchi S. Quantitative electron microscopy of the human cruciate and meniscofemoral ligaments. Trans Orthop Res Soc 40, 1994.

Mow VC, Arnoczky SP, Jackson DW. *Knee Meniscus: Basic and Clinical Foundations.* New York: Raven Press, 1992.

Noyes FR, Butler DL, Grood ES, et al. Biomechanical analysis of human ligament grafts used in knee-ligament repairs and reconstructions. J Bone Joint Surg 66A:344–352, 1984.

Rodrigo JJ, Jackson CW, Simon TM, Muto KN. The immune response to freeze dried bone tendon bone ACL allografts in humans. Am J Knee Surg 6:47–53, 1993.

Schultz RA, Miller DC, Kerr CS, Micheli L. Mechanoreceptors in human cruciate ligaments. J Bone Joint Surg 66A:1072–1076, 1984.

Seebacher JR, Inglis AE, Marshall JL, Warren RF. The structure of the posterolateral aspect of the knee. J Bone Joint Surg 64A:536–541, 1982.

Thompson WO, Theate FL, Fu FH, Dye SF. Tibial meniscal dynamics using three-dimensional reconstruction of magnetic resonance images. Am J Sports Med 19:210–216, 1991.

Warren LF, Marshall JL. The supporting structures and layers of the medial side of the knee. J Bone Joint Surg 61A:56–62, 1979.

Warren R, Arnoczky SP, Wickiewicz TL. Anatomy of the knee. In Nicholas JA, Hershman EB (eds). The Lower Extremity and Spine in Sports Medicine. St Louis: CV Mosby, 1986, pp 657–694.

Weber W, Weber E. Kinematics. In Muller W (ed) *The Knee: Form, Function and Ligament Reconstruction.* New York: Springer-Verlag 1983, pp 8–28.

Wiberg, G. Roentgenographic and anatomic studies on the femoropatellar joint. Acta Orthop Scand 12:319, 1941.

Woo SL-Y, Hollis JM, Adams DJ, et al. Tensile properties of the human femur-anterior cruciate ligament-tibia complex: the effect of specimen age and orientation. Am J Sports Med 19:217–225, 1991.

History and Physical Examination

Back BR Jr, Warren RF, Wickiewicz TL. The pivot shift phenomenon: results and description of a modified clinical test for anterior cruciate ligament insufficiency. Am J Sports Med 16:571–576, 1988.

Cooper DE. Tests for posterolateral instability of the knee in normal subjects. Results of examination under anesthesia. J Bone Joint Surg 73A:30–36, 1991.

Daniel DM, Malcom LL, Losse G, et al. Instrumented measurement of anterior laxity of the knee. J Bone Joint Surg 67A:720–726, 1985.

Daniel DM, Stone ML, Barnett P, Sachs R. Use of the quadriceps active test to diagnose posterior cruciate ligament disruption and measure posterior laxity of the knee. J Bone Joint Surg 70A:386–391, 1988.

Fetto JF, Marshall JL. Inquiry to the anterior cruciate ligament producing the pivot shift sign. J Bone Joint Surg 61A:710–714, 1979.

Fulkerson JP, Kalenak A, Rosenberg TD, Cox JS. Patellofemoral pain. Instr Course Lect 41:57–71, 1992.

Galway RD, Beaupre A, MacIntosh DL. Pivot shift. J Bone Joint Surg 54B:763, 1972.

Hosea TM, Tria AJ. Physical examination of the knee: clinical. In Scott WN (ed). *Ligament and Extensor Mechanism Injuries of the Knee: Diagnosis and Treatment.* St Louis: CV Mosby, 1991.

Hughston JC. Subluxation of the patella. J Bone Joint Surg 50A:1003–1026, 1968.

Hughston JC, Andrews JR, Cross MJ, Moschi A. Classification of knee ligament instabilities (I & II). J Bone Joint Surg 58A:159–180, 1976.

Hughston JC, Norwood LA Jr. The posterolateral drawer test and external rotational recurvatum test for posterolateral rotatory instability of the knee. Clin Orthop 147:82–87, 1980.

Insall JN. Examination of the knee. In Insall JN (ed). *Surgery of the Knee.* New York: Churchill Livingstone, 1984.

Jakob RP, Hassler H, Staeubli HU. Observations on rotatory instability of the lateral compartment of the knee. Experimental studies on the functional anatomy and pathomechanics of the true and the reversed pivot shift sign. Acta Orthop Scand 52(suppl 2191):1–32, 1981.

Losee RE, Johnson TR, Southwick WO. Anterior subluxation of the lateral tibial plateau: a diagnostic test and operative repair. J Bone Joint Surg 60A:1015–1030, 1978.

Muller W. Examination of the injured knee. In Muller W (ed). *The Knee.* Berlin: Springer-Verlag, 1983.

Powell JW, Shootman M. A multivariate risk analysis of selected playing surfaces in the national football league: 1980 to 1989. Am J Sports Med 20:686–694, 1992.

Ritchie JR, Miller MD, Harner CD. History and physical examination of the knee. In Fu FH, Harner CD, Vince KG (eds). *Knee Surgery.* Baltimore: Williams & Wilkins, 1994.

Rubinstein RA Jr, Shelbourne KD. Diagnosis of posterior cruciate ligament injuries and indications for nonoperative and operative treatment. Op Tech Sports Med 1:99–103, 1993.

Slocum DB, Larson RL. Rotatory instability of the knee. J Bone Joint Surg 50A:211, 1968.

Torg JS, Conrad W, Kalen V. Clinical diagnosis of anterior cruciate ligament instability in the athlete. Am J Sports Med 4:84, 1976.

Imaging

Aspelin P, Ekberg O, Thorsson O, et al. Ultrasound examination of soft tissue injury of the lower limb in athletes. Am J Sports Med 20:601–603, 1992.

Blackburne JS, Peel TE. A new method of measuring patellar height. J Bone Joint Surg 59B:241–242, 1977.

Blumensaat C. Die lageabweichunger und verrenkungen der kniescheibe. Ergeb Chir Orthop 31:149–223, 1938.

Boden SD, Davis DO, Dina TS, et al. The prospective and blinded investigation of magnetic resonance imaging of the knee: abnormal findings in asymptomatic subjects. Clin Orthop 282:208–212, 1992.

Cobby MJ, Schweitzer ME, Resnick D. The deep lateral femoral notch: an indirect sign of a torn anterior cruciate ligament. Radiology 184:855–858, 1992.

Danzig LA, Newell JD, Guerra J Jr, Resnick D. Osseous landmarks of the normal knee. Clin Orthop 156:201–206, 1981.

Dye SF. Special procedures. In Fu FH, Harner CD, Vince KG (eds). Knee Surgery. Baltimore, Williams & Wilkins, 1994.

Dye SF, McBride JT, Chew M, et al. Unrecognized abnormal osseous metabolic activity in patients with documented meniscal pathology. Am J Sports Med 17:723–724, 1989.

Dye SF, Peartree PK. Sequential radionuclide imaging of the patellofemoral joint in symptomatic young adults. Am J Sports Med 17:727, 1989.

Fairbank TJ. Knee joint changes after meniscectomy. J Bone Joint Surg 30B:664–670, 1948.

Fischer SP, Fox JM, DelPizzo W, et al. Accuracy of diagnoses from magnetic resonance imaging of the knee. J Bone Joint Surg 73A:2–10, 1991.

Graf BK, Cook DA, DeSmet AA, Keene JS. "Bone bruises" on magnetic resonance imaging evaluation of anterior cruciate ligament injuries. Am J Sports Med 21:220–223, 1993.

Gross ML, Grover JS, Bassett LW, et al. Magnetic resonance imaging of the posterior cruciate ligament. Clinical use to improve diagnostic accuracy. Am J Sports Med 20:732–737, 1992.

Harms SE, Flamig DP, Fisher CF, Fulmer M. New method for fast MR imaging of the knee. Radiology 173:743–750, 1989.

Insall J, Salvati E. Patella position in the normal knee joint. Radiology 101:101–104, 1971.

Jackson DW, Jennings LD, Maywood RM, Bergere PE. Magnetic resonance imaging of the knee. Am J Sports Med 16:29–38, 1988.

Kaplan PA, Walker CW, Kilcoyne RF, et al. Occult fracture patterns of the knee associated with anterior cruciate ligament tears: assessment of MR imaging. Radiology 183:835–838, 1992.

Lotysch M, Mink J, Crues JV, Schwartz A. Magnetic resonance in the detection of meniscal injuries (abstr). Magn Reson Imaging 4:185, 1986.

McCauley TR, Kier R, Lynch KJ, Jokl P. Chondromalacia patellae: diagnosis with MR imaging. AJR 158:101–105, 1992.

Merchant AC, Mercer RL, Jacobsen RH, Cool CR. Roentgenographic analysis of patellofemoral congruence. J Bone Joint Surg 56A:1391–1396, 1974.

Mink JH, Deutsch AL. Magnetic resonance imaging of the knee. Clin Orthop 244:29–47, 1989.

Murphy BJ, Smith RL, Uribe JW, et al. Bone signal abnormalities in the posterolateral tibia and lateral femoral condyle in complete tears of the anterior cruciate ligament: a specific sign? Radiology 182:221–224, 1992.

Nachlas IW, Olpp JL. Para-articular calcification (Pellegrini-Stieda) in affections of the knee. Surg Gynecol Obstet 81:206–212, 1945.

Newhouse KE, Rosenberg TD. Basic radiographic examination of the knee. In Fu FH, Harner CD, Vince KG (eds). Knee Surgery. Baltimore: Williams & Wilkins, 1994.

Rosen MA, Jackson DW, Berger PE. Occult osseous lesions documented by magnetic resonance imaging associated with anterior cruciate ligament ruptures. Arthroscopy 7:45–51, 1991.

Rosenberg TD, Paulos LE, Parker RD, et al. The forty-five-degree posteroanterior flexion weight-bearing radiograph of the knee. J Bone Joint Surg 70A:1479–1483, 1988.

Rogers LF, Jones S, Davis AR, Dietz G. Clipping injury. Fracture of the epiphysis in the adolescent football player: an occult lesion of the knee. Am J Roentgenol 121:69–78, 1974.

Schutzer SF, Ramsby GR, Fulkerson JP. The evaluation of patellofemoral pain using computerized tomography. Clin Orthop 204:286–293, 1986.

Scuderi JR. The femoral intercondylar roof angle: radiographic and MRI measurement. Am J Knee Surg 6:10–14, 1993.

Segond P. Recherches cliniques et experimentales sur lees epanchements sanguins du genou par entorse. Prog Med VII, 1879.

Speer KP, Spritzer CE, Bassett FA III, et al. Osseous injury associated with acute tears of the anterior cruciate ligament. Am J Sports Med 20:382–389, 1992.

Stoller DW, Martin C, Cruees JV, et al. Meniscal tears: pathologic correlation with MR imaging. Radiology 163:731–735, 1987.

Thaete FL, Britton CA. Magnetic resonance imaging. In Fu FH, Harner CD, Vince KG (eds). Knee Surgery. Baltimore: Williams & Wilkins, 1994.

Woods GW, Stanley RF, Tullos HS. Lateral capsular sign: x-ray clue to a significant knee instability. Am J Sports Med 7:27–33, 1979.

Knee Arthroscopy

Coward DB. General principles and instrumentation of arthroscopic surgery. In Chapman MW (ed). Operative Orthopaedics. Philadelphia: JB Lippincott, 1988, pp 1549–1559.

DeLee JC. Complications of arthroscopy and arthroscopic surgery: Results of a national survey. Arthroscopy 4:214–220, 1988.

DiGiovine NM, Bradley JP. Arthroscopic equipment and set-up. In Fu FH, Harner CD, Vince KG (eds). Knee Surgery. Baltimore: Williams & Wilkins, 1994.

Gillquist J. Arthroscopy of the posterior compartments of the knee. Contemp Orthop 10:39–45, 1985.

Halbrecht JL, Jackson DW. Office arthroscopy: a diagnostic alternative. Arthroscopy 8:320–326, 1992.

Johnson LL. Arthroscopic Surgery: Principles and Practice. 3rd ed. St Louis: CV Mosby, 1986.

O'Connor RL. Arthroscopy in the diagnosis and treatment of acute ligament injuries of the knee. J Bone Joint Surg 56A:333–337, 1974.

Rosenberg TD, Paulos LE, Parker RD, Abbott PJ. Arthroscopic surgery of the knee. In Chapman MW (ed). *Operative Orthopaedics*. Philadelphia: JB Lippincott, 1988, pp 1585–1604.

Schreiber SN. Proximal superomeedial portal in arthroscopy of the knee. Arthroscopy 7:246–251, 1991.

Small NC. Complications in arthroscopy: the knee and other joints. Arthroscopy 2:253–258, 1986.

Wantanabe M, Takeda S. The number 21 arthroscope. J Jpn Orthop Assoc 34:1041, 1960.

Meniscus

Aichroth PM, Patel DV, Marx CL. Congenital discoid lateral meniscus in children. A follow-up study and evolution of management. J Bone Joint Surg 73B:932–936, 1991.

Annandale T. An operation for displaced semilunar cartilage. Br Med J 1:779, 1885.

Arnoczky SP, Warren RF. Microvasculature of the human meniscus. Am J Sports Med 10:90–95, 1982.

Arnoczky SP, Warren RF. The microvasculature of the meniscus and its response to injury—an experimental study in the dog. Am J Sports Med 11:131–141, 1983.

Arnoczky SP, DiCarlo EF, O'Brien SJ, Warren RF. Cellular repopulation of deep frozen meniscal autografts. An experimental study in the dog. Arthroscopy 8:428–436, 1992.

Arnoczky SP, Warren RF, McDevitt CA. Meniscal replacement using a cryopreserved allograft. Clin Orthop 252:121–128, 1992.

Arnoczky SP, Warren RF, Spivak JM. Meniscal repair using an exogenous fibrin clot—an experimental study in dogs. J Bone Joint Surg 70A:1209–1220, 1988.

Baratz ME, Fu FH, Mengato R. Meniscal tears: the effect of meniscectomy and of repair on intra-articular contact areas and stresses in the human knee. Am J Sports Med 14:270–275, 1986.

Barrie HJ. The pathogenesis and significance of meniscal cysts. J Bone Joint Surg 61B:184, 1979.

Bolano LE, Grana EA. Isolated arthroscopic partial meniscectomy. Functional radiographic evaluation at five years. Am J Sports Med 21:432–437, 1993.

Cabaud HE, Rodkey WG, Fitzwater JE. Medial meniscus repairs. An experimental and morphologic study. Am J Sports Med 9:129–134, 1981.

Cannon WD Jr. Arthroscopic meniscal repair. In McGinty JB (ed). *Operative Arthroscopy*. New York: Raven Press, 1991, pp 237–251.

Cannon WD, Vittori JM. The incidence of healing in arthroscopic meniscal repairs in anterior cruciate ligament reconstructed knees versus stable knees. Am J Sports Med 20:176–181, 1992.

Cassidy RE, Shaffer AJ. Repair of peripheral meniscus tears. A preliminary report. Am J Sports Med 9:209–214, 1981.

Clancy WG, Graf BK. Arthroscopic meniscal repair. Orthopedics 6:1125–1129, 1983.

Cooper DE, Arnoczky SP, Warren RF. Arthroscopic meniscal repair. Clin Sports Med 9:589–607, 1990.

Cox JS, Nye CE, Schaeffer WW, et al. The degenerative effects of partial and total resection of the medial meniscus in dogs' knees. Clin Orthop 109:178–183, 1975.

DeHaven KE. Peripheral meniscal repair: an alternative to meniscectomy. J Bone Joint Surg 63B:463, 1981.

DeHaven KE. Decision making factors in the treatment of meniscus lesions. Clin Orthop 252:49–54, 1990.

DeHaven KE. Meniscectomy versus repair: Clinical experience. In Mow VW, Arnoczky SP, Jackson DW (eds). *Knee Meniscus: Basic and Clinical Foundations*. New York: Raven Press, 1992, pp 131–139.

DeHaven KE, Black KP, Griffiths HJ. Open meniscus repair. Technique and two to nine year results. Am J Sports Med 17:788–795, 1989.

DeHaven KE, Stone RC. Meniscal repair. In Sahiaree H (ed). *O'Connor's Textbook of Arthroscopic Surgery*. Philadelphia: Lippincott, 1992, pp 327–338.

Dickhaut SC, DeLee JC. The discoid lateral meniscus syndrome. J Bone Joint Surg 64A:1068–1073, 1982.

Fairbank TJ. Knee joint changes after meniscectomy. J Bone Joint Surg 30B:664–670, 1948.

Fauno P, Nielsen AD. Arthroscopic partial meniscectomy, a long term follow-up. Arthroscopy 8:345–349, 1992.

Ferriter PJ, Nisonson B. Role of arthroscopy in the treatment of lateral meniscal cysts. Arthroscopy 2:142, 1985.

Fukubayashi T, Kurasawa H. The contact area and pressure distribution pattern of the knee. A study of normal and osteoarthritic knee joints. Acta Orthop Scand 51:871–880, 1980.

Garrett JC, Stevensen RW. Meniscal transplantation in the human knee: a preliminary report. Arthroscopy 7:57–62, 1991.

Gershuni DH, Skyhar MJ, Danzig LA, et al. Experimental models to promote healing of tears in the avascular segment of canine knee menisci. J Bone Joint Surg 71A:1363–1370, 1989.

Gillquist J, Hagberg G, Oretorp N. Arthroscopic examination of the posteromedial compartment of the knee joint. Int Orthop 3:313, 1979.

Glasgow MMS, Allen PW, Blakeway C. Arthroscopic treatment of cysts of the lateral meniscus. J Bone Joint Surg 75B:299–302, 1993.

Hashimoto J, Kurosaka M, Yoshiya S, Hirohata K. Meniscal repair using fibrin sealant and endothelial cell growth factor. An experimental study in dogs. Am J Sports Med 20:537–541, 1992.

Heatley FW. The meniscus—can it be repaired? An experimental investigation in rabbits. J Bone Joint Surg 62B:397–402, 1980.

Henning CE. Arthroscopic repair of meniscus tears. Orthopedics 6:1130–1132, 1983.

Henning CE. Current status of meniscal salvage. Clin Sports Med 9:567–576, 1990.

Henning CE, Lynch MA, Yearout KM, et al. Arthroscopic meniscal repair using an exogenous fibrin clot. Clin Orthop 252:64, 1990.

Henning CE, Lynch MA, Clark JR. Vascularity for healing of meniscus repairs. Arthroscopy 3:13–18, 1987.

Hughston JC, Filers AF. The role of the posterior oblique ligament in repairs of acute medial (collateral) ligament tears of the knee. J Bone Joint Surg 55A:923–940, 1973.

Ikeuchi H. Surgery under arthroscopic control. Proceedings of the Societe Internationale d'Arthroscopie 1975. Rheumatology 31:57–62, 1976.

Ishimura M, Tamai S, Fujisawa Y. Arthroscopic meniscal repair with fibrin glue. Arthroscopy 7:177–181, 1991.

Jackson DW, McDevitt CA, Simon TM et al. Meniscal transplantation using fresh and cryopreserved allografts: an experimental study in goats. Am J Sports Med 20:644–656, 1992.

Jackson DW, Whelan J, Simon TM. Cell survival after transplantation of fresh meniscal allografts. DNA probe analysis in a goat model. Am J Sports Med 21:540–550, 1993.

Johnson LL. *Diagnostic and Surgical Arthroscopy: The Knee and Other Joints.* 2nd ed. St Louis: CV Mosby, 1981.
King D. The healing of semilunar cartilages. J Bone Joint Surg 18A:333–342, 1936.
King D. The function of the semilunar cartilages. J Bone Joint Surg 18A:1069–1076, 1936.
Levy M, Torzilli PA, Warren RF. The effect of medial meniscectomy on anterior-posterior motion of the knee. J Bone Joint Surg 64A:883–888, 1982.
McConville OR. The effect of meniscal status on knee stability and function after anterior cruciate ligament reconstruction. Arthroscopy 9:394–405, 1993.
McGinty JB, Guess LF, Marvin RA. Partial or total meniscectomy. J Bone Joint Surg 59A:763–766, 1977.
Miller MD, Ritchie JR, Royster RM, et al. Meniscal repair: an experimental study in the goat. Am J Sports Med (in press).
Miller MD, Warner JJP, Harner CD. Mensical repair. In Fu FH, Harner CD, Vince KG (eds). *Knee Surgery.* Baltimore: Williams & Wilkins, 1994.
Morgan CD. The "all-inside" meniscus repair. Technical note. Arthroscopy 7:120–125, 1991.
Morgan CD, Casscells SW. Arthroscopic meniscus repair: a safe approach to the posterior horns. Arthroscopy 2:3–12, 1986.
Morgan CD, Wojtys EM, Casscells CD, Casscells SW. Arthroscopic meniscal repair evaluated by second-look arthroscopy. Am J Sports Med 19:632–638, 1991.
Mullhollan JS. Inside/inside meniscus repair technique: sewing and tying through punctures. Instructional Course. Arthroscopy Association of North America, 11th Annual Meeting, Boston, MA, April 1992.
Neuschwander DC, Drez D, Finney TP. Lateral meniscal variant with absence of the posterior coronary ligament. J Bone Joint Surg 74A:1186–1190, 1992.
Newman AP, Daniels AU, Burks RT. Principles and decision making in meniscal surgery. Arthroscopy 9:33–51, 1993.
O'Brien SJ, Miller DV, Fealy SV, et al. Lasers in the meniscus. In Mow VC, Arnoczky SP, Jackson DW (eds). *Knee Meniscus.* New York: Raven Press, 1992, pp 153–164.
O'Connor RL. The history of partial meniscectomy. In Shahriaree J (ed). *Arthroscopic Surgery.* Philadelphia: JB Lippincott, 1984, pp 93–97.
Parisien JS. Arthroscopic treatment of cysts of the menisci. A preliminary report. Clin Orthop 257:154–158, 1990.
Phemister DB. Cysts of the external semilunar cartilage of the knee. JAMA 80:593, 1923.
Pisani AJ. Pathognomonic sign for cyst of the knee cartilage. Arch Surg 54:188, 1947.
Reagan WB, McConkey JP, Loomer RL, Davidson RG. Cysts of the lateral meniscus: arthroscopy versus arthroscopy plus open cystectomy. Arthroscopy 5:274–281, 1989.
Rosenberg TD, Scott SM, Coward DB, et al. Arthroscopic meniscal repair evaluated with repeat arthroscopy. Arthroscopy 2:14–20, 1986.
Ryu RKN, Dunbar WH. Arthroscopic meniscal repair with two-year follow up. A clinical review. Arthroscopy 4:168–173, 1988.
Scott GA, Jolly BL, Henning CE. Combined posterior incision and arthroscopic intra-articular repair of the meniscus: an examination of factors affecting healing. J Bone Joint Surg 68A:847, 861, 1986.
Seger BM, Woods WG. Arthroscopic management of lateral meniscal cysts. Am J Sports Med 14:105, 1986.
Siegel MG, Roberts CS. Meniscal allografts. Clin Sports Med 12:59–80, 1993.
Smillie IS. The congenital discoid meniscus. J Bone Joint Surg 30B:671–682, 1948.
Smillie IS. *Injuries of the Knee Joint.* 4th ed. New York: Churchill Livingstone, 1971.
Sommerlath K. The prognosis of repaired and intact menisci in unstable knees—a comparative study. Arthroscopy 4:93–95, 1988.
Sommerlath K, Gillquist J. The effect of a meniscal prosthesis on knee biomechanics and cartilage. Am J Sports Med 20:73–81, 1992.
Stone KR, Rodkey WA, Weber R, et al. Meniscal regeneration with copolymeric collagen scaffolds. Am J Sports Med 20:104–111, 1992.
Stone KR, Rosenberg T. Surgical technique of meniscus replacement. Technical note. Arthroscopy 9:234–237, 1993.
Stone RG, Frewin PR, Gonzales S. Long term assessment of arthroscopic meniscus repair: a two to six year follow-up study. Arthroscopy 6:73–78, 1990.
Sutton JB. *Ligaments: Their Nature and Morphology.* London: MK Lewis, 1897.
Thompson WO, Theate FL, Fu FH, Dye SF. Tibial meniscal dynamics using three-dimensional reconstruction of magnetic resonance images. Am J Sports Med 19:210–216, 1991.
Walker PS, Erkman MJ. The role of the menisci in force transmission across the knee. Clin Orthop 109:184–192, 1975.
Wang CJ, Walker PS. Rotatory laxity of the human knee joint. J Bone Joint Surg 56A:161–170, 1974.
Warren RF. Arthroscopic meniscal repair. Arthroscopy 1:170, 1985.
Warren RF. Meniscectomy and repair in the anterior cruciate ligament-deficient patient. Clin Orthop 252:55–63, 1990.
Webber RJ, York L, VanderSchilden JL, et al. An organ culture model for assaying wound repair of the fibrocartilaginous knee joint mensicus. Am J Sports Med 17:393, 1989.
Weiss CB, Lundberg M, DeHaven KE, Gillquist J: Nonoperative treatment of meniscal tears. J Bone Joint Surg 71A:811–821, 1989.
Wirth C. Meniscal repair. Clin Orthop 157:153–160, 1981.

Osteochondral Lesions

Aichroth P. Osteochondritis dissecans of the kneee. J Bone Joint Surg 53B:440, 1971.
Aichroth PM. Osteochondral fracture and osteochondritis dissecans in sportsmen's knee injuries. J Bone Joint Surg 59B:108, 1977.
Bauer M, Jackson RW. Chondral lesions of the femoral condyles. A system of arthroscopic classification. Arthroscopy 4:97–102, 1988.
Burks RT. Arthroscopy and degenerative arthritis of the knee: a review of the literature. Arthroscopy 6:43–47, 1990.

Clanton TO, DeLee JC. Osteochondritis dissecans: history, pathophysiology, and current treatment concepts. Clin Orthop 167:50–64, 1982.

Dzioba RB. The classification and treatment of acute articular cartilage lesions. Arthroscopy 4:72–80, 1988.

Garrett JC. Treatment of osteochondral defects of the distal femur with fresh osteochondral allografts. Preliminary results. Arthroscopy 2:222–226, 1986.

Garrett JC. Osteochondritis dissecans. Clin Sports Med 10:569, 1991.

Guhl J. Arthroscopic treatment of osteochondritis dissecans. Clin Orthop 167:65–74, 1982.

Hubbard MJS. Arthroscopic surgery for chondral flaps in the knee. J Bone Joint Surg 69B:794–796, 1987.

Hughston JC, Hergenroeder PT, Courtenay BG. Osteochondritis dissecans of the femoral condyles. J Bone Joint Surg 66A:1340, 1984.

Johnson LL. Arthroscopic abrasion arthroplasty. Historical and pathologic perspective: present status. Arthroscopy 2:54, 1986.

Kennedy JC, Grangier RW, McGraw RW. Osteochondral fractures of the femoral condyles. J Bone Joint Surg 48B:437–440, 1966.

Linden B. Osteochondritis dissecans of the femoral condyles: a long-term follow-up study. J Bone Joint Surg 59A:769, 1977.

Lotke PA, Ecker ML. Transverse fractures of the patella. Clin Orthop 158:180–184, 1981.

Mesgarzadeh M, Sapega AA, Bonakdarpour A, et al. Osteochondritis dissecans: analysis of mechanical stability with radiography, scintigraphy, and MRI imaging. Radiology 165:775, 1987.

Paletta GA, Arnoczky SP, Warren RF. The repair of osteochondral defects using an exogenous fibrin clot. An experimental study in dogs. Am J Sports Med 20:725–731, 1992.

Rand JA. Arthroscopic diagnosis and management of articular cartilage pathology. In Scott WN (ed). *Arthroscopy of the Knee*. Philadelphia: WB Saunders, 1990, pp 113–128.

Rorabeck CH, Bobechko WP. Acute dislocation of the patella with osteochondral fracture: a review of eighteen cases. J Bone Joint Surg 58A:237–240, 1976.

Rosenberg TD, Paulos LE, Parker RD, Abbott PJ. Arthroscopic surgery of the knee. In Chapman MW. *Operative Orthopaedics*. Philadelphia: JB Lippincott, 1988, pp 1585–1604.

Smillie IS. *Osteochondritis Dissecans: Loose Bodies in Joints. Etiology, Pathology, Treatment*. London: E & S Livingstone, 1960.

Sprague NF III. Arthroscopic debridement for degenerative knee joint disease. Clin Orthop 160:118, 1981.

Terry GC, Flandry F, Van Manen JW, Norwood LA. Isolated chondral fractures of the knee. Clin Orthop 234:170–177, 1988.

Vince KG. Osteochondritis dissecans of the knee. In Scott WN (ed). *Arthroscopy of the Knee*. Philadelphia: WB Saunders, 1990.

Wilson JN. A diagnostic sign in osteochondritis dissecans of the knee. J Bone Joint Surg 49A:477, 1967.

Synovial Lesions

Amatuzzi MM, Gazzi A, Varella MH. Pathologic synovial plica of the knee: results of conservative treatment. Am J Sports Med 18:466–469, 1990.

Brashear HR. Pigmented villonodular synovitis. South Med J 49:679, 1956.

Byers PD, Cotton RE, Deacon OW, Lowy M. The diagnosis and treatment of pigmented villonodular synovitis. J Bone Joint Surg 50B:290, 1968.

Collican MR, Dandy DJ. Arthroscopic management of synovial chondromatosis of the knee: findings and results in 18 cases. J Bone Joint Surg 71B:498, 1989.

Flandry F, Hughston JC. Current concepts review: pigmented villonodular synovitis. J Bone Joint Surg 69A:942, 1987.

Granowitz SP, Mankin HJ. Localized pigmented villonodular synovitis of the knee: report of five cases. J Bone Joint Surg 49A:122, 1967.

Higgenbothen CL. Arthroscopic synovectomy. Arthroscopy 1:190, 1985.

Jackson RW, Marshall DJ, Fujisawa Y. The pathological medial shelf. Orthop Clin North Am 13:307, 1982.

Johnson DP, Eastwood DM, Witherow PJ. Symptomatic synovial plicae of the knee. J Bone Joint Surg 75A:1485–1496, 1993.

Koshino T, Okamoto R. Resection of the painful shelf (plica synovialis mediopatellaris) under arthroscopy. Arthroscopy 1:136, 1985.

Mandelbaum BR, Grant TT, Hartzman S, et al. The use of MRI to assist in diagnosis of pigmented villonodular synovitis of the knee joint. Clin Orthop 231:135, 1988.

Milgram JW. Synovial chondromatosis: a histopathological study of thirty cases. J Bone Joint Surg 59A:792, 1977.

Miller WE. Villonodular synovitis: pigmented and nonpigmented variations. South Med J 75:1084, 1982.

Murphy FP, Dahlin DC, Sullivan RC. Articular synovial chondromatosis. J Bone Joint Surg 44A:77, 1962.

Muse GL, Grana WA, Hollingsworth S. Arthroscopic treatment of medial shelf syndrome. Arthroscopy 1:63, 1985.

Rao AS, Vigorita VJ. Pigmented villonodular synovitis: a review of eighty one cases. J Bone Joint Surg 66A:76, 1984.

Robinson DL, Blair DW, Lee SS, Ho PK. Pigmented villonodular synovitis presenting as a large lateral knee mass: case report and review of the literature. Orthop Rev 17:59, 1988.

Sims FH. Synovial proliferative disorders. Role of synovectomy. Arthroscopy 1:198, 1985.

Weiss C, Averbuch PF, Steiner GC, Rusoff JH. Synovial chondromatosis and instability of the proximal tibiofibular joint. Clin Orthop 198:187, 1975.

Wilson WJ, Parr TJ. Synovial chondromatosis. Orthopedics 11:1179, 1988.

Wu KK, Ross PM, Guise ER. Pigmented villonodular synovitis: a clinical analysis of twenty four cases treated at Henry Ford Hospital. Orthopedics 3:751, 1980.

Knee Ligament Injuries

Abe EA. Light and electron microscopic study of the remodelling and maturation process in autogenous graft for anterior cruciate ligament reconstruction. Arthroscopy 9:394–405, 1993.

Almeekinders LC, Logan TC. Results following treatment of traumatic dislocations of the knee joint. Clin Orthop 284:203–207, 1992.

Anderson AF. Evaluation of knee ligament rating systems. Am J Knee Surg 6:67–73, 1993.

Andersson C, Odensten M, Gillquist J. Knee function after surgical or non-surgical treatment of acute ACL tears: a randomized study with a long-term follow-up period. Clin Orthop 264:255–263, 1991.

Bessette GC, Hunter RE. The anterior cruciate ligament. Orthopedics 13:553–562, 1990.

Beynon EA. The effect of functional knee braces on strain in the anterior cruciate ligament. J Bone Joint Surg 74A:1298–1312, 1992.

Buckley SL, Barrack RL, Alexander AH. The natural history of conservatively treated partial anterior cruciate ligament tears. Am J Sports Med 17:221–225, 1989.

Butler DL, Noyes FR, Grood ES: Ligamentous restraints to anterior-posterior drawer in the human knee. A biomechanical study. J Bone Joint Surg 62A:259–270, 1980.

Cain TE, Schwab GH. Performance of an athlete with straight posterior knee instability. Am J Sports Med 9:203–208, 1981.

Castle TH, Noyes FR, Grood ES. Posterior tibial subluxation of the posterior cruciate-deficient knee. Clin Orthop 284:203–207, 1992.

Cawley PW, France EP, Paulos LE. The current state of functional knee bracing research. Am J Sports Med 19:226–233, 1991.

Clancy WG, Ray JM, Zoltan DJ. Acute tears of the anterior cruciate ligament. Surgical versus conservative treatment. J Bone Joint Surg 70A:1483–1488, 1988.

Clancy WG, Shelbourne KD, Zoellner GB, et al. Treatment of knee joint instability secondary to rupture of the posterior cruciate ligament. Report of a new procedure. J Bone Joint Surg 65A:310–322, 1983.

Clendenin MB, DeLee JC, Heckman JD: Interstitial tears of the posterior cruciate ligament of the knee. Orthopedics 3:764–772, 1980.

Cooper DE, Speer KP, Wickiewicz TL, Warren RF. Complete knee dislocation without posterior cruciate disruption: a report of four cases and reeview of the literature. Clin Orthop 284:228–233, 1992.

Cooper DE, Warren RF, Warner JJP. The posterior cruciate ligament and posterolateral structures of the knee: anatomy, function, and patterns of injury. Instr Course Lect 40:249–270, 1991.

Cross MJ, Powell JF. Long-term followup of posterior cruciate ligament rupture: a study of 116 cases. Am J Sports Med 12:292–297, 1984.

Dandy DJ, Pusey RJ. The long term results of unrepaired tears of the posterior cruciate ligament. J Bone Joint Surg 64B:92–94, 1982.

Daniel DM, Akeson WH, O'Connor JJ (eds). *Knee Ligaments: Structure, Function, Injury and Repair.* New York: Raven Press, 1990.

Dejour H, Neyret P, Boileau P, Donnel ST. Anterior cruciate reconstruction combined with valgus tibial osteotomy. Clin Orthop 299:220–228, 1994.

Dejour H, Walch G, Peyrot J, Eberhard P. The natural history of rupture of the posterior cruciate ligament. Fr J Orthop Surg 2:112–120, 1988.

Feagin JA (ed). *The Crucial Ligaments: Diagnosis and Treatment of Ligamentous Injuries About the Knee.* New York: Churchill Livingstone, 1988.

Fetto JF, Marshall JL. The natural history and diagnosis of anterior cruciate ligament insufficiency. Clin Orthop 147:29–38, 1980.

Fisher SE, Shelbourne KD. Arthroscopic treatment of symptomatic extension block complicating anterior cruciate ligament construction. Am J Sports Med 21:558–564, 1993.

Fowler PJ, Messieh SS: Isolated posterior cruciate ligament injuries in athletes. Am J Sports Med 15:553–557, 1987.

Frassica FJ, Sim FH, Staeheli JW, Pairolero PC. Dislocation of the knee. Clin Orthop 263:200–205, 1991.

Fruensgaard S, Johannsen HV. Incomplete ruptures of the anterior cruciate ligament. J Bone Joint Surg 71B:526–530, 1989.

Fukibayashi T, Torzilli PA, Sherman MF, Warren RF. An in vitro biomechanical evaluation of anterior-posterior motion of the knee. Tibial displacement, rotation, and torque. J Bone Joint Surg 64A:258–264, 1982.

Gillquist J, Good L. The value of intraoperative isometry measurements in anterior cruciate ligament reconstruction: an in vivo correlation between substitute tension and length change. Arthroscopy 9:525–532, 1993.

Giove TP, Miller SJ, Kent BE, et al. Nonoperative treatment of the torn anterior cruciate ligament. J Bone Joint Surg 65A:184–192, 1983.

Girgis FG, Marshall JL, Al Monajem ARS: The cruciate ligaments of the knee joint. Anatomical, functional and experimental analysis. Clin Orthop 106:216–231, 1975.

Grood ES, Hefzy MS, Lindenfield TN. Factors affecting the region of most isometric femoral attachments. Part I. The posterior cruciate ligament. Am J Sports Med 17:197–207, 1989.

Grood ES, Stowers SF, Noyes FR: Limits of movement in the human knee: effect of sectioning the posterior cruciate ligament and posterolateral structures. J Bone Joint Surg 70A:88–97, 1988.

Harner CD, Irrgang JJ, Paul J, et al. Loss of motion following anterior cruciate ligament reconstruction. Am J Sports Med 20:507–515, 1992.

Harner CD, Paulos LE, Greenwald AE, et al. Detailed analysis of patients with bilateral anterior cruciate ligament injuries. Am J Sports Med 22:37–43, 1994.

Hefzy MS, Grood ES, Noyes FR. Factors affecting the region of most isometric femoral attachments. Part II. the anterior cruciate ligament. Am J Sports Med 17:208–216, 1989.

Howell SM, Taylor MA. Failure of reconstruction of the anterior cruciate ligament due to impingement by the intercondylar roof. J Bone Joint Surg 75A:1044–1055, 1993.

Huegel M, Indelicato PA. Trends in rehabilitation following anterior cruciate ligament reconstruction. Clin Sports Med 7:801–811, 1988.

Hughston JC, Norwood LA. Acute tears of the posterior cruciate ligament. J Bone Joint Surg 62A:438–450, 1980.

Indelicato PA, Hermansdorfer J, Huegel M. Nonoperative management of complete tears of the medial collateral ligament of the knee in intercollegiate football players. Clin Orthop 256:174–177, 1990.

Johnson RJ, Beynnon BD, Nichols CE, Renstrom PAFH. Current concepts review: the treatment of injuries of the anterior cruciate ligament. J Bone Joint Surg 74A:140–151, 1992.

Kannus P, Jarvinen M. Conservatively treated tears of the anterior cruciate ligament. Long term results. J Bone Joint Surg 69A:1007–1012, 1987.

Keene GC, Bickerstaff D, Rae PJ, Paterson RS. The natural history of meniscal tears in anterior cruciate ligament insufficiency. Am J Sports Med 21:672–679, 1993.

Keller PM, Shelbourne D, McCarroll JR, Rettig AC. Nonoperatively treated isolated posterior cruciate ligament injuries. Am J Sports Med 21:132–136, 1993.

Kennedy JC. Complete dislocation of the knee joint. J Bone Joint Surg 45A:889–904, 1963.

Kennedy JC, Grainger RW. The posterior cruciate ligament. J Trauma 7:367–377, 1967.

Linn RM, Fischer DA, Smith JP, et al. Achilles tendon allograft reconstruction of the anterior cruciate ligament-deficient knee. Am J Sports Med 21:825–831, 1993.

Lipscomb AB Jr, Anderson AF, Norwig ED, et al. Isolated posterior cruciate ligament reconstruction. Long-term results. Am J Sports Med 21:490–496, 1993.

Marder RA, Rasking JR, Carroll M. Prospective evaluation of arthroscopically assisted ACL reconstruction. Patellar tendon versus semitendinosus and gracilis tendons. Am J Sports Med 19:478–483, 1991.

Marshall JL, Warren RF, Wickewicz TL. Primary surgical treatment of anterior cruciate ligament lesions. Am J Sports Med 10:103–107, 1982.

Marzo JM, Bowen MK, Warren RF, et al. Intraarticular fibrous nodule as a cause of loss of extension following anterior cruciate ligament reconstruction. Arthroscopy 8:10–18, 1992.

McCarroll JR, Rettig AC, Shelbourne KD. Anterior cruciate ligament injuries in the young athlete with open physes. Am J Sports Med 16:44–47, 1988.

McDaniel WJ, Dameron TB. The untreated ACL rupture. Clin Orthop 172:158–163, 1983.

Melby A, Noble JS, Askew MJ, et al: The effects of graft tensioning on the laxity and kinematics of the anterior cruciate ligament reconstructed knee. Arthroscopy 7:257–266, 1991.

Meyers MH, Harvey JP. Traumatic dislocation of the knee joint. A study of eighteen cases. J Bone Joint Surg 53A:16–29, 1971.

Miller MD, Fu FH. The role of osteotomy in the anterior cruciate ligament deficient knee. Clin Sports Med 12:697–708, 1993.

Miller MD, Harner CD. The use of allograft. Techniques and results. Clin Sports Med 12:757–770, 1993.

Muller W. *The Knee: Form, Function, and Ligament Reconstruction.* New York: Springer-Verlag, 1983.

Noyes FR, Barber SD. The effect of a ligament-augmentation device on allograft reconstructions for chronic ruptures of the anterior cruciate ligament. J Bone Joint Surg 74A:960–973, 1992.

Noyes FR, Barber SD, Manginee RE. Bone-patellar ligament-bone and fascia lata allografts for reconstruction of the anterior cruciate ligament. J Bone Joint Surg 72A:1125–1136, 1990.

Noyes FR, Barber SD, Simon R. High tibial osteotomy and ligament reconstruction in varus angulated, anterior cruciate ligament-deficient knees. A two to seven year follow-up study. Am J Sports Med 21:2–12, 1993.

Noyes FR, Mooar LA, Moorman CT, McGinniss GH. Partial tears of the anterior cruciate ligament. Progression to complete ligament deficiency. J Bone Joint Surg 66A:825–833, 1989.

O'Brien SJ, Warren RF, Pavlov H, et al. Reconstruction of the chronically insufficient anterior cruciate ligament with the central third of the patellar ligament. J Bone Joint Surg 73A:278–286, 1991.

O'Brien SJ, Warren RF, Wickiewicz TL, et al. The iliotibial band lateral sling procedure and its effect on the results of anterior cruciate ligament reconstruction. Am J Sports Med 19:21–25, 1991.

O'Donoghue DH. *Treatment of Injuries to Athletes.* 3rd ed. Philadelphia: WB Saunders, 1976.

Olson EJ, Kang JD, Fu FH, et al. The biomechanical and histological effects of artificial ligament wear particles in vitro and in vivo studies. Am J Sports Med 16:558–570, 1988.

Otero AL, Hutcheson LA. A comparison of the doubled semitendinosus and central third patellar tendon autografts in arthroscopic anterior cruciate ligament reconstruction. Arthroscopy 9:143–148, 1993.

Pagnani MJ, Warner JJP, O'Brien SJ, Warren RF. Anatomic considerations in harvesting the semitendinosus and gracilis tendons and a technique of harvest. Am J Sports Med 21:565–571, 1993.

Paulos LE, Rosenberg TD, Drawbert J, et al. Infrapatellar contracture syndrome: an unrecognized cause of knee stiffness with patellar entrapment and patella infera. Am J Sports Med 15:331–341, 1987.

Quinlan AG, Sharrard WJW. Posterolateral dislocation of the knee with capsular interposition. J Bone Joint Surg 40B:660–663, 1958.

Reid JS, Hanks GA, Kalenak A, et al. The Ellison iliotibial-band transfer for a torn anterior cruciate ligament. Long-term follow-up. J Bone Joint Surg 74A:1392–1402, 1992.

Robins AJ, Newman AP, Burks RT. Postoperative return of motion in anterior cruciate ligament and medial collateral ligament injuries. The effect of medial collateral ligament rupture location. Am J Sports Med 21:20–24, 1993.

Sachs RA, Daniel DM, Stone ML, Garfein RF. Patellofemoral problems after anterior cruciate ligament reconstruction. Am J Sports Med 17:760–765, 1989.

Sapega AA, Moyer RA, Schneck C, Komalahiranya N. Testing for isometry during reconstruction of the ACL. J Bone Joint Surg 72A:259–267, 1990.

Satku K, Chew CN, Seow H: Posterior cruciate ligament injuries. Acta Orthop Scand 55:26–29, 1984.

Scaglioni NA, DelPizzo W, Fox JM, et al. Arthroscopic-assisted anterior cruciate ligament reconstruction with the semi-tendinosus tendon: comparison of results with and without braided polypropylene augmentation. Arthroscopy 8:65–77, 1992.

Scott WN (ed). *Ligament and Extensor Mechanism of the Knee: Diagnosis and Treatment.* St Louis: CV Mosby, 1991.

Shelbourne KD, Nitz P. Accelerated rehabilitation after anterior cruciate ligament reconstruction. Am J Sports Med 18:292–299, 1990.

Shelbourne KD, Nitz PA. The O'Donoghue triad revisited. Combined injuries involving the anterior cruciate and medial collateral ligament tears. Am J Sports Med 19:474–477, 1991.

Shelbourne KD, Porter DA. Anterior cruciate ligament-medial collateral ligament injury: Nonoperative management of medial collateral ligament tears with anterior cruciate ligament reconstruction. A preliminary report. Am J Sports Med 20:283–286, 1992.

Shelbourne KD, Wilckens JH. Intraarticular anterior cruciate ligament reconstruction in the symptomatic arthritic knee. Am J Sports Med 21:685–689, 1993.

Shields L, Mital M, Cave EF. Complete dislocation of the knee: experience at the Massachusetts General Hospital. J Trauma 6:192–212, 1969.

Sisto DJ, Warren RF. Complete knee dislocation. A follow-up study of operative treatment. Clin Orthop 198:94–101, 1985.

Sitler N, Ryan J, Hopkinson W, et al. The efficacy of a prophylactic knee brace to reduce knee injuries in football: a prospective, randomized study at West Point. Am J Sports Med 18:310–315, 1990.

Skyhar MJ, Warren RF, Orits GS, et al. The effects of sectioning of the posterior cruciate ligament and posterolateral complex on the articular contact pressures within the knee. J Bone Joint Surg 75A:694–699, 1993.

Sommerlath K, Lysholm J, Gillquist J. The long-term course after treatment of acute ACL ruptures. Am J Sports Med 19:156–162, 1991.

Sommerlath K, Odensten M, Lysholm J. The late course of acute partial anterior cruciate ligament tears: a nine to 15-year follow-up evaluation. Clin Orthop 281:152–158, 1992.

Souryal TO, Freeman TR. Intercondylar notch size and anterior cruciate ligament injuries in athletes. A prospective study. Am J Sports Med 21:535–539, 1993.

Speer KP, Spritzer CE, Bassett FH, et al. Osseous injury associated with acute tears of the anterior cruciate ligament. Am J Sports Med 20:382–389, 1992.

Taylor AR, Arden GP, Rainey HA. Traumatic dislocation of the knee. A report of forty-three cases with special reference to conservative treatment. J Bone Joint Surg 54B:96–102, 1972.

Torg JS, Barton TM, Pavlov H, Stine R. Natural history of the posterior cruciate ligament-deficient knee. Clin Orthop 246:208–216, 1989.

Tria AJ, Alicea JA, Cody RP. Patella baja in anterior cruciate ligament reconstruction of the knee. Clin Orthop 299:229–234, 1994.

Van Dommelen BA, Fowler PR. Anatomy of the posterior cruciate ligament. A review. Am J Sports Med 17:24–29, 1989.

Warner JJP, Warren RF, Cooper DE. Management of acute anterior cruciate ligament injury. Instr Course Lect 40:219–232, 1991.

Wascher DC, Grauer JD, Markoff KL. Biceps tendon tenodesis for posterolateral instability of the knee. An in vitro study. Am J Sports Med 21:400–406, 1993.

Wasilewski SA, Covall DJ, Cohen S. Effect of surgical timing on recovery and associated injuries after anterior cruciate ligament reconstruction. Am J Sports Med 21:338–342, 1993.

Whipple TL. Posterior cruciate ligament injuries. Clin Sports Med 10:515–517, 1991.

Woodhouse MI. Evaluative testing of functional knee braces in anterior cruciate ligament deficient limbs. An in vivo study. Am J Knee Surg 5:108–116, 1992.

Woods GA, Indelicato PA, Prevott TJ. The Gore-Tex anterior cruciate ligament prosthesis. Two versus three year results. Am J Sports Med 19:48–55, 1991.

Anterior Knee Pain

Abraham E, Washington E, Huang TL. Insall proximal realignment for disorders of the patella. Clin Orthop 248:61–65, 1989.

Agleitti P, Insall JN, Cerulli G. Patellar pain and incongruence I: measurements of incongruence. Clin Orthop 176:217–224, 1983.

Busch MT, DeHaven KE. Pitfalls of the lateral retinacular release. Clin Sports Med 8:279–290, 1989.

Cooper DE, DeLee JC. Reflex sympathetic dystrophy. In Fu FH, Harner CD, Vince KG (ed). Knee Surgery. Baltimore: Williams & Wilkins, 1994.

Cox JS. Evaluation of the Roux-Emslie-Trillat procedure for knee extensor realignment. Am J Sports Med 10:303–310, 1982.

Dandy DJ, Griffiths D. Lateral release for recurrent dislocation of the patella. J Bone Joint Surg 71B:121–125, 1989.

DeHaven KE, Dolan WA, Mayer PJ. Chondromalacia patellae in athletes. Clinical presentation and conservative management. Am J Sports Med 7:5–11, 1979.

Ferguson AB, Brown TD, Fu FH, et al. Relief of patellofemoral contact stress by anterior displacement of the tibial tubercle. J Bone Joint Surg 61A:159–166, 1979.

Fulkerson JP. Awareness of the retinaculum in evaluating patellofemoral pain. Am J Sports Med 10:147–149, 1982.

Fulkerson JP. Anteromedialization of the tibial tuberosity for patellofemoral malalignment. Clin Orthop 177:176–181, 1983.

Fulkerson JP, Hungerford DS. Disorders of the Patellofemoral Joint. 2nd ed. Baltimore: Williams & Wilkins, 1990.

Fulkerson JP, Shea KP. Disorders of patellofemoral alignment. Current concepts review. J Bone Joint Surg 72A:1424–1429, 1990.

Grelsamer RP, Meadows S. The modified Insall-Salvati ratio for assessment of patellar height. Clin Orthop 282:170–176, 1992.

Hauser EW. Total tendon transplant for slipping patella. A new operation for recurrent dislocation of the patella. Surg Gynecol Obstet 66:199–214, 1941.

Henry JH, Goletz TH, Williamson B. Lateral retinacular release in patellofemoral subluxation. Indications, results, and comparison to open patellofemoral reconstruction. Am J Sports Med 14:129, 1986.

Hoffa A. The influence of the adipose tissue with regard to the pathology of the knee joint. JAMA 43:795, 1904.

Holmes JC, Pruitt AL, Whalen NJ. Iliotibial band syndrome in cyclists. Am J Sports Med 21:419–424, 1993.

Hughston JC. Patella subluxation: a recent history. Clin Sports Med 8:153–162, 1989.

Hughston JC, Walsh WM. Proximal and distal reconstuction of the extensor mechanism for patellar subluxation. Clin Orthop 144:36–42, 1979.

Insall J. Patellar pain. Current concepts review. J Bone Joint Surg 64A:147, 1982.

Jacobsen KE, Flandry FC. Diagnosis of anterior knee pain. Clin Sports Med 8:179–196, 1989.

Kilowich P, Paulos L, Rosenberg T, Farnsworth S. Lateral release of the patella: indications and contraindications. Am J Sports Med 18:361, 1990.

Lancourt JE, Cristini JA. Patella alta and patella infera: their etiological role in patellar dislocation, chondromalacia, and apophysitis of the tibial tubercle. J Bone Joint Surg 57A:1112–1115, 1975.

Larson RL, Cabaud HE, Slocum DB, et al. The patellar compression syndrome. Surgical treatment by lateral retinacular release. Clin Orthop 134:158–167, 1978.

Maquet P. Advancement of the tibial tuberosity. Clin Orthop 115:225–230, 1976.

McGinty JB, McCarthy NC. Endoscopic lateral retinacular release. A preliminary report. Clin Orthop 158:120–125, 1981.

Merchant A. Classification of patellofemoral disorders. Arthroscopy 4:235–240, 1988.

Merchant AC, Mercer RL. Lateral release of the patella: a preliminary report. Clin Orthop 103:40–45, 1974.

Merchant AC, Mercer RL, Jacobsen RJ, Cool CR. Roentgenographic analysis of patello-femoral congruence. J Bone Joint Surg 56A:1391–1396, 1974.

Miller BJ, LaRochelle PJ. The treatment of patellofemoral pain by combined rotation and elevation of the tibial tubercle. J Bone Joint Surg 68A:419–423, 1986.

Morshius WJ, Pavlov PW, De Rooy KP. Anteromedialization of the tibial tuberosity in the treatment of patellofemoral pain and malalignment. Clin Orthop 255:242–250, 1990.

O'Neill DB, Micheli LJ, Warner JP. Patellofemoral stress: a prospective analysis of exercise treatment in adolescents and adults. Am J Sports Med 20:151–156, 1992.

Radin EL, Pan HQ. Long term follow-up study on the Maquet procedure with special reference to the causes of failure. Clin Orthop 290:253–258, 1993.

Rasul AT, Fischer DA. Primary repair of quadriceps tendon ruptures: results of treatment. Clin Orthop 289:205–207, 1993.

Ray JM, Clancy WG, Lemon RA. Semimembranosus tendinitis. An overlooked cause of medial knee pain. Am J Sports Med 16:347–351, 1988.

Riegler HF. Recurrent dislocations and subluxations of the patella. Clin Orthop 227:201–209, 1988.

Scuderi G, Cuomo F, Scott WN. Lateral release and proximal realignment for patellar subluxation and dislocation. J Bone Joint Surg 70A:856–861, 1988.

Simmons E, Cameron JC. Patella alta and recurrent dislocation of the patella. Clin Orthop 274:265–269, 1992.

Trillat A, DeJour H, Couette A. Diagnostic et traitement des subluxation recidevantes die la rotule. Rev Chir Orthop 50:813–824, 1964.

Wiberg G. Roentgenographic and anatomic studies on the femoral patellar joint: with special reference to chondromalacia patella. Acta Orthop Scand 12:319–332, 1941.

Childhood and Adolescent Knee Disorders

Adams JD, Leonard RD. A developmental anomaly of the patella frequently diagnosed as a fracture. Surg Gynecol Obstet 41:601–604, 1925.

Angel KR, Hall DJ. Anterior cruciate ligament injury in children and adolescents. Arthroscopy 4:197–201, 1989.

Baxter MP, Wiley JJ. Fractures of the tibial spine in children: an evaluation of knee stability. J Bone Joint Surg 70B:228–230, 1988.

Binazzi R, Felli L, Vaccari V, Borelli P. Surgical treatment of unresolved Osgood-Schlatter lesions. Clin Orthop 289:202–204, 1993.

Clanton TO, DeLee JC, Sanders B, et al. Knee ligament injuries in children. J Bone Joint Surg 61A:1195–1201, 1979.

Glynn MK, Regan BF. Surgical treatment of Osgood-Schlatter's disease. J Pediatr Orthop 3:216–219, 1983.

Green WT. Painful bipartite patellae. A report of three cases. Clin Orthop 110:197–200, 1975.

Hawkins RJ, Bell RH, Anisette G. Acute patellar dislocations: the natural history. Am J Sports Med 14:117–120, 1986.

Jaramillo D, Hoffer FA, Shapiro F, et al. MR imaging of fractures of the growth plate. Am J Roentgenol 155:1261–1265, 1990.

Krause BL, Williams JP, Catterall A. Natural history of Osgood-Schlatter disease. J Pediatr Orthop 10:65–68, 1990.

Lipscomb AB, Anderson AF. Tears of the anterior cruciate ligament in adolescents. J Bone Joint Surg 68A:19–28, 1986.

Lombardo SJ, Harvey JP. Fractures of the distal femoral epiphysis. Factors influencing prognosis: A review of 34 cases. J Bone Joint Surg 59A:742–751, 1977.

Matz SO, Jackson DW. Anterior cruciate ligament surgery in children. Am J Knee Surg 1:59–65, 1988.

McCarroll JR, Rettig AC, Shelbourn KD. Anterior cruciate ligament injuries in the young athlete with open physes. Am J Sports Med 16:44–47, 1988.

McManus F, Rang M, Heslin DJ. Acute dislocation of the patella in children: the natural history. Clin Orthop 139:88–91, 1979.

Medlar RC, Lyne ED. Sinding-Larsen-Johansson disease: its etiology and natural history. J Bone Joint Surg 60A:1113–1116, 1978.

Meyers MH, McKeever FM. Fractures of the intercondylar eminence of the tibia. J Bone Joint Surg 41A:209–222, 1959.

Micheli LJ. Overuse injuries in children's sports: the growth factor. Orthop Clin North Am 14:337–360, 1983.

Micheli LJ, Foster TE. Acute knee injuries in the immature athlete. Instr Course Lect 42:473–481, 1993.

Ogden JA. *Skeletal Injury in the Child*. 2nd ed. Philadelphia: WB Saunders, 1990.

Ogden JA, McCarthy SM, Jokl P. The painful bipartite patella. J Pediatr Orthop 2:263–269, 1982.

Ogden JA, Tross RB, Murphy MJ: Fractures of the tibial tuberosity in adolescents. J Bone Joint Surg 62A:205–215, 1980.

Osgood RB. Lesions of the tibial tubercle occurring during adolescence. Boston Med Surg J 145:114–117, 1903.

Parker AW, Drez D, Cooper JL. Anterior cruciate ligament injuries in patients with open physes. Am J Sports Med 22:44–47, 1994.

Riseborough EJ, Barrett IR, Shapiro F. Growth disturbances following distal femoral physeal fracture-separations. J Bone Joint Surg 65A:885–893, 1983.

Sinding-Larsen MF. A hitherto unknown affliction of the patella. Acta Radiol 1:171–174, 1921.

Sroble RR, Henderson RC, Campion ER, et al. Meniscectomy in children and adolescents: a long-term follow-up study. Clin Orthop 279:180–189, 1992.

Stanitski CL. Knee overuse disorders in the pediatric and adolescent athlete. Instr Course Lect 42:483–495, 1993.

CHAPTER 2

Leg, Foot, and Ankle

I. Introduction
  A. Overview—Because of increasing emphasis on fitness in our society, the number of athletic injuries, particularly of the foot and ankle, has escalated. Advances in treatment range from a better understanding of the most common injury in sports, the ankle sprain, to diagnosis and treatment recommendations for disorders never previously described. Injuries to the foot and ankle tend to be somewhat sport specific:

Sport	Common Injuries
Aerobic dance	Sesamoid fractures, tendinitis, stress fractures
Ballet	Sesamoid fractures, tendinitis, stress fractures
Baseball	Talonavicular joint injury, ankle sprains, osteophytes
Basketball	Fifth metatarsal base fractures, stress fractures, tendinitis
Bicycling	Lacerations, strains, sprains
Football	Sesamoid fractures, ankle fractures, sprains, turf toe, tarsometatarsal fractures/dislocations
Hockey	Puck injuries/fractures, contusions, ankle and hindfoot injuries, exostoses, bursitis
Racket sports	Ankle sprains, Achilles injuries, tendinitis
Running	Ankle sprains, overuse injuries, stress fractures
Skiing	Ankle fractures, peroneal tendon dislocation
Soccer	Forefoot injuries, tendinitis, ankle sprains
Wrestling	Fifth metatarsal base fractures, Achilles tendinitis, ankle sprains

  B. History and Physical Examination—Key historical points include the mechanism of injury, location and onset of pain and swelling, ability to return to sport, and functional deficits. The physical examination should include inspection of stance and gait, palpation, assessment of range of motion, and specialized tests, described in individual sections that follow. A thorough understanding of the underlying anatomy assists in the physical examination.
  C. Anatomy—The foot and ankle comprise 28 bones: the tibia, fibula, 7 tarsal bones, 5 metatarsals, and 14 phalanges. These bones are interconnected by a series of ligaments (Table 2–1 and Figs. 2–1 and 2–2). The muscles of the foot are arranged in four layers (Table 2–2 and Fig. 2–3). Common approaches to the foot and ankle include the anterior approach (through the extensor hallucis longus–extensor digitorum longus interval) (Fig. 2–4), the lateral approach (Fig. 2–5), and the medial approach (Fig. 2–6).
  D. Radiographs—Important standard radiographs include weight-bearing anteroposterior (AP) views, oblique views, and specialized views for other problems (e.g., sesamoid views, axial views). Computed tomography, magnetic resonance imaging (MRI), and bone scans are often helpful in the workup of specific disorders.

II. Chronic/Exertional Compartment Syndrome
  A. Introduction—Compartment syndrome, caused by elevated pressures within a confined space, has been well described in the trauma literature. Chronic or exertional compartment syndrome associated with sports participation (especially in runners), however, has been recognized only within the past decade. The anterior and deep posterior compartments of the leg are most frequently involved.
  B. History and Physical Examination—Athletes typically complain of pain that has a gradual onset during exercise and that gradually reaches a level where it restricts further performance. Some patients may complain of numbness, tightness, or weakness, but most do not. Nuclear imaging sometimes demonstrates diffuse linear uptake along the posteromedial border of the tibia, although this is more consistent with periostitis (shin splints).

TABLE 2–1. ANKLE AND INTERTARSAL LIGAMENTS

Ligament	Origin	Insertion
Deltoid:		
Tibionavicular	MM	Talus
Tibiocalcaneal	MM	Sustentaculum tali
Posterior tibiotalar	MM	Inner talus
Deep	MM	Medial talus
ATFL	LM	Transversely to talus anteriorly
PTFL	LM	Transversely to talus posteriorly
CFL	LM	Obliquely posteriorly to calcaneus
TC interosseous (cervical)	Talus	Calcaneus
CC CN (bifurcate)	Calcaneus	Cuboid and navicular
CC-MT (long plantar)	Calcaneus	Cuboid and metatarsals
Plantar CC (short plantar)	Calcaneus	Cuboid
Plantar CN (spring)	Sustentaculum tali	Navicular
TMT (Lisfranc)	Medial cuneiform	Second metatarsal base

Abbreviations: MM = medial malleolus; LM = lateral malleolus; ATFL = anterior talofibular ligament; PTFL = posterior talofibular ligament; CFL = calcaneofibular ligament; TC = talocalcaneal; CC = calcaneocuboid; CN = calcaneonavicular; TMT = tarsometatarsal; MT = metatarsal.

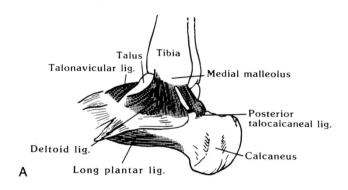

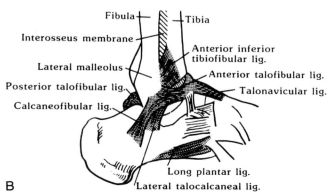

FIGURE 2–1. Ankle ligaments. *A*, Medial. *B*, Lateral. (From Weissman BN, Sledge CB. *Orthopedic Radiology*. Philadelphia: WB Saunders, 1986, pp 593, 594.)

Compartment pressure measurements taken before, during, and immediately after exercise can be helpful in confirming the diagnosis. Although the magnitude of pressure measurements necessary to make this diagnosis is uncertain, most authorities agree that resting pressures >15 mm Hg or delay in normalization after exercise (pressure >20 mm Hg 5 minutes after exercise) is consistent with chronic exertional compartment syndrome.

C. Differential Diagnosis—The differential diagnosis of lower extremity compartment syndrome includes stress fractures, periostitis, and popliteal artery entrapment syndrome. Stress fractures are discussed later. A careful history regarding previous trauma should be obtained. Although popliteal artery entrapment syndrome is unusual, failure to recognize it can have disastrous consequences. Popliteal artery entrapment syndrome can cause calf pain similar to compartment syndrome. The pain is caused by calf claudication secondary to decreased popliteal artery flow and is often associated with an anatomic variation of the popliteal artery along its course. Patients have a reduced pulse with knee extension and foot dorsiflexion and with treadmill testing. Workup includes ultrasonography and MRI evaluation; however, an arteriogram after exercise is most helpful. Initial treatment includes avoiding precipitating

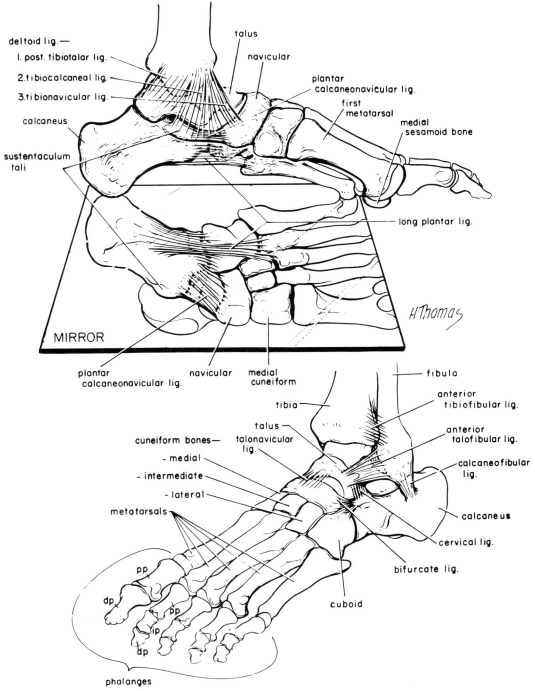

deltoid lig.—
1. post. tibiotalar lig.
2. tibiocalcaneal lig.
3. tibionavicular lig.
calcaneus
sustentaculum tali
talus
navicular
plantar calcaneonavicular lig.
first metatarsal
medial sesamoid bone
long plantar lig.
MIRROR
plantar calcaneonavicular lig.
navicular
medial cuneiform
tibia
talus
talonavicular lig.
cuneiform bones—
- medial
- intermediate
- lateral
metatarsals
pp
dp
pp
ip
dp
phalanges
cuboid
fibula
anterior tibiofibular lig.
anterior talofibular lig.
calcaneofibular lig.
calcaneus
cervical lig.
bifurcate lig.

FIGURE 2–2. Foot ligaments. (From Jahss MH. *Disorders of the Foot and Ankle.* 2nd ed. Philadelphia: WB Saunders, 1991, p 15.)

activities. Surgery is indicated if ischemic symptoms are present. If the syndrome is diagnosed early, treatment involves release of the offending structure (usually the medial head of the gastrocnemius). Late diagnosis usually results in arterial damage requiring venous bypass graft or endarterectomy. The latter procedures are associated with a worse prognosis.

D. Treatment—Nonoperative management (e.g., activity modification, nonsteroidal medica-

tions) is sometimes successful, especially in borderline cases. Orthotics with a medial wedge may be helpful in treating posterior compartment syndrome. Studies have demonstrated that compartment pressures after maximal exercise were significantly greater in runners than in cyclists and suggested that cycling may be an effective cross-training technique for symptomatic runners. For patients who do not respond to these measures, fasciotomies are sometimes required. One

TABLE 2–2. MUSCLES OF THE ANKLE AND FOOT

Muscle	Origin	Insertion	Action	Innervation
Dorsal Layer				
Extensor digitorum brevis	Superolateral calcaneus	Base of proximal phalanges	Extend	Deep peroneal
First Plantar Layer				
Abductor hallucis	Calcaneal tuberosity	Base of great toe proximal phalanx	Abduct great toe	Medial plantar
Flexor digitorum brevis	Calcaneal tuberosity	Distal phalanges of 2nd–5th toes	Flex toes	Medial plantar
Abductor digiti minimi	Calcaneal tuberosity	Base of 5th toe	Abduct small toe	Medial plantar
Second Plantar Layer				
Quadratus plantae	Medial & lateral calcaneus	Flexor digitorum longus tendon	Helps flex digital phalanges	Lateral plantar
Lumbrical	Flexor digitorum longus tendon	Extensor digitorum longus tendons	Flex metatarsophalangeal, extend interphalangeal	Medial & lateral plantar
Flexor digitorum longus and flexor hallucis longus	Tibia/fibula	Distal phalanges of digits	Flex toes/invert foot	Tibial
Third Plantar Layer				
Flexor hallucis brevis	Cuboid/lateral cuneiform	Proximal phalanx of great toe	Flex great toe	Medial plantar
Adductor hallucis	Oblique: 2nd–4th metatarsals/ transverse: metatarsophalangeal	Proximal phalanx of great toe laterally	Adduct great toe	Lateral plantar
Flexor digiti minimi brevis	Base of 5th metatarsal head	Proximal phalanx of small toe	Flex small toe	Lateral plantar
Fourth Plantar Layer				
Dorsal interosseous	Metatarsals	Dorsal extensors	Abduct	Lateral plantar
Plantar interosseous	3rd–5th metatarsals	Proximal phalanges medially	Adduct toes	Lateral plantar
(Peroneus longus and tibialis posterior)	Fibula/tibia	Medial cuneiform/ navicular	Everts/invert foot	Superficial peroneal/ Tibial

Note: For abduction and adduction in the foot, the second toe serves as the reference. (From Miller MD. *Review of Orthopaedics*. Philadelphia: WB Saunders, 1992, p 353.)

group of investigators reported 78% good to excellent results with surgical release. In performing this procedure for posterior compartment syndrome, it is important to release not only the deep posterior compartment but also the posterior tibial compartment (Fig. 2–7).

III. Stress/Fatigue Fractures
   A. Introduction—Stress or fatigue fractures are common in athletes and represent 6% of all injuries to runners. Pain, exacerbated by exercise and partially relieved by rest, is typical. Patients may relate a history of recent change in activity or training. A brief menstrual history is appropriate for women athletes because of the association of amenorrhea or oligomenorrhea with osteoporosis. One study of stress fractures in ballet dancers identified amenorrhea and heavy training schedules as factors predisposing to stress fractures.
   B. History and Physical Examination—Patients often relate a history of overuse or a recent change in training. Questioning patients about running shoe wear is appropriate. Studies have shown that shoes used for 500 miles retain only approximately 70% of their initial shock absorption. Examination may reveal localized tenderness or induration. Radio-

graphs may demonstrate established fractures, but bone scan is most helpful in establishing the diagnosis. Stress fracture location tends to be somewhat sport specific (Table 2–3).
   C. Treatment—Stress fractures generally resolve with activity modification and rest. Improved shoe shock attenuation may have a preventive role in overuse injuries of the foot. Recalcitrant fractures, such as transverse anterior tibial stress fractures and tarsal navicular stress fractures, may require operative treatment. Transverse anterior tibial stress fractures merit special emphasis. Persistence of "the dreaded black line," especially with a positive bone scan, for more than 6 months is an indication for excision and bone grafting (Fig. 2–8). This recommendation is based on the frequency with which anterior tibial stress fractures eventually develop into complete fractures. Other authorities have described treatment with pulsing electromagnetic fields as having some success.
   Stress fractures of the tarsal navicular can also be difficult to manage. The importance of immobilization and abstaining from weight bearing in the initial treatment of navicular stress fractures cannot be overemphasized.

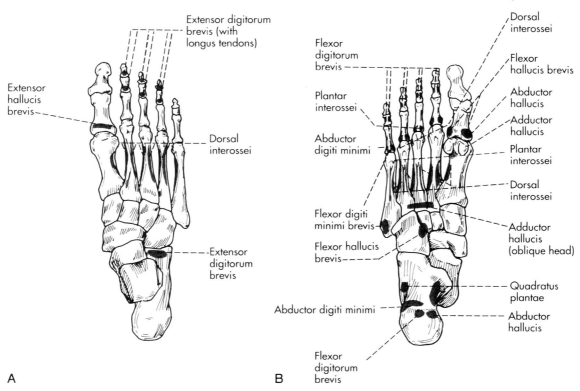

FIGURE 2–3. Origins and insertions of muscles of the foot. *A,* Dorsal. *B,* Plantar. (From Jenkins DB. *Hollinshead's Functional Anatomy of the Limbs and Back.* 6th ed. Philadelphia: WB Saunders, 1991, Fig. 20–7.)

This treatment resulted in healing in 86% of patients, versus healing in only 26% of patients with continued weight bearing and activity limitation. Autologous bone grafting for complete fractures, nonunion, cysts, and incomplete fractures that do not heal when weight bearing has been avoided should be considered. Preinjury activity level was regained within a year in 12 of 15 patients treated with this procedure.

Forefoot and hindfoot fractures are relatively common. Stress fractures in the forefoot most commonly involve the metatarsals, especially in the distal second and third metatarsal shafts. Stress fractures can also involve the proximal phalanx of the great toe. Fifth metatarsal base stress fractures should be treated by abstaining from weight bearing. Open reduction and internal fixation of fifth metatarsal base stress fractures (and navicular stress fractures) is indicated for chronic injuries that demonstrate adjacent sclerosis. Hindfoot fatigue fractures usually involve the calcaneus; however, talar fractures, usually involving the dome of the talus, have also been reported. Patients with calcaneal stress fractures often have pain and tenderness on both sides of the heel. Radiographs may show subtle areas of increased density posteriorly, but bone scans are most helpful. Treatment

consists of activity modification with or without immobilization.

  D. Freiberg Infraction—This disorder, which most commonly involves the second metatarsal head, is probably related to stress overloading of an adolescent's foot. Radiographs typically demonstrate irregularity and flattening of the metatarsal head. Initial treatment includes activity modification, casting, and orthotics. Surgical treatment for refractory symptoms includes debridement of loose bodies, partial synovectomy, and limited resection of the dorsal portion of the metatarsal head.

IV. Tendon Injuries
  A. Peroneal Tendon Injuries—These injuries include subluxation/dislocation, tenosynovitis, and tendon splitting/rupture.
    1. Subluxation/Dislocation—Traumatic subluxation or dislocation of the peroneal tendons has been reported to result from various sports-related injuries. The mechanism of injury is violent dorsiflexion of the ankle with the foot everted. The peroneal muscles contract reflexively during the injury and break through their fibro-osseous sheath (Fig. 2–9). The tendons may spontaneously relocate; however, if activation of the peroneal muscles reproduces the

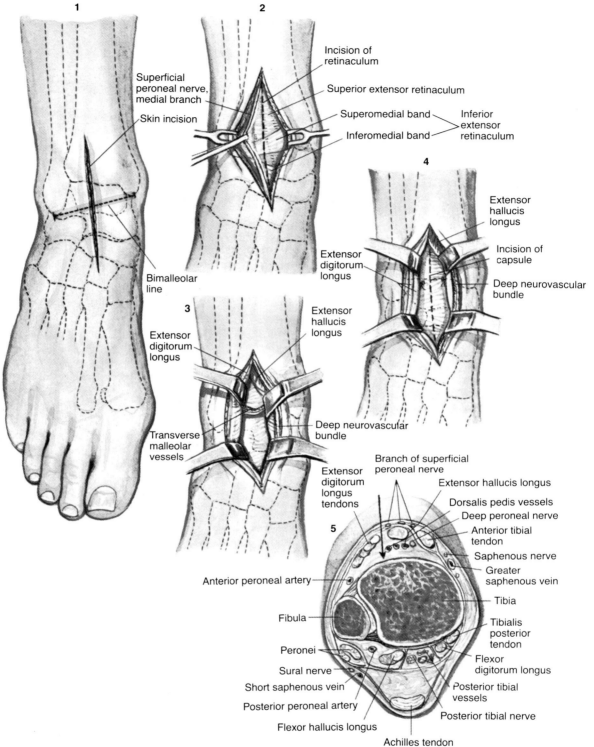

FIGURE 2–4. Anterior approach to the ankle. *1–4,* Sequential steps. *5,* Cross-sectional view. (From Jahss MH. *Disorders of the Foot and Ankle.* 2nd ed. Philadelphia: WB Saunders, 1991, p 291.)

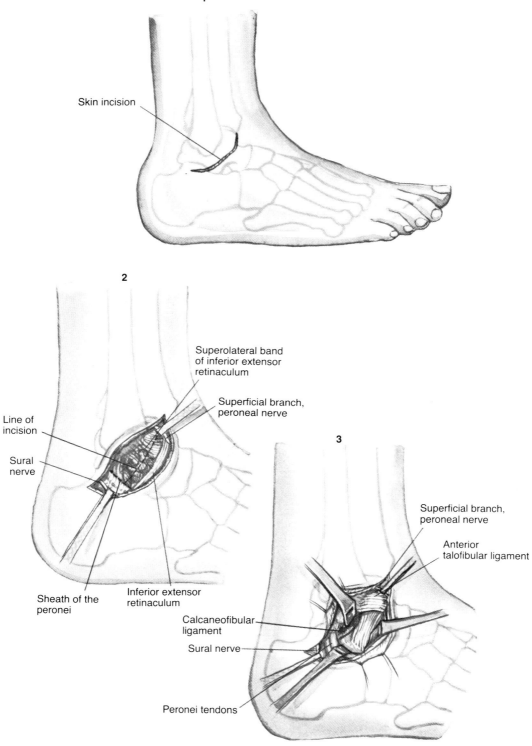

FIGURE 2–5. Lateral approach to the ankle. (From Jahss MH. *Disorders of the Foot and Ankle*. 2nd ed. Philadelphia: WB Saunders, 1991, p 303.)

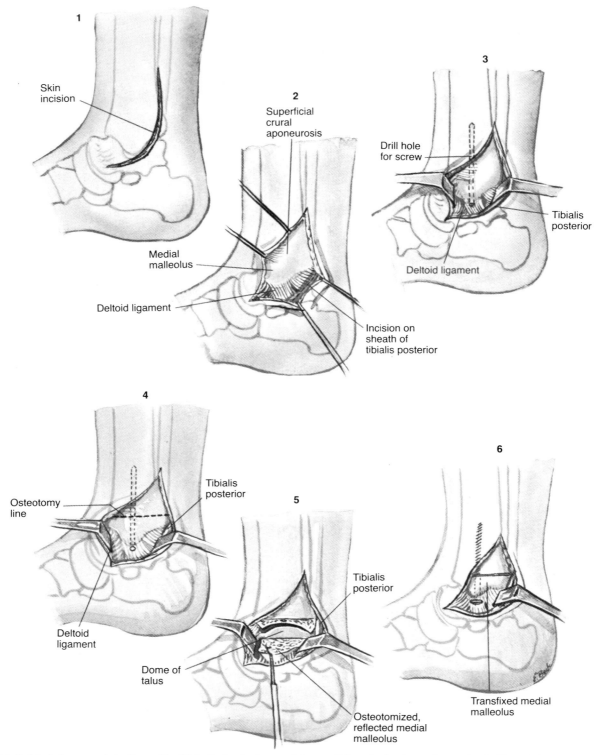

1
Skin incision

2
Superficial crural aponeurosis
Medial malleolus
Deltoid ligament
Incision on sheath of tibialis posterior

3
Drill hole for screw
Tibialis posterior
Deltoid ligament

4
Osteotomy line
Tibialis posterior
Deltoid ligament

5
Tibialis posterior
Dome of talus
Osteotomized, reflected medial malleolus

6
Transfixed medial malleolus

FIGURE 2–6. Medial approach to the ankle. Note that osteotomy of the medial malleolus is rarely required. (From Jahss MH. *Disorders of the Foot and Ankle.* 2nd ed. Philadelphia: WB Saunders, 1991, p 300.)

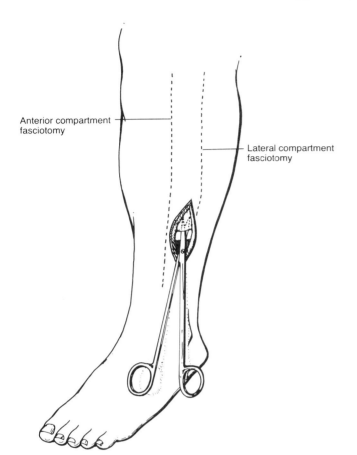

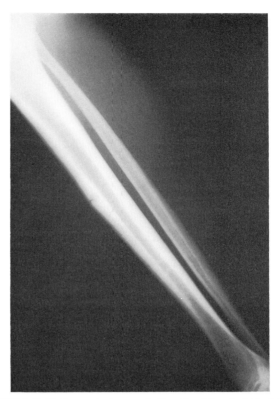

FIGURE 2–8. Radiograph demonstrating the "dreaded black line" associated with impending complete fracture from an anterior tibial stress fracture.

FIGURE 2–7. Anterior and lateral compartment release. (From DeLee JC, Drez D. *Orthopaedic Sports Medicine: Principles and Practice.* Philadelphia: WB Saunders, 1994, p 1618.)

pain or overtly dislocates the tendons, the diagnosis is confirmed. Additionally, a rim fracture of the distal fibula (Fig. 2–10), which represents an avulsion of the superior peroneal retinaculum, is diagnostic of peroneal tendon subluxation or dislocation. Despite the high specificity of this finding, it is encountered in fewer than 50% of cases.

Acute treatment of peroneal tendon dislocation/subluxation is controversial; however, chronic, painful lesions require operative treatment. Procedures that have been advocated include soft tissue reconstruction, bone block techniques, tissue transfer procedures, rerouting of the tendons, and groove-deepening procedures (Fig. 2–11).

TABLE 2–3. LOCATION OF SPORT-SPECIFIC STRESS FRACTURES

Sport	Location of Most Common Stress Fractures
Running	Tibia (distal), fibula, metatarsals
Basketball	Tarsal navicular, tibia (midshaft)
Football	Metatarsals, first metatarsophalangeal sesamoids
Dancing	Metatarsal (base), tibia (midshaft)
Recruits	Metatarsal (distal shaft), calcaneus, tibia (proximal)

Acute injuries can usually be repaired to bone primarily. It is generally advisable to treat acute injuries surgically because of the excellent results and the high rate of recurrent dislocation with nonoperative treatment.

2. Tenosynovitis, Tendinitis, and Tendinosis of the Peroneal Tendons—These conditions may be more common than is reported. Longitudinal splitting of the peroneus brevis tendon has been increasingly recognized. This appears to be a result of prolonged mechanical attrition within the fibular groove after ankle trauma and may be associated with peroneal subluxation. Repair and decompression is generally recommended for chronic lesions. If longitudinal tearing is extensive, excision of one tendon with suture to the adjacent tendon is acceptable. Complete tears of the peroneal tendons are unusual, especially in athletes. Primary repair is recommended if possible; however, if the tendons have retracted, tenodesis of the proximal tendon to the adjacent intact peroneal muscle is effective.

B. Posterior Tibialis Tendon Injury—Injuries to the posterior tibialis tendon are most commonly a result of chronic degenerative processes in nonathletic middle-aged women.

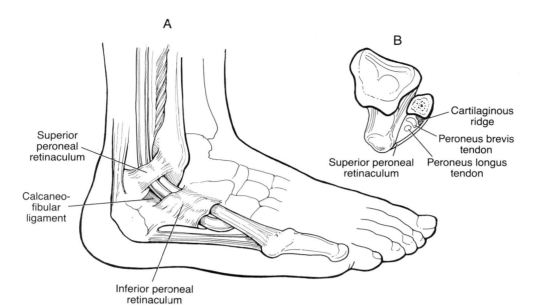

FIGURE 2–9. Normal relationship of peroneal tendons. Note the superior and inferior retinacula and the cartilaginous ridge on the posterolateral fibula. *A*, Lateral view. *B*, Superior view.

Complete or partial posterior tibial tendon rupture can also occur in older athletes. The investigators noted that the patients described pain in the midarch region, had difficulty pushing off, and had a pronated, flattened longitudinal arch. They recommend early recognition and debridement of partial ruptures. Chronic complete ruptures may require excision of the damaged posterior tibialis tendon and suturing of the tendon to the flexor digitorum longus tendon, which is used to reconstruct the posterior tibialis tendon (Fig. 2–12). Dislocation of the posterior tibial tendon has also been described. Treatment is similar to the more common peroneal tendon dislocation—that is, reduction and repair/reconstruction of the groove and retinaculum.

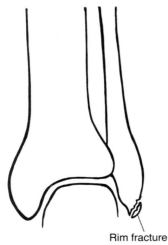

FIGURE 2–10. Rim fracture of the lateral aspect of the distal fibula associated with dislocating peroneal tendons.

C. Anterior Tibialis Tendon Injury—Acute spontaneous rupture of the tibialis anterior tendon is uncommon but has been reported. Diagnosis is confirmed by noting localized tenderness, inversion/dorsiflexion weakness, and normal findings on neurologic examination. Recommended treatment for acute rupture is surgical repair; however, treatment of chronic ruptures is controversial.

D. Achilles Tendon Injury—Achilles tendon disorders are among the most common athletic injuries. These disorders represent a continuum from tendinitis to complete rupture.
1. Tendinitis—This is often a result of overuse, with running being the sport most frequently implicated. It is important to differentiate peritendinitis from actual tendinitis. The "painful arc sign" can be helpful in making this distinction. In peritendinitis, the area of localized tenderness remains fixed with dorsiflexion and plantar flexion of the foot; however, with tendinitis (and partial rupture), the point of tenderness moves (with the tendon) (Fig. 2–13). Treatment includes rest and physical therapy modalities. Soft tissue massage and mobilization techniques are useful in the treatment of fibrosing peritendinitis. Surgery is rarely indicated but may be considered in an athlete with symptoms that have not responded to 4 months of treatment. This consists of exploration and debridement of necrotic tendon.
2. Partial Ruptures of the Tendon—Partial ruptures of the tendon have escaped detection in the past but are being recognized with increasing frequency. Most authorities favor initial treatment as outlined earlier for tendinitis. Because of the long-term

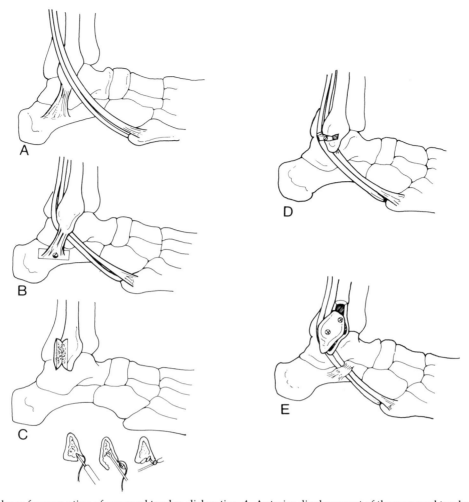

FIGURE 2–11. Procedures for correction of peroneal tendon dislocation *A,* Anterior displacement of the peroneal tendons. *B,* Pöll and Duijftes bone block method. *C,* Groove-deepening procedure. *D,* DuVries procedure. *E,* Kelly bone block procedure.

morbidity associated with chronic partial Achilles tendon ruptures, surgical excision of scar and granulation tissue with or without osteotomy of the calcaneal tuberosity has been recommended. Approximately 80% of athletes can return to their former level of activity after this treatment. Because the diagnosis of partial ruptures can be difficult, some researchers have advocated special imaging modalities. European studies suggest sensitivity of 94% and specificity of 100% using ultrasonography in the diagnosis of partial ruptures. Other European studies characterized Achilles tendon injuries as being one of four types according to MRI findings:

I Inflammatory reaction
II Degenerative change
III Incomplete (partial) rupture
IV Complete rupture

3. Complete Rupture of the Achilles Tendon— This is caused by maximal plantar flexion contraction of the gastrocnemius-soleus muscles while the foot is planted during the push-off phase in running or jumping. This contraction overloads the Achilles tendon (which commonly has asymptomatic antecedent degenerative changes). It may be associated with a painful "pop" that occurs after landing or jumping on the foot. Patients may relate that they thought that they had been "shot" or kicked in the heel. The Thompson test (squeezing the calf passively plantar flexes the foot with an intact Achilles tendon) is commonly used to diagnose Achilles tendon ruptures. Because the other flexor tendons can plantarflex the ankle, active plantar flexion does not allow adequate assessment of Achilles tendon integrity. A clinical test using a sphygmomanometer cuff has been

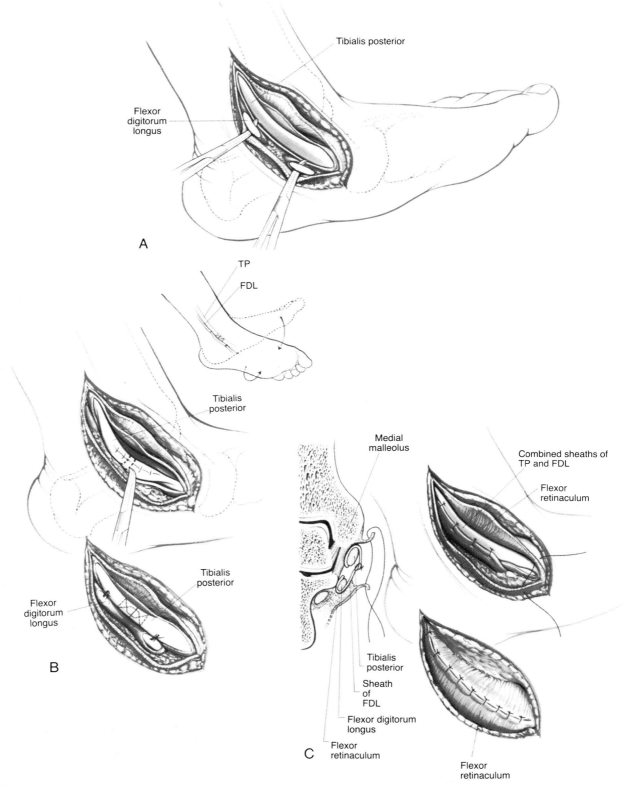

FIGURE 2–12. Treatment of a damaged posterior tibialis tendon may require debridement of the damaged portion, repair of the defect, and suture of the tendon to that of the flexor digitorum longus. *A,* Exposure of the tibialis position and flexor digitorum longus. *B,* Excision of damaged or redundant tendon and repair with suturing to flexor tendon proximal and distal. *C,* Repair of the sheaths and retinaculum. (From Jahss MH. *Disorders of the Foot and Ankle.* 2nd ed. Philadelphia: WB Saunders, 1991, pp 1495–1496.)

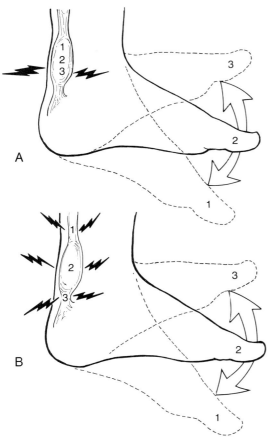

FIGURE 2–13. Painful arc sign. *A,* Peritendinitis—the location of tenderness does not vary with foot movement. *B,* Tendinitis—the location of tenderness varies with foot position.

described as useful both for diagnosis and for quantification of treatment progress.

Treatment of complete Achilles tendon ruptures remains controversial. However, all authorities agree that the rate of rerupture is much lower with surgical treatment. Although percutaneous repair, was popular initially, most surgeons now advocate conventional open repair. This may be because of reports of higher rerupture rates and the potential for sural nerve injury associated with percutaneous repair. Open repair for athletes with Achilles tendon ruptures is routinely performed (Fig. 2–14). Direct posterior incisions should be avoided, and atruamatic soft tissue technique should be used.

Treatment of chronic defects, particularly those with large gaps, can be challenging. Several techniques have been advocated for these cases. One technique, popular in Europe, involves transforming pedicled muscle-tendon flaps from the triceps surae muscle into free flaps or transplants. Another technique uses the tendon of the flexor digitorum longus as a bridging graft and has had good to excellent results in six of seven patients. The semitendinosus can also be used in a box configuration as a free graft.

E. Gastrocnemius-Soleus Strain—Injury of the tendinous origin of the triceps surae is relatively common. In the past, these injuries were often attributed to rupture of the plan-

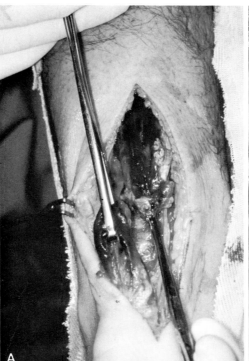
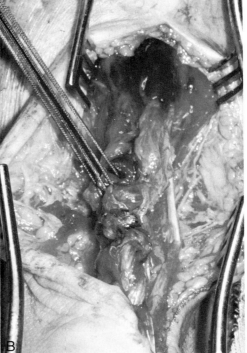

FIGURE 2–14. Clinical example of an Achilles tendon rupture. *A,* Exposure. *B,* Surgical repair.

taris; however, most of these injuries were more likely to be gastrocnemius-soleus strains. This injury has been nicknamed "tennis leg" because of its high incidence in this sport. The mechanism of injury consists of forced plantar flexion of the ankle while pushing off. Treatment is conservative, consisting of rest, ice, elevation, and relative immobilization. Early compressive dressings may help minimize hematoma formation. Surgery is rarely necessary.

V. Nerve Entrapment
  A. Introduction—A number of nerve entrapment syndromes have been described on the basis of their anatomic location (Fig. 2–15). Of these, the most common entrapment syndrome in athletes involves the superficial peroneal nerve. Many nerve problems are functional (i.e., the nerve is compressed only during athletic activity); therefore, special considerations in history taking, examination, and testing (e.g., nerve conduction studies in conjunction with treadmill examination) may be necessary.

  B. Saphenous Nerve—The saphenous nerve can be entrapped as it pierces the Hunter canal. It can also be compressed as it pierces the fascia lata between the tendons of the sartorius and gracilis muscles. The infrapatellar branch of this nerve is commonly injured with medial approaches to the knee, sometimes resulting in a painful neuroma.

  C. Common Peroneal Nerve—The common peroneal nerve can be compressed as it passes between the biceps tendon and the lateral head of the gastrocnemius muscle and behind the neck of the fibula between the two heads of the peroneus longus muscle. This nerve is commonly injured by a direct blow to the lateral aspect of the knee or by stretching as a result of a varus knee injury.

  D. Superficial Peroneal Nerve—The superficial peroneal nerve, which innervates the peroneus brevis and longus, pierces the deep fascia of the anterolateral compartment about 12 cm proximal to the tip of the lateral malleolus. It is at this point that the nerve can be entrapped by fascial defects, fibrous bands, and local muscle herniation. The nerve is com-

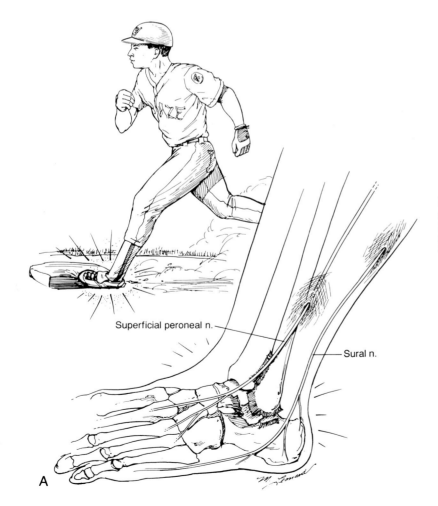

Superficial peroneal n.

Sural n.

FIGURE 2–15. *A*, Superfical peroneal nerve and sural nerve entrapment can result from inversion injuries. (From Schon LC: Nerve entrapment, neuropathy, and nerve dysfunction in athletes. Orthop Clin North Am 25:55, 1994.)

A

monly entrapped or compressed in skating and skiing as a result of the type of footwear. Patients may have pain over the lateral border of the distal calf and dorsum of the foot that is worse with activity and relieved by rest. Local tenderness, fascial defects, and provocative tests can be helpful in establishing the diagnosis. Specifically, active dorsiflexion and eversion of the foot against resistance or passive plantar flexion and eversion causes tenderness at the site of impingement. Concomitant anterolateral compartment syndrome should be considered and fasciotomy performed at the time of decompression if it is indicated. Simple exploration and decompression is usually effective.

E. Deep Peroneal Nerve (Anterior Tarsal Tunnel)—Although the deep peroneal nerve can be compressed at several locations, the most common entrapment is under the inferior extensor retinaculum, commonly referred to as the anterior tarsal tunnel syndrome. The nerve may be entrapped at the superior edge of the retinaculum, where the extensor hallucis longus tendon crosses over it. Patients may complain of dorsal foot pain with occasional radiation into the first web space. Findings on examination may include localized tenderness, decreased sensation in the first web space, and weakness of the extensor digitorum brevis in more proximal entrapments. Conservative measures (e.g., avoiding provocative maneuvers, loosening external constraints, activity modification) should be tried initially. If these fail, exploration and surgical release of the offending structures may be indicated.

F. Tibial Nerve (Tarsal Tunnel)—The tibial nerve can be entrapped behind the medial malleolus under the laciniate ligament (flexor retinaculum), leading to what is commonly referred to as tarsal tunnel syndrome. Diagnosis may

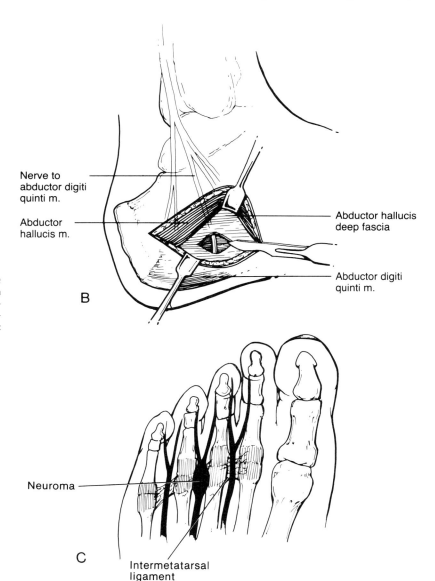

FIGURE 2–15. *Continued B*, Release of the nerve to the abductor digiti quinti. *C*, Entrapment of the common digital nerve beneath the intermetatarsal ligament (Morton neuroma). *B* and *C* from DeLee JC, Drez D. *Orthopaedic Sports Medicine: Principles and Practice*. Philadelphia: WB Saunders, 1994, pp 1834, 1894.)

be confirmed with electrodiagnostic testing, and release of the retinaculum is curative in the majority of cases. Entrapment has been described distal to this point, involving the first branch of the lateral plantar nerve. This branch is entrapped between the deep fascia of the abductor hallucis longus and the medial margin of the quadratus plantae muscle. Patients have burning pain and tenderness along the course of the nerve and may be unable to abduct the small toe. Conservative treatment (e.g., stretching, contrast baths, nonsteroidal anti-inflammatory drugs [NSAIDs], orthotics) is usually successful. Surgical release of the deep fascia of the abductor hallucis has been successful in cases that failed to resolve with extended conservative management. The location of symptoms and physical examination findings suggest the exact location and guide release of the nerve entrapment.

G. Medial Plantar Nerve (Jogger's Foot)—Entrapment of the medial plantar nerve usually occurs near where the flexor digitorum longus tendon crosses over the flexor hallucis longus tendon (knot of Henry). This entrapment can often be caused by external compression, such as by the use of arch supports. Symptoms may include pain radiating into the medial toes, and patients may have localized tenderness, pain with walking on the toes, and decreased sensation after activity. If conservative measures fail, surgical release is often successful.

H. Sural Nerve—The sural nerve can be entrapped anywhere along its course. It can be irritated by injuries, ganglia, postsurgical scarring, and even Achilles peritendinitis. Localized tenderness can usually be elicited. Surgical release is usually effective. Resection is required for postsurgical entrapment.

I. Interdigital Nerve (Morton Neuroma)—Interdigital nerve entrapment can occur in athletes during the push-off phase while running. Typically this occurs between the third and fourth metatarsals, plantar to the deep transverse metatarsal ligament. Conservative management including wider shoes, metatarsal pads, and occasionally injection can be helpful. Surgical excision of the neuroma is usually successful if these measures fail.

VI. Plantar Fasciitis
A. Introduction—Plantar fasciitis, or inflammation of the plantar fascia in the central to medial subcalcaneal region, is easy to diagnose but difficult to manage. It can be exacerbated by excessive or prolonged pronation. It is important to rule out other causes of heel pain in athletes, such as stress fractures, nerve entrapment, S1 radiculopathy, and seronegative spondyloarthropathy.

B. Treatment—Plantar fasciitis is best treated initially with rest, orthotics, stretching, and NSAIDs. This condition is common in runners. Treatment several times per day consisting of ice massage, heel cord stretching, posterior tibial and peroneal strengthening, heel cushioning, and NSAIDs is recommended. In cases with symptoms lasting more than 6 weeks, casting may be required for absolute rest. Plantar fasciotomy has been advocated for intractable symptoms. Good results have been reported with this procedure. The researchers did point out, however, that the recovery was often prolonged, additional treatment was often required, and abnormalities in foot function often persisted despite satisfactory clinical results.

VII. Os Trigonum
A. Introduction—An unfused or fractured os trigonum can cause impingement in certain sporting activities. The patient can have pain with dorsiflexion of the foot (Fig. 2–16). The condition is becoming increasingly recognized, especially in ballet dancers. A 15-year-old basketball player had posterior ankle pain that was refractory to rest, casting, NSAIDs, and other conservative measures. Radiographs demonstrated what appeared to be a fracture of a fused os trigonum. Technetium bone scan demonstrated increased uptake in this area.

B. Treatment—Injection of anesthetic (not steroids because of risk of flexor hallucis longus tendon rupture) in the area can relieve symptoms temporarily. Other supportive treatment is also effective. Removal of the offending bone may occasionally be necessary. This generally yields excellent results. Subtalar arthroscopic resection of the lesion has been tried but is still experimental.

VIII. Ankle Instability
A. Introduction—Ankle injuries are the most common joint injury encountered in sports medicine, general orthopaedics, and family practice. The anterior talofibular ligament (ATFL) is the most commonly injured ankle ligament. Other lateral ligaments, including the calcaneofibular ligament (CFL) and the posterior talofibular ligament (PTFL), can also be injured (Fig. 2–17). Both the ATFL and CFL function to restrict excessive adduction of the ankle; however, because of its orientation, the ATFL serves this function only with plantar flexion of the foot. Ankle sprains may be more common in larger athletes and in those with a previous history of an ankle sprain. The type of footwear (high-top versus low-top shoes) does not appear to affect the incidence of ankle sprains. Strain measurements have confirmed that the ATFL is most com-

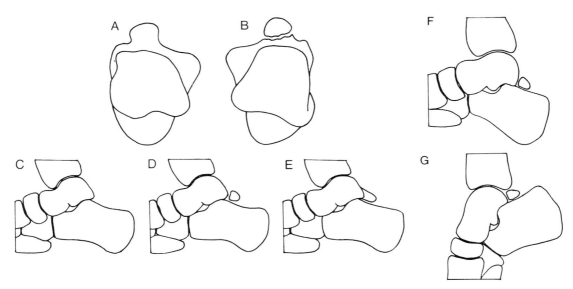

FIGURE 2–16. Os trigonum nonunions can cause symptoms with dorsiflexion of the foot. *A*, Normal fused os trigonum. *B*, Fracture of fused os trigonum. *C*, Absent os trigonum. *D*, Large os trigonum. *E*, Symptomatic fused os trigonum. *F*, Os trigonum in dorsiflexion. *G*, Impingement of os trigonum in plantar flexion. (From Quirk R. Common foot injuries in dance. Orthop Clin North Am 25:127, 1994.)

monly injured with ankle inversion, plantar flexion, and internal rotation. Primary tears of the CFL occur with dorsiflexion or with severe inversion after ATFL tears. The ATFL contributes to ankle stability in plantar flexion; however, the CFL appears to contribute to ankle stability in all positions. In addition, there is high incidence of articular cartilage lesions in ankles with lateral ligament injury, occurring exclusively in chronic ankle sprains, suggesting a more aggressive approach for significant primary ankle sprains.

B. History and Physical Examination—Patients usually have point tenderness over the area of the torn ligaments. It is essential to palpate all bony areas to help rule out a fracture. This includes the proximal fibula because of the associated incidence of high fibular fractures with syndesmosis injuries (Maisonneuve fracture). Instability can be assessed on the basis of examination of talar tilt and anterior drawer testing (Fig. 2–18).

Plain films should include a lateral and a mortise view. The mortise view should be ex-

FIGURE 2–17. *A*, Lateral ankle sprains result from inversion injuries. *B*, The ligament injured most commonly is the anterior talofibular (atf) ligament, followed in order of frequency by the calcaneofibular (cf) ligament and the posterior talofibular (ptf) ligament. (From DeLee JC, Drez D. *Orthopaedic Sports Medicine: Principles and Practice.* Philadelphia: WB Saunders, 1994, pp 1706, 1707.)

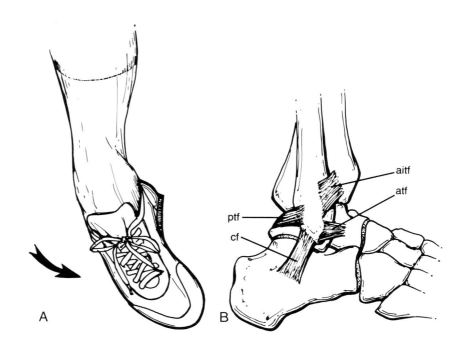

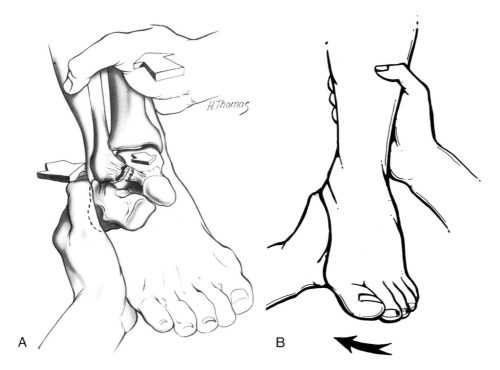

FIGURE 2–18. *A,* Anterior drawer test for assessment of the integrity of the anterior talofibular ligament. (From Jahss MH. *Disorders of the Foot and Ankle.* 2nd ed. Philadelphia: WB Saunders, 1991, p 56.) *B,* Varus stress (tilt) test for assessment of the integrity of the calcaneofibular ligament. (From DeLee JC, Drez D. *Orthopaedic Sports Medicine: Principles and Practice.* Philadelphia: WB Saunders, 1994, pp 1706, 1707.)

amined to ensure that there is at least 1 mm of overlap between the tibia and fibula, no more than 4 mm of medial clear space, and an intact tibiofibular line (Fig. 2–19). Several studies have confirmed that the use of stress radiography may be of benefit in the evaluation of patients with chronic ankle instability. Lesser degrees of anterior instability are consistent with isolated ATFL injuries, whereas greater degrees of instability may denote combined injuries to the AFTL and the CFL.

Greater than 5 mm of anterior displacement of the talus on drawer stress testing is consistent with injury to the ATFL. Greater than 15 mm of tibiotalar tilt or greater than 5° of side-to-side difference in tibiotalar tilt with varus stressing is consistent with injury to the CFL.

C. Treatment—Initial treatment of ankle sprains includes rest, ice, elevation, and protection. This should be followed by supervised therapy including peroneal strengthening and proprioception training. The effect of ankle taping on mechanical stability is insignificant; however, the use of a semirigid orthosis may provide enough external support to prevent ankle sprains and protect ligament reconstructions. Surgical treatment is reserved for recurrent, symptomatic ankle instability in patients who have objective findings and who have not responded to extended nonoperative treatment. The role of early surgery in elite athletes with an acute injury is controversial, and most of even these athletes fare quite well and return to sports earlier with conservative treatment. Most authorities currently favor a modified Bröstrom procedure for surgical treatment of ankle instability in athletes who have failed to respond to nonoperative measures. Other authorities have suggested reinforcing this repair with a periosteal flap; however, this has not been found to be necessary. The technique, which is an anatomic reinforcement and tightening of the lateral ligaments, is illustrated in Figure 2–20. The use of the inferior arm of the extensor retinaculum (Gould) can reinforce the repair. In more se-

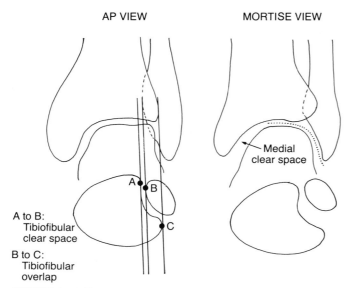

AP VIEW   MORTISE VIEW

Medial clear space

A to B: Tibiofibular clear space

B to C: Tibiofibular overlap

FIGURE 2–19. Drawing of lines that should be evaluated on the AP and mortise views.

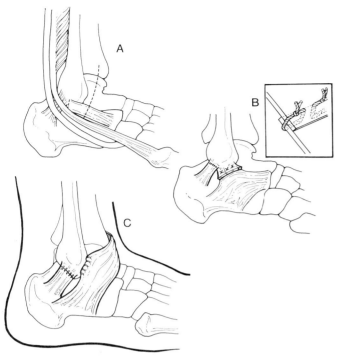

FIGURE 2–20. Bröstrom procedure for lateral ankle reconstruction. *A*, Incision. *B*, Imbrication. *C*, Reinforcement.

vere ankle injuries and for revisions, it may be necessary to reinforce the repair with tendon graft, usually from the peroneus brevis. Various procedures have been proposed but can severely restrict subtalar motion (Fig. 2–21).

D. Syndesmotic Ankle Injuries—Increased emphasis is being placed on recognition and treatment of "high" ankle sprains. These injuries are especially common in professional athletes who have incurred repetitive injuries. The mechanism of injury is commonly related to excessive external rotation. Radiographs may demonstrate calcification of the distal syndesmosis with injuries that are recognized late. Injuries to the syndesmosis are often associated with a recovery time almost twice that of patients with severe ankle sprains. We

recommend incorporation of a squeeze test into the standard ankle examination to identify these patients (Fig. 2–22*A*). Another test that has been proposed is the abduction–external rotation stress test (Fig. 2–22*B*). Some authorities recommend that this test be used radiographically to diagnose latent syndesmotic injuries. Treatment of these injuries requires immobilization in a non–weight-bearing cast for 4 weeks. Treatment of frank injuries to the syndesmosis, which can be diagnosed on plain radiographs (>1-mm reduction in the medial clear space), may require closed reduction and fixation with one to two syndesmotic screws.

E. Subtalar Instability—This can commonly occur in conjunction with ankle injuries. Acutely, patients may have tenderness in the area of the sinus tarsi. Broden stress radiographs with the heel in varus and foot internally rotated and the beam directed 20° caudally can demonstrate instability. Surgical treatment if nonoperative management fails involves ankle reconstruction to include the subtalar joint.

IX. Ankle Arthroscopy

A. Introduction—The indications for ankle arthroscopy have rapidly expanded from diagnostic to therapeutic procedures. Currently, arthroscopic treatment of osteochondral lesions of the talus, posttraumatic synovitis, posttraumatic osteoarthritis, and many other conditions of the ankle is well accepted. Follow-up studies of ankle arthroscopy demonstrate consistently good results.

B. Arthroscopic Setup—Most surgeons prefer to perform arthroscopy with patients supine with a setup similar to that for knee arthroscopy. Some surgeons recommend a distractor that is mounted similarly to an external fixator; however, manual traction by an assistant or with a noninvasive distraction device is usually adequate (Fig. 2–23). Other surgeons prefer a lateral decubitus position without

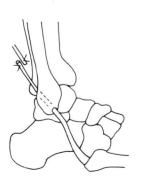

Evan's procedure

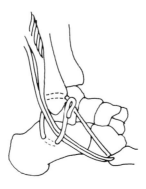

Chrisman-Snook procedure

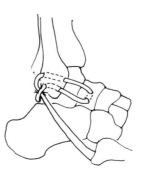

Watson-Jones procedure

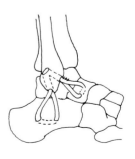

Elmslie procedure

FIGURE 2–21. Other ligament reconstructions for lateral and subtalar instability.

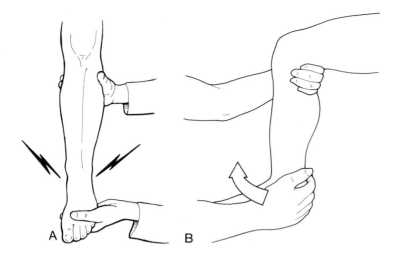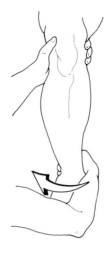

FIGURE 2–22. A, Squeeze test used to diagnose syndesmotic injury. B, Abduction–external rotation stress test.

lowering the end of the operating table. The standard 4.0-mm arthroscope is used, although smaller scopes (2.7 mm) may occasionally be helpful for areas that are more difficult to reach. Five arthroscopic portals have been described (Fig. 2–24):

Portal	Location	Risk
Anterolateral	Lateral to peroneus tertius and extensors	Superior peroneal nerve
Anterocentral	Medial or lateral to external hallucis longus	Dorsalis pedis, deep peroneal nerve
Anteromedial	Medial to tibialis anterior	Saphenous nerve/vein

Portal	Location	Risk
Posterolateral	Lateral to Achilles, 2 cm proximal to lateral malleolus	Sural nerve
Posteromedial	Medial to Achilles	Posterior tibial artery/ tibial nerve

Because of the significant neurovascular risk associated with the posteromedial portal, most arthroscopists do not use this portal. Surgical pathology is usually addressed through the ipsilateral portal, and the contralateral portal is used for visualization (Fig. 2–25).

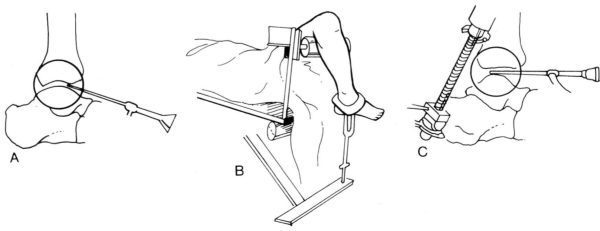

FIGURE 2–23. A, Lateral view of arthroscopy without distraction. B, Setup for ankle arthroscopy with noninvasive distraction. C, Lateral view of ankle arthroscopy with distraction.

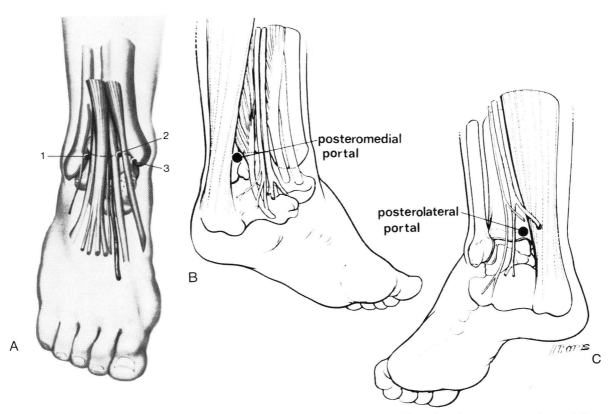

FIGURE 2–24. Portals for ankle arthroscopy. *A,* Anterior portals. (1 = anterolateral portal lateral to the peroneus tertius and the extensor digitorum communis tendons; 2 = anterocentral portal medial or lateral to the extensor hallucis longus tendon; 3 = anteromedial portal medial to the tibialis anterior tendon.) *B,* Posteromedial portal, just medial to the Achilles tendon. *C,* Posterolateral portal, just lateral to the Achilles tendon. (From Jahss MH. *Disorders of the Foot and Ankle.* 2nd ed. Philadelphia: WB Saunders, 1991, p 206.)

C. Osteochondral Lesions—Treatment of osteochondral lesions of the talus can often be performed arthroscopically. Loomer and colleagues noted that anterior and midtalar lesions, which represent most of the lesions, can be treated arthroscopically (Fig. 2–26). These investigators added a fifth type to the Berndt and Harty classification scheme (Fig. 2–27). This newly described type, which was the most common variety in their series, is a radiolucent fibrous defect in the talus.

Curettage and drilling of the osteochondral lesions resulted in good to excellent results in 74% of their patients. A long-term follow-up study of patients with osteochondral lesions of the talus treated with open drilling demonstrated that the initial good results of surgery deteriorated with time, and pain and swelling were noted in more than half of the patients. Nevertheless, the researchers noted that only one patient in their series (18 patients) had significant pain at 9- to 15-year follow-up.

The transmalleolar approach, developed by Guhl, may be helpful for hard-to-reach areas. A guide is used to place the drill into the desired position for chondral drilling. It may occasionally be necessary to resort to open techniques via an osteotomy of the medial malleolus (Fig. 2–28). A posteromedial approach through the posterior tibial flexor tendon sheath may allow access to this area without an osteotomy.

D. Tibiotalar Spurs—Arthroscopy is also useful in the treatment of anterior tibiotalar spurs. These osteophytes, which can form on both the anterior tibia and the talar neck, result in reduction of motion. When the tibiotalar angle is <60°, arthroscopic treatment may be indicated (Fig. 2–29). A decreased length of hospitalization and recovery time in patients treated arthroscopically versus with open techniques can be expected, and patients with advanced arthritis and tibiotalar narrowing (type IV degeneration) are not suitable candidates for arthroscopic debridement.

E. Arthroscopically Assisted Tibiotalar Arthrodesis—Arthroscopic tibiotalar fusion has been successful in early follow-up studies. Debridement of the articular cartilage is followed by placement of two to three 6.5-mm cannulated screws from the tibia to the talus under arthrosopic control. This procedure is

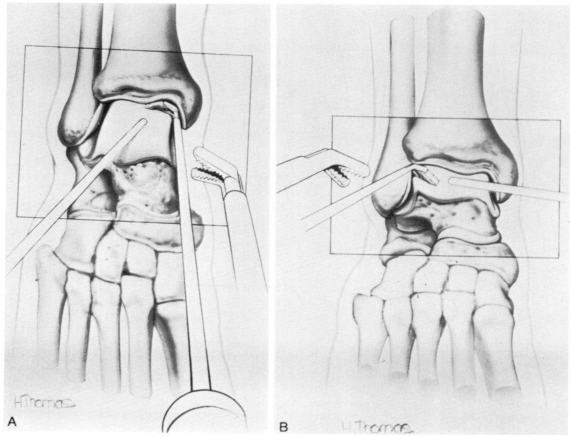

FIGURE 2–25. Arthroscopic visualization and instrumentation techniques. The grasper is placed in the portal opposite the arthroscope. *A,* Medial talar lesion. *B,* Lateral talar lesion. (From Jahss MH. *Disorders of the Foot and Ankle.* 2nd ed. Philadelphia: WB Saunders, 1991, p 219.)

indicated only for degenerative arthritis without severe angular deformities.

F. Soft Tissue Lesions—Arthroscopy has also been advocated for the treatment of anterolateral synovial impingement after injury (Fig. 2–30). Excellent results and debridement of scar tissue in patients treated with arthroscopic partial synovectomy have been reported. Arthroscopic excision of fibrous

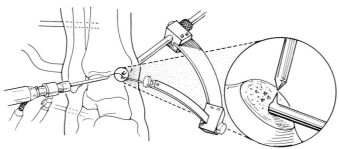

FIGURE 2–26. Transmalleolar drilling of an osteochondral lesion. Note the use of an arthroscopic anterior cruciate ligament drill guide.

bands located between the talus and fibula ("meniscoid" lesions), which can follow ankle sprains, has also been reported to be effective. Unfortunately, arthroscopic treatment of these cases has not been uniformly successful. Arthroscopic treatment of talar impingement by the anteroinferior tibiofibular ligament, the so-called Duke lesion, resulted in good to excellent results in six of seven patients after arthroscopic resection of this ligament.

X. Ankle and Foot Fractures

A. Introduction—Ankle fractures are common in athletics. Early management of ankle fractures includes acute reduction and immobilization. Displaced ankle fractures have an increased incidence of skin complications in fractures that are not reduced acutely. Treatment of ankle fractures does not necessarily require open reduction and internal fixation. Type II supination-eversion injuries treated nonoperatively have clinical results at least equal to those of operative treatment.

B. Fixation Techniques—Reports of complications associated with absorbable internal fixa-

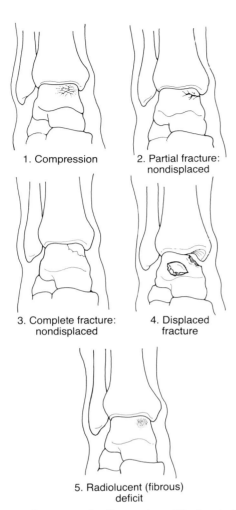

1. Compression

2. Partial fracture: nondisplaced

3. Complete fracture: nondisplaced

4. Displaced fracture

5. Radiolucent (fibrous) deficit

FIGURE 2–27. Loomer and colleagues' modification to the Berndt and Harty classification of osteochondral lesions of the talus.

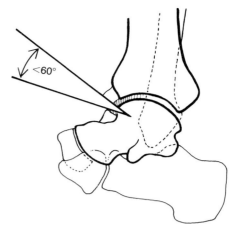

FIGURE 2–29. Osteophytes on the distal tibia or talar neck can result in reduction of the tibiotalar angle to <60°.

tion necessitate judicious use of these implants. Of most concern are osteolysis and granulomatous reactions associated with the use of these devices. The use of the posterior antiglide plate for fixation of lateral malleolar fractures has been advocated in several studies. This technique uses a buttress-type effect to stabilize the fracture during fixation (Fig. 2–31).

C. Postoperative Management—Two current studies of postoperative immobilization after open reduction and internal fixation of ankle fractures noted no functional difference between a cast, an orthosis, or no cast or orthosis as long as patients abstained from weight bearing for 6 weeks postoperatively. Sports activities can usually begin between the 10th and 20th week.

D. Foot Injuries—Most fractures of the foot can be successfully treated nonoperatively. Significantly displaced fractures and intra-

FIGURE 2–28. Osteotomy of the medial malleolus is rarely required for access to the posteromedial talus. *A*, Predrilling of the osteotomy site. *B*, Osteotomy. Note that the deltoid ligament is left attached, and the osteotomy is hinged on its distal attachment. *C1*, Drilling the base of the lesion. *C2*, Fixation of the loose fragment. *D*, Reduction and fixation of the osteotomy.

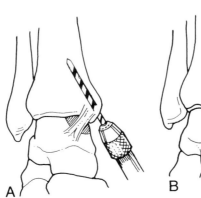
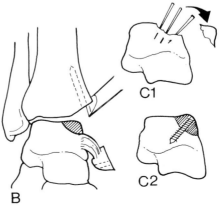
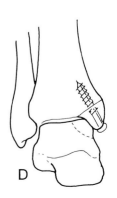

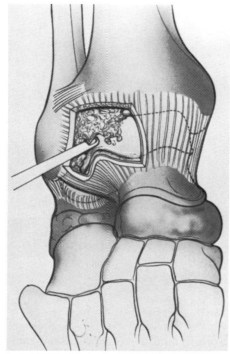

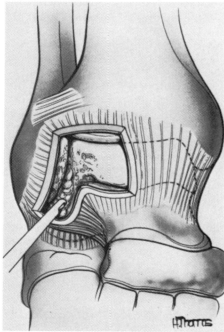

FIGURE 2–30. Synovial excision through the scope. (From Jahss MH. *Disorders of the Foot and Ankle*. Philadelphia: WB Saunders, 1991, p 228.)

articular fractures may require more aggressive treatment. Tarsometatarsal injuries in athletes have been diagnosed with increasing frequency. Passive pronation and abduction of the forefoot may aid in the diagnosis. Injuries with diastasis of the metatarsal bases (Lisfranc joint) require open reduction and internal fixation.

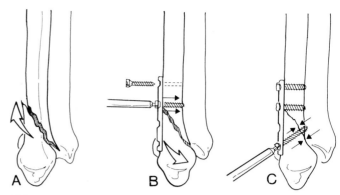

FIGURE 2–31. Antiglide plate for distal fibular fractures. *A*, Fracture. *B*, Indirect reduction. *C*, Interfragmentary fixation.

XI. Injuries to the Great Toe
  A. Introduction—Injuries to the great toe, especially "turf toe," have become increasingly frequent. This is probably at least partly because of the popularity of artificial turf and more flexible shoes. The injury, which is more common in offensive linemen and receivers, is related to severe dorsiflexion of the metatarsophalangeal joint of the great toe (Fig. 2–32). Diagnosis is made by the clinical picture of a dorsally tender, red, stiff, swollen joint. Dorsiflexion stress lateral radiographs can detect traumatic disruption of the plantar plate/flexor hallucis brevis complex or a bipartite sesamoid.
  B. Treatment—Rehabilitation consists of range of motion exercises, ice, and taping. Special shoes designed for artificial turf may help reduce the incidence of these injuries. If symptoms persist, the athlete should be carefully evaluated to rule out a stress fracture of the proximal phalanx. Acute complete disruption of the plantar complex is unusual and should be treated surgically.

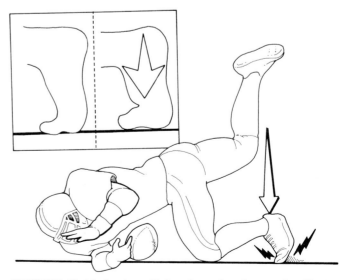

FIGURE 2–32. Mechanism of injury for turf toe is acute dorsiflexion of the first metatarsophalangeal joint.

Selected References

Introduction

Baxter DE. The foot in running. In Mann RA, Coughlin MJ (eds). *Surgery of the Foot and Ankle*. 2nd ed. St Louis: Mosby–Year Book, 1993.

Clanton TO, Schon LC. Athletic injuries to the soft tissues of the foot and ankle. In Mann RA, Coughlin MJ (eds). *Surgery of the Foot and Ankle*. 2nd ed. St Louis: Mosby–Year Book, 1993, pp 1095–1224.

Garrick JG, Requa RK. The epidemiology of foot and ankle injuries in sports. Clin Sports Med 7:29–36, 1988.

Compartment Syndrome

Beckham SG, Grana WA, Buckley P, et al. A comparison of anterior compartment pressures in competitive runners and cyclists. Am J Sports Med 21:36–40, 1993.

Bourne RB, Rorabeck CH. Compartment syndromes of the lower leg. Clin Orthop 240:97–104, 1989.

Clanton TO, Schon LC. Athletic injuries to the soft tissues of the foot and ankle. In Mann RA, Coughlin MJ (eds). *Surgery of the Foot and Ankle*. 2nd ed. St Louis: Mosby–Year Book, 1993, pp 1095–1224.

Delaney TA, Gonzalez LL. Occlusion of the popliteal artery due to muscular entrapment. Surgery 69:97–101, 1971.

Eisele SA, Sammarco GJ. Chronic exertional compartment syndrome. Instr Course Lect 42:213–217, 1993.

Holder LE, Michael RH. The specific scintigraphic pattern of "shin splints in the lower leg." J Nucl Med 25:865–869, 1984.

Insua JA, Young JR, Humphries AW. Popliteal artery entrapment syndrome. Arch Surg 101:771–775, 1970.

James SL, Bates BT, Osternig LR. Injuries to runners. Am J Sports Med 6:40–50, 1978.

Jarvinnen M, Aho H, Niittmymaki S. Results of the surgical treatment of the medial tibial syndrome in athletes. Int J Sports Med 10:55–57, 1989.

Love JW, Wheler TJ. Popliteal artery entrapment syndrome. Am J Surg 109:620–624, 1965.

Martens MA, Moeyersoons JP. Acute and recurrent effort-related compartment syndrome in sports. Sports Med 9:62–68, 1990.

Pedowitz RA, Horgens AR, Mubarak SJ, et al. Modified criteria for the objective diagnosis of compartment syndrome of the leg. Am J Sports Med 18:35–40, 1990.

Pellegrini VD, Evarts CM. Complications. In Rockwood CA, Green DP, Bucholz RW (eds). *Rockwood and Green's Fractures and Dislocations*. 3rd ed. Philadelphia: JB Lippincott, 1991, pp 355–416.

Rorabeck CH. Exertional tibialis posterior compartment syndrome in athletes. Clin Orthop 208:61–64, 1986.

Rorabeck CH, Bourne RB, Fowler PJ. The surgical treatment of exertional compartment syndromes in athletes. J Bone Joint Surg 65A:1245, 1983.

Rorabeck CH, Fowler PJ, Nitt L. The results of fasciotomy in the management of chronic exertional compartment syndrome. Am J Sports Med 16:224–227, 1986.

Stress/Fatigue Fractures

Anderson EG. Fatigue fractures of the foot. Injury 21(5):275–279, 1990.

Cook S, Kester M, Brunet M. Shock absorption characteristics of running shoes. Am J Sports Med 13:248–253, 1985.

Eisele SA, Sammarco GJ. Fatigue fractures of the foot and ankle in the athlete. Instr Course Lect 42:175–183, 1993.

Fitch KD, Blackwell JB, Gilmour WN. Operation for non-union of stress fracture of the tarsal navicular. J Bone Joint Surg 71B:105–110, 1989.

Green NE, Rogers RA, Lipscomb AB. Nonunions of stress fractures of the tibia. Am J Sports Med 13:171–176, 1985.

Kadel NJ, Teitz CC, Kronmal RA. Stress fractures in ballet dancers. Am J Sports Med 20:445–449, 1992.

Khan KM, Fuller PJ, Brukner PD, et al. Outcome of conservative and surgical management of navicular stress fracture in athletes. Eight-six cases proven with computerized tomography. Am J Sports Med 20:657–661, 1992.

McBryde AM. Stress fractures in runners. Clin Sports Med 4:737–752, 1985.

Milgrom C, Finestone A, Shlamkovitch N, et al. Prevention of overuse injuries of the foot by improved shoe shock attenuation. A randomized prospective study. Clin Orthop 281:189–192, 1992.

Rettig AC, Shelbourne KD, McCarroll JR, et al. The natural history and treatment of delayed union stress fractures of the anterior cortex of the tibia. Am J Sports Med 16:250–255, 1988.

Shiraishi M, Mizuta H, Kubota K, et al. Stress fracture of the proximal phalanx of the great toe. Foot Ankle 14:28–34, 1993.

Sproul J, Klaaren H, Mannarino F. Surgical treatment of Freiberg's infraction in athletes. Am J Sports Med 21:381–384, 1993.

Tendon Injuries

Aracil J, Pina A, Lozano JA, et al. Percutaneous suture of Achilles tendon ruptures. Foot Ankle 13:350–351, 1992.

Arrowsmith SR, Flemming LL, Allman FL. Traumatic dislocations of the peroneal tendons. Am J Sports Med 11:142, 1983.

Bassett FH, Speer KP. Longitudinal rupture of the peroneal tendons. Am J Sports Med 21:354–357, 1993.

Biedert R. Dislocation of the tibialis posterior tendon. Am J Sports Med 20:775–776, 1992.

Bradley JP, Tibone JE. Percutaneous and open surgical repairs of Achilles tendon ruptures. A comparative study. Am J Sports Med 18:188–195, 1990.

Brage ME, Hansen ST. Traumatic subluxation/dislocation of the peroneal tendons. Foot Ankle 13:423–430, 1992.

Clanton TO, Schon LC. Athletic injuries to the soft tissues of the foot and ankle. In Mann RA, Coughlin MJ (eds). *Surgery of the Foot and Ankle*. 2nd ed. St Louis: Mosby–Year Book, 1993, pp 1095–1224.

Copeland SA. Rupture of the Achilles tendon: a new clinical test. Ann R Coll Surg 72:270–271, 1990.

Frosmon A. Tennis leg. JAMA 209:415–416, 1969.

Hardaker WT Jr. Foot and ankle injuries in classical ballet dancers. Orthop Clin North Am 20:621–627, 1989.
Kalebo P, Allenmark C, Peterson L, Sward L. Diagnostic value of ultrasonography in partial ruptures of the Achilles tendon. Am J Sports Med 20:378–380, 1992.
Leach RE, Schepsis AA, Takai H. Long term results of surgical management of Achilles tendinitis in runners. Clin Orthop 282:208–212, 1992.
Leitner A, Voigt CH, Rahmanzadeh R. Treatment of extensive aseptic defects in old Achilles tendon ruptures: methods and case reports. Foot Ankle 13:176–180, 1992.
Lutter LD. Hindfoot problems. Instruct Course Lect 42:195–200, 1993.
Ma GWC, Griffith TG. Percutaneous repair of acute closed ruptured Achilles tendon: A new technique. Clin Orthop 128:247–255, 1977.
Mann RA, Holmes GB, Seale KS, Collins DN. Chronic rupture of the Achilles tendon: a new technique of repair. J Bone Joint Surg 73A:214–219, 1991.
Marti R. Dislocation of the peroneal tendons. Am J Sports Med 5:19–22, 1977.
Millar AP. Strains of the posterior calf musculature ("tennis leg"). Am J Sports Med 7:172–174, 1979.
Ouzounian TJ, Myerson MS. Dislocation of the posterior tibial tendon. Foot Ankle 13:215–219, 1992.
Rask MR, Steinberg LH. The pathognostic sign of tendoperoneal subluxation; report of a case treated conservatively. Orthop Rev 8:65–68, 1979.
Renstrom PAFH. Mechanism, diagnosis, and treatment of running injuries. Instr Course Lect 42:225–234, 1993.
Rimoldi RL, Oberlander MA, Waldrop JI, Hunter SC. Acute rupture of the tibialis anterior tendon: a case report. Foot Ankle 12(3):176–177, 1991.
Sobel M, Bohne WHO, Markisz JA. Longitudinal attrition of the peroneus brevis tendon in the fibular groove; an anatomic study. Foot Ankle 11:124–128, 1990.
Sobel M, Geppert MJ, Olson EJ, et al. The dynamics of peroneus brevis tendon splits: a proposed mechanism, technique of diagnosis, and classification of injury. Foot Ankle 13:413–421, 1992.
Thompson FM, Patterson AH. Rupture of the peroneus longus tendon. Report of three cases. J Bone Joint Surg 71:293–295, 1989.
Weinstabl R, Stiskal M, Neuhold A, et al. Classifying calcaneal tendon injury according to MRI findings. J Bone Joint Surg 73B:683–685, 1991.
Williams JGP. Achilles tendon lesions in sport. Sports Med 3:114–135, 1986.
Woods L, Leach RE. Posterior tibial tendon rupture in athletic people. Am J Sports Med 19:495–498, 1991.

Nerve Entrapment Syndromes

Baxter DE. Functional nerve disorders in the athlete's foot, ankle, and leg. Instr Course Lect 42:185–194, 1993.
Baxter DE, Pfeffer GB. Treatment of chronic heel pain by surgical release of the first branch of the lateral plantar nerve. Clin Orthop 279:229–236, 1992.
Baxter DE, Pfeffer GB, Thigpen M. Chronic heel pain treatment rationale. Orthop Clin North Am 20:563–570, 1989.
Borges LF, Hallett HM, Selkoe DJ, et al. The anterior tarsal tunnel syndrome: report of two cases. J Neurosurg 54:89–92, 1981.
Jordan BD, Tsairis P, Warren RF. Sports Neurology. Rockville, MD: Aspen Press, 1989.
Styf J. Entrapment of the superficial peroneal nerve: diagnosis and results of decompression. J Bone Joint Surg 71B:131–135, 1989.

Plantar Fascitis

Daly PJ, Kitaoka HB, Chao EYS. Plantar fasciotomy for intractable plantar fasciitis: clinical results and biomechanical evaluation. Foot Ankle 13:188–196, 1992.
Kwong PK, Kay D, Voner RT, White MW. Plantar fascitis: mechanics and pathomechanics of treatment. Clin Sports Med 7:119–126, 1988.

Os Trigonum

Marotta JJ, Micheli LJ. Os trigonum impingement in dancers. Am J Sports Med 20:533–536, 1992.

Ankle Instability

Barrett JR, Tanji JL, Drake C, et al. High- versus low-top shoes for the prevention of ankle sprains in basketball players. A prospective randomized study. Am J Sports Med 21:582–585, 1993.
Colville MR, Marder RA, Boyle JJ, Zarins B. Strain measurement in lateral ankle ligaments. Am J Sports Med 18:196–200, 1990.
Hamilton WG, Thompson FM, Snow SW. The modified Bröstrom procedure for lateral ankle instability. Foot Ankle 14:1–7, 1993.
Hopkinson WJ, St Pierre P, Ryan JB, Wheeler JH. Syndesmosis sprains of the ankle. Foot Ankle 10:325–330, 1990.
Karlsson J, Andreasson GO. The effect of external ankle support in chronic lateral ankle joint instability: an electromyographic study. Am J Sports Med 20:257–261, 1992.
Lofvenberg R, Karrholm J. The influence of an ankle orthosis on the talar and calcaneal motions in chronic lateral instability of the ankle. Am J Sports Med 21:224–227, 1993.
Milgrom C, Shlamkovitch N, Finestone A, et al. Risk factors for lateral ankle sprain: a prospective study among military recruits. Foot Ankle 12:26–29, 1992.
Myasa M, Amir H, Porath A, Dekel S. Radiological assessment of a modified anterior drawer test of the ankle. Foot Ankle 13:400–403, 1992.
Raatikainen T, Putkonen M, Puranen J. Arthrography, clinical examination, and stress radiograph in the diagnosis of acute injury to the lateral ligaments of the ankle. Am J Sports Med 20:2–6, 1992.
Rasmussen O. Stability of the ankle joint; analysis of the function and traumatology of the ankle ligaments. Acta Orthop Scand Suppl 211:1–75, 1985.
Sjolin SU, Dons-Jensen J, Simonser O. Reinforced anatomical reconstruction of the anterior talofibular ligament in chronic anterolateral instability using a periosteal flap. Foot Ankle 12:15–18, 1991.

Sobel M, Geppert MJ. Repair of concomitant lateral ankle ligament instability and peroneus brevis splits through a posteriorly modified Bröstrom Gould. Foot Ankle 13:224–225, 1992.

Stephens MM, Sammarco GJ. The stabilizing role of the lateral ligament complex around the ankle and subtalar joints. Foot Ankle 12:130–134, 1992.

Wilkerson LA. Ankle injuries in athletes. Primary Care 19:377–392, 1992.

Ankle Arthroscopy

Angermann P, Jensen P. Osteochondritis dissecans of the talus: long term results of surgical treatment. Foot Ankle 10:161–163, 1989.

Bassett FH, Billys JB, Gates HS. A simple surgical approach to the posteromedial ankle. Am J Sports Med 21:144–146, 1993.

Bassett FH, Gates HS, Billys JB, et al. Talar impingement by the anteroinferior tibiofibular ligament. J Bone Joint Surg 72A:55–59, 1990.

Feder KS, Schonholtz GJ. Ankle arthroscopy: review and long-term results. Foot Ankle 13:382–385, 1992.

Ferkel RD, Scranton PE. Current concepts review. Arthroscopy of the ankle and foot. J Bone Joint Surg 75A:1233–1243, 1993.

Guhl J. *Ankle Arthroscopy. Pathology and Surgical Techniques.* Thorofare, NJ: Slack, 1988, pp 49–117.

Loomer R, Fisher C, Lloyd-Smith R, et al. Osteochondral lesions of the talus. Am J Sports Med 21:13–19, 1993.

McCarroll JR, Schrader JW, Shelbourne KD, et al. Meniscoid lesions of the ankle in soccer players. Am J Sports Med 15:257, 1987.

Meislin RJ, Rose DJ, Parisien S, Springer S. Arthroscopic treatment of synovial impingement of the ankle. Am J Sports Med 21:186–189, 1993.

Ogilvie-Harris DJ, Lieverman I, Fitsalos D. Arthroscopically assisted arthrodesis for osteoarthritic ankles. J Bone Joint Surg 75A:1167–1174, 1993.

Scranton PE, McDermott JE. Anterior tibiotalar spurs: a comparison of open versus arthroscopic debridement. Foot Ankle 13:125–129, 1992.

Taga I, Shino K, Inoue M, et al. Articular cartilage lesions in ankles with lateral ligament injury: an arthroscopic study. Am J Sports Med 21:120–124, 1993.

Thein R, Eichenblat M. Arthroscopic treatment of sports-related synovitis of the ankle. Am J Sports Med 20:496–499, 1992.

Ankle and Foot Fractures

Bostman OM. Osteolytic changes accompanying degradation of absorbable fracture fixation implants. J Bone Joint Surg 73B:679–682, 1991.

Bostman OM. Intense granulomatous inflammatory lesions associated with absorbable internal fixation devices made of polyglycolide in ankle fractures. Clin Orthop 278:193–199, 1992.

Boytim MJ, Fischer DA, Neumann L. Syndesmotic ankle sprains. Am J Sports Med 19:294–298, 1991.

Chandler RW. Management of complex ankle fractures in athletes. Clin Sports Med 7:127–141, 1988.

Cimino W, Ichtertz D, Slabaugh P. Early mobilization of ankle fractures after open reduction and internal fixation. Clin Orthop 267:152–156, 1991.

Curtis MJ, Myerson M, Scura B. Tarsometatarsal joint injuries in the athlete. Am J Sports Med 21:497–502, 1992.

Edwards GS Jr, DeLee JC. Ankle diastasis without fracture. Foot Ankle 4:305–312, 1984.

Finsen V, Saetermo R, Kibsgaard L, et al. Early postoperative weight-bearing in patients who have a fracture of the ankle. J Bone Joint Surg 71A:23–27, 1991.

Frokjaer J, Moller BN. Biodegradable fixation of ankle fractures: complications in a prospective study of 25 cases. Acta Orthop Scand 63:434–436, 1992.

Ryd L, Bengtsson S. Isolated fracture of the lateral malleolus requires no treatment. Acta Orthop Scand 63:443–446, 1992.

Watson JAS, Hollingdale JP. Early management of displaced ankle fractures. Injury 23:87–88, 1992.

Winkler B, Weber BG, Simpson LA. The dorsal antiglide plate in the treatment of Danis-Weber type B fractures of the distal fibula. Clin Orthop 259:204–209, 1990.

Wissing JC, Van Laarhoven CJHM, Van Der Werken C. The posterior antiglide plate for fixation of fractures of the lateral malleolus. Injury 23:94–96, 1992.

Great Toe Injuries

Rodeo SA, O'Brien S, Warren RF, et al. Turf toe: an analysis of metatarsal phalangeal joint pain in professional football players. Am J Sports Med 18:280–285, 1990.

Sammarco GJ. Turf toe. Instr Course Lect 42:207–212, 1993.

CHAPTER 3

Thigh, Hip, and Pelvis

I. Introduction
  A. Overview—Although injuries above the knee are not particularly common in sports medicine, certain problems and disorders bear special emphasis.
  B. Relevant Anatomy—The hip is constrained by the bony anatomy much more than are the other joints of the lower extremity. The acetabulum is relatively deep, and the labrum provides additional stability to its contour. The hip capsule (including the iliofemoral ligament anteriorly and the ischiofemoral ligament posteriorly) is more stout anteriorly and further restrains the hip joint. In addition to the hip joint, the sacroiliac joint and symphysis pubis, both supported by stout ligamentous structures, make up the pelvis. Several muscles cross the hip joint, providing additional stability to the hip and pelvis (Fig. 3–1). The femur is the largest bone in the body. The femoral neck is angled approximately 130° from the shaft and is anteverted 14°. The femur flares distally at the metaphysis to form the condyles of the knee. Nerves that supply the lower extremity are roots of the lumbosacral plexus and include the sciatic nerve (tibial and peroneal portions), femoral nerve (supplies the anterior thigh muscles), obturator nerve (supplies the adductor muscles), and various smaller branches.
  C. Nerve Entrapment Syndromes—Lower extremity nerve entrapment above the knee is distinctly unusual, but an understanding of the course of the nerves and vessels can be helpful (Fig. 3–2). The ilioinguinal nerve can be entrapped by hypertrophied abdominal muscles as a result of intensive training. Hyperextension of the hip may exacerbate the pain, and patients commonly have hyperesthesia. Surgical treatment may occasionally be necessary. Obturator nerve entrapment may occur and should be considered in the differential diagnosis of chronic medial thigh pain in an athlete. This is especially true in athletes with well-developed hip adductor muscles (e.g., in skaters). Electromyographic studies can confirm the diagnosis. The genitofemoral nerve can also be entrapped, causing similar symptoms. Entrapment of the lateral femoral cutaneous nerve of the thigh can lead to a painful condition termed *meralgia paresthetica*. Tight belts, pads, or long periods of hip flexion can result in this condition. Release of compressive devices, posture exercises, and anti-inflammatory medications are often helpful, but surgical release may occasionally be necessary.

II. Contusions
  A. Iliac Crest Contusion—Direct trauma to the iliac crest, known as a "hip pointer" in football, can cause pain and loss of motion. These injuries are usually a result of a fall directly onto the pelvis or a collision with a direct blow to this area. These injuries can occasionally result in periostitis or exostosis formation. In adolescent athletes, radiographs should be carefully reviewed to rule out avulsion of the iliac apophysis. Treatment of these injuries and all contusions begins with early efforts to control swelling with ice, compression, pain control, and positioning of the extremity to put the affected muscles on maximum stretch. The recovery phase of treatment should emphasize motion, strengthening, mobilization, maintenance of strength, and then avoidance of recurrent injury. An injection of a long-acting local anesthetic with or without steroid may occasionally be efficacious. Additional padding is helpful to prevent recurrence in football players.
  B. Groin Contusions—Groin contusions can have serious consequences, including traumatic phlebitis, phlebothrombosis, and femoral neuropathy. Fortunately, one of the most common groin injuries, iliopsoas strain, is less serious. Radiographs should be obtained and carefully reviewed to rule out an avulsion of the lesser trochanter. Treatment includes activity modification, physical therapy including modalities (e.g., ultrasound), and gradual return to athletic participation.
  C. Quadriceps Contusions—These injuries are common in contact sports and are usually caused by a direct blow to the thigh. Injury to the muscle can cause hemorrhage, muscle fiber disruption, and late myositis ossificans. Classi-

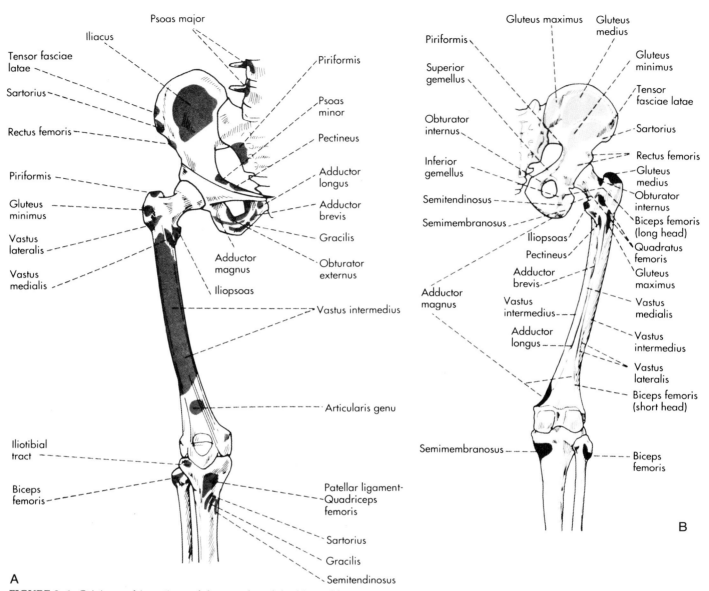

FIGURE 3–1. Origins and insertions of the muscles of the hip and leg. *A*, Anterior. *B*, Posterior. (From Jenkins DB. *Hollinshead's Functional Anatomy of the Limbs and Back*. 6th ed. Philadelphia: WB Saunders, 1991, Figs. 16–7 and 17–3.)

fication is based on the severity of the injury (Jackson and Feagin):

Class	Symptoms	Knee Flexion	Gait Alterations
Mild	Localized tenderness	>90°	None
Moderate	Tenderness, swelling	45–90°	Antalgic gait
Severe	Pain, with or without knee effusion	<45°	Severe limp

Acute treatment includes cold compression and rest (*in flexion*). Thigh girth is measured and monitored serially. Passive motion is initiated once swelling has stabilized. Crutches are used until at least 90° of flexion is regained and the patient has good quadriceps control and can walk without a limp. After the acute period has passed, quadriceps rehabilitation should be started and the thigh protected. The incidence of late myositis ossificans is related to the severity of the trauma. Surgical treatment of this condition is usually not necessary; however, if indicated, it should be delayed until the lesion has matured to prevent exacerbation of the condition. Patients with quadriceps contusions should be closely monitored in the acute period to ensure that they do not develop thigh compartment syndrome, although such a sequela is unusual. One study reported eight cases of compartment syndrome associated with anterior thigh contusions. These patients have severe pain at rest that does not respond

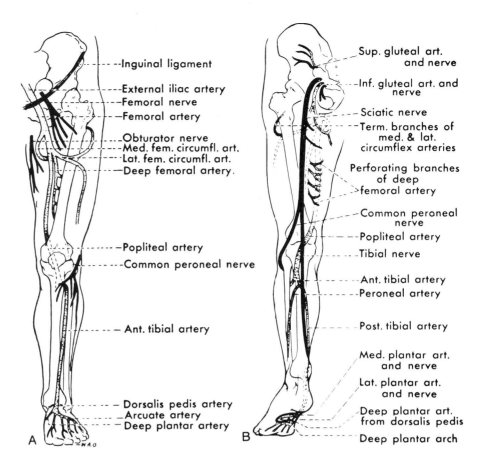

FIGURE 3–2. Nerves and vessels of the lower extremity. *A*, Anterior view. *B*, Posterior view. (From Jenkins DB. *Hollinshead's Functional Anatomy of the Limbs and Back.* 6th ed. Philadelphia: WB Saunders, 1991, p 221.)

to narcotic analgesia. Compartment pressures should be monitored if there is any question. All patients in the foregoing study had elevated compartment pressures, and most had both edema and hematoma in the rectus femoris or vastus intermedius muscles on exploration.

III. Muscle Strains
  A. Hamstring Strain—The hamstring is one of the most commonly injured muscles. The mechanism of injury is usually sudden, forced change in the musculotendinous length, usually during active sprinting with hip flexion and knee extension. Because of the variable locations of the musculotendinous junctions of the hamstring muscles (Fig. 3–3), strains can occur anywhere in the posterior thigh. Symptoms are proportional to the severity of the injury and include muscle spasm, variable loss of knee extension, and swelling. In severe injuries, a defect may be palpable before onset of hematoma. Treatment includes ice, elevation, and compression. Stretching and isometric exercises are initiated after subsidence of swelling, with a gradual return to isotonic and isokinetic exercise and resumption of activities after full range of motion and 90% strength are restored. Hamstring heating and stretching

before sports participation and limitation of hyperextension can help prevent injury recurrence. Reinjury after a hamstring strain is generally more severe and has a longer recovery time. Therefore, good judgment is necessary in determining when an athlete should return to play.
  B. Adductor Strain—This injury is common in soccer players and is very common in Europe. The adductor longus is most often injured in most sports. The mechanism of injury can be either powerful abduction stress during leg adduction or overuse. Acutely, localized tenderness is usual. In chronic cases, pain may be elicited with resisted leg adduction. Most injuries respond to conservative management. Rest, anti-inflammatory medication, and monitored exercises are initiated. Several procedures have been described for chronic groin injuries, including adductor release, rectus tightening, and other procedures popularized in Europe. Because of the proximity of the adductor muscle origin to the abdominal wall structures (Fig. 3–4), diagnosis is sometimes difficult. Chronic strains of the abdominal muscles' insertion into the pubis have been reported in soccer and hockey players. These generally require surgical treatment. The Basini repair has been proposed for rectus abdo-

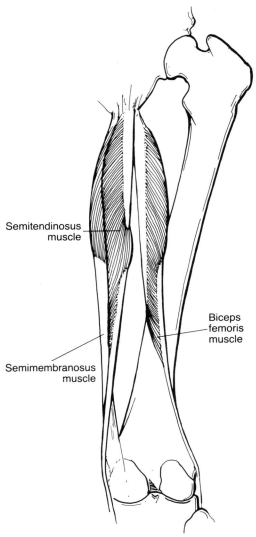

FIGURE 3–3. Variable locations of the musculotendinous junctions of the hamstring muscles. (From DeLee JC, Drez D. *Orthopaedic Sports Medicine: Principles and Practice.* Philadelphia: WB Saunders, 1994, p 1091.)

minis injuries. This is sometimes combined with an adductor release. Inguinal and femoral hernias can cause hip pain and mimic the pain associated with contusions and muscle strains. In subtle cases, herniography can be helpful in making the diagnosis. Herniorrhaphy is usually successful, with return to athletics in 6 to 8 weeks.

C. Rectus Femoris Strain—The rectus femoris is commonly susceptible to disruptions. Injuries are usually located more distally on the thigh. Chronic injuries are often near the origin above the hip. Pain is exacerbated by resisted hip flexion or knee extension. Conservative management is usually successful. For rectus and other muscle strains, magnetic resonance imaging can sometimes be a useful adjunct if the diagnosis of a soft tissue injury is in doubt.

D. Avulsion Fractures—Avulsion fractures around the pelvis and hip are relatively common, particularly in immature athletes. These injuries result from excessive strain at the apophyseal origin/insertion of the affected muscle (Fig. 3–5A). Avulsion fractures of the lesser trochanter can occur as a result of hip hyperextension (Fig. 3–5B). Avulsion fractures of the ischial tuberosity can also occur with forced contraction or overstretching of the hamstring muscles, such as in jumping hurdles. Avulsion of the anterior inferior iliac spine due to powerful quadriceps contraction with subsequent pain has been reported in soccer players. Most of these injuries occurred in players in their midteens. Treatment is nonoperative, and the prognosis is excellent. Similar avulsion injuries in adults may require surgical intervention.

IV. Bursitis
   A. Introduction—Bursitis can be disabling in an athlete. Bursitis most commonly involves the trochanteric bursa, but the ischial bursa and iliopectineal bursa can also be involved (Fig. 3–6).
   B. Greater Trochanteric Bursitis—This condition can cause localized tenderness and pain with external rotation and adduction. Running on

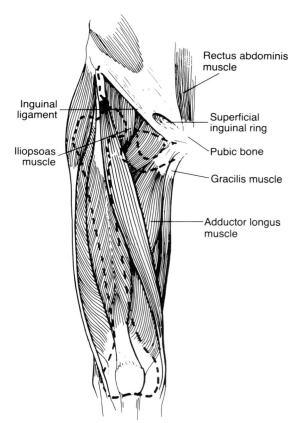

FIGURE 3–4. Adductor muscle origin is immediately adjacent to the abdominal wall structures. (From DeLee JC, Drez D. *Orthopaedic Sports Medicine: Principles and Practice.* Philadelphia: WB Saunders, 1994, p 1103.)

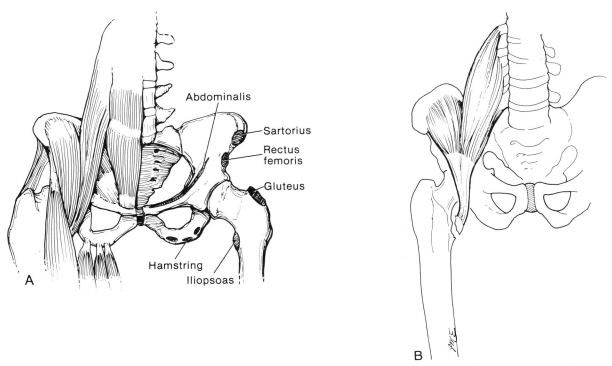

FIGURE 3–5. *A*, Muscular origins and insertions of the pelvis associated with avulsion fractures of the apophysis in adolescents from lesser trochanteric avulsion. (From DeLee JC, Drez D. *Orthopaedic Sports Medicine: Principles and Practice.* Philadelphia: WB Saunders, 1994, p 1069.) *B*, Avulsion of the lesser trochanter by the iliopsoas.

banked surfaces can exacerbate trochanteric bursitis. *Snapping iliotibial band syndrome* can also be related to this problem. In this condition, the tensor fascia lata slides over the trochanter, causing an uncomfortable snap. The condition occurs more commonly in female athletes with a wide pelvis and prominent tro-

chanter. Examination reveals that, with the knee extended and the hip adducted, flexion of the hip produces a snap. Conservative management includes stretching and strengthening, as well as local modalities or injections. It is occasionally necessary to divide the iliotibial band to relieve the symptoms (Fig. 3–7).

FIGURE 3–6. Location of pelvic bursae. (Modified from DeLee JC, Drez D. *Orthopaedic Sports Medicine: Principles and Practice.* Philadelphia: WB Saunders, 1994, p 1067.)

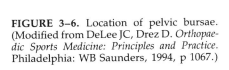

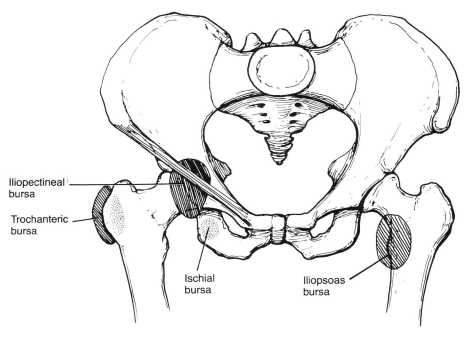

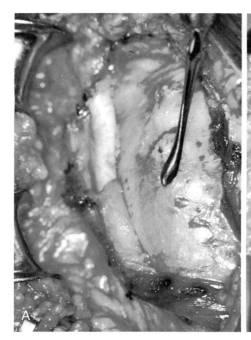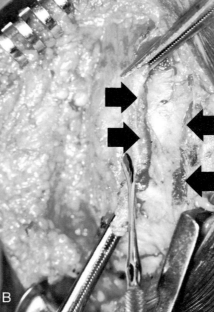

FIGURE 3–7. Operative case demonstrating technique of proximal iliotibial band release in a case of snapping iliotibial band. *A,* Before and *B,* after iliotibial band release. *Arrows* demonstrate the edge of the released iliotibial band. Z lengthening of the iliotibial band has also been described.

C. Iliopsoas Bursitis—This is another cause of anterior hip pain in athletes. It may occasionally improve with fluoroscopically guided corticosteroid injection with bursography to confirm the location. The snapping iliopsoas tendon is a less common cause of the snapping hip and should be distinguished from a snapping iliotibial band (located over the greater trochanter). Surgical lengthening of the iliopsoas tendon has been reported to be successful in treating this disorder if conservative treatment fails.

D. Ischial Bursitis—Ischial bursitis can be caused by direct trauma or by prolonged sitting. Conservative treatment is usually successful.

E. Iliopectineal Bursitis—This condition can cause disabling pain of the anterior hip and an antalgic gait. Patients attempt to flex and externally rotate the hip to relieve the pain. Conservative management is usually successful.

V. Stress Fractures

A. Introduction—Although stress fractures of the lower extremity are more common below the knee, several important fractures can occur more proximally. A history of overuse with an insidious onset is common. Physical examination may demonstrate localized pain and swelling. As with all stress fractures, a bone scan can be diagnostic even if radiographs show no abnormality. Basic treatment includes rest, activity modification including avoidance of impact, cross training, analgesics, and therapeutic modalities. Female athletes with amenorrhea and stress fractures should receive a

full endocrine evaluation and appropriate hormone therapy.

B. Femoral Neck Stress Fractures—The classification of these injuries includes tension or transverse (distraction) fractures and compression fractures. Tension or transverse fractures are more serious and may require internal fixation. However, this distinction is not always clear, and the presence of inferior neck sclerosis does not preclude the possibility of completion of the fracture to the superior aspect of the neck. Clinical findings in femoral neck stress fractures include groin pain, limp, and painful range of motion. Most fractures can be treated by abstinence from bearing weight.

C. Femoral Shaft Stress Fractures—These are described on the basis of their anatomic location. Again, bone scans can be very helpful in diagnosis (Fig. 3–8). Patients may complain of deep thigh pain, similar to a quadriceps contusion. Treatment includes crutches for 4 to 8 weeks. Complications include completion of the fracture or an undiagnosed fracture at another location.

D. Osteitis Pubis—Although this may not be a stress fracture in the true sense of the word, it is often a result of overuse. It is commonly encountered in soccer players, hockey players, and runners. Radiographic findings, which are the hallmark of the disease, include resorption of the medial pubic bones and a widened or unstable symphysis pubis. Patients may complain of gradual onset of localized pain, antalgic gait, and occasionally adductor spasm. Treatment includes rest and anti-inflammatory drugs. Moist heat and other modalities can be

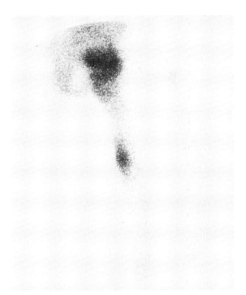

FIGURE 3–8. Technetium bone scan of a midshaft femur stress fracture.

helpful. Three months is usually required for complete resolution.

VI. Injuries to the Hip
    A. Osteonecrosis of the Hip—Traumatic hip injuries can result in serious late sequelae. Traumatic subluxation of the hip can interrupt or damage the arterial supply to the femoral head and has been reported to have led to osteonecrosis in two professional football players. Early recognition of these injuries is critical.

    B. Osteoarthritis of the Hip—Although this condition is not common in younger athletes, one study demonstrated a 4.5-fold increase in hip arthritis in patients with extensive participation in sports. Sports presenting the most risk included track and field sports and racket sports. Men with both high occupational and sports exposure had a relative risk that was 8.5 times normal. Impact loading activities are obviously not appropriate for total hip replacement recipients. One study noted a higher rate of aseptic loosening in patients who participate in high-impact activities.

    C. Fractures of the Hip—Although hip fractures are more common in the elderly, they can occur in athletes. Cross-country skiing has been implicated in several cases of proximal femoral fractures ("skier's hip"). Release bindings have been suggested to reduce the incidence of these injuries.

VII. Hip Arthroscopy
    A. Overview—Hip arthroscopy is relatively new, and indications are somewhat limited. The most common indications for hip arthroscopy include removal of loose bodies or foreign bodies and synovectomy. Other relative indications include unresolved pain, articular cartilage lesions, and soft tissue injuries (e.g., torn labrum, impingement of the ligamentum teres).

    B. Arthroscopic Setup—Most surgeons advocate performance of the procedure with a patient in the lateral decubitus position with the involved hip on top. Approximately 50 pounds (20–25 kg) of traction is necessary to distract the hip. A fracture table with a well-padded pero-

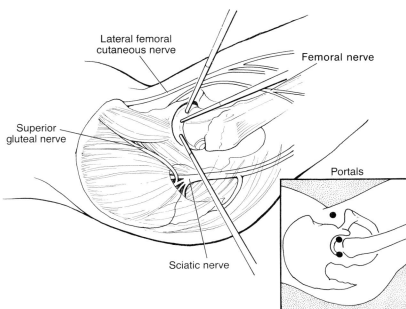

FIGURE 3–9. Portals for hip arthroscopy include the anterior portal and two portals adjacent to the greater trochanter.

neal post is usually recommended. Image intensification is helpful to verify that adequate distraction has been obtained (at least 8 mm is usually necessary) and to help guide instruments into the joint. Longer instruments and telescoping cannulas are often helpful as well.

C. Portals—The three portals that are most commonly used include the direct anterior portal and the anterior and posterior edges of the greater trochanter (Fig. 3–9). The portal at the anterior edge of the greater trochanter is established first with a spinal needle. Injection of 10 to 15 mL of air breaks the suction in the joint, allowing additional distraction. The joint

can then be aspirated, and saline can be injected into the joint. The other portals are then selected by placing spinal needles and allowing fluid to egress before making a skin incision. The cannulas are inserted by progressive dilation.

D. Complications—Most of the complications reported for hip arthroscopy include nerve traction palsies and articular cartilage scuffing. Neurapraxias are usually temporary and can be reduced with careful padding and special hip distractors. Adequate care should be taken in and around the joint to avoid articular cartilage injury. Neurovascular injury can be avoided with careful portal placement.

Selected References

Introduction

Renstrom PAHF. Tendon and muscle injuries in the groin area. Clin Sports Med 11:815–831, 1992.

Contusions

Campbell JD. Injuries of the pelvis, hip and thigh. Clin Sports Med 10(2):305–312, 1991.
Colosimo AJ, Ireland, ML. Thigh compartment syndrome in a football athlete: a case report and review of the literature. Med Sci Sports Exerc 24:958–963, 1992.
Ekberg O, Blomquist P, Olsson S. Positive contrast herniography in adult patients with obscure groin pain. Surgery 89:532–535, 1981.
Jackson DW, Feagin JA. Quadriceps contusions in young athletes. J Bone Joint Surg 55A:95–105, 1973.
Rooser B, Bengston S, Hagglund G. Acute compartment syndrome from anterior thigh muscle contusion: a report of eight cases. J Orthop Trauma 5:57–59, 1991.
Ryan JB, Wheeler JH, Hopkinson WJ, et al. Quadriceps contusions. West Point update. Am J Sports Med 19:299–304, 1991.
Smedberg SGG, Broome AEA, Gullmo A, et al. Herniography in athletes with groin pain. Am J Surg 140:378–382, 1985.

Muscle Strains

Akermark C, Johansson C. Tenotomy of the adductor longus tendon in the treatment of chronic groin pain in athletes. Am J Sports Med 20:640–643, 1992.
Burkett LN. Investigation into hamstring strains: the case of the hybrid muscle. J Sports Med 3:228, 1975.
Renstrom PAHF. Tendon and muscle injuries in the groin area. Clin Sports Med 11:815–831, 1992.
Speer KP, Lohnes J, Garrett WE. Radiographic imaging of muscle strain injury. Am J Sports Med 21:89–93, 1993.
Tegner Y, Heenriksson A, Lorentzon R, et al. Avulsion of the anterior-inferior iliac spine in young soccer players. Clin Sports Med 2:143–148, 1990.
Zarins B, Ciullo JV. Acute muscle and tendon injuries in athletes. Clin Sports Med 2:167, 1983.

Bursitis

Brignall CG, Stainsby GD. The snapping hip. Treatment by z-plasty. J Bone Joint Surg 73B:253–254, 1991.
Holmes JC, Pruitt AL, Whalen NJ. Iliotibial band syndrome in cyclists. Am J Sports Med 21:419–424, 1993.
Jacobs M, Young B. Snapping hip phenomenon among dancers. Am Correct Ther J 32:92, 1973.
Martens M, Libbrecht P, Burssens A. Surgical treatment of the iliotibial band friction syndrome. Am J Sports Med 17:651–654, 1989.
Renne JW. The iliotibial band friction syndrome. J Bone Joint Surg 57A:1110–1111, 1975.

Stress Fractures

Bargren JH, Tilson DH, Bridgeford OE. Prevention of displaced fatigue fractures of the femur. J Bone Joint Surg 53A:1115, 1971.
Blickenstaff LD, Morris JM. Fatigue fracture of the femoral neck. J Bone Joint Surg 48A:1031, 1966.
Cochrand JM. Osteitis pubis in athletes. Br J Sports Med 5:233, 1971.
Gilbert RS, Johnson HA. Stress fractures in military recruits: a review of twelve years' experience. Milit Med 131:716, 1966.
Hajek MR, Noble HB. Stress fractures of the femoral neck in joggers. Case reports and review of the literature. Am J Sports Med 10:112, 1982.
Janson PG, Angevine M, Juhl JH. Osteitis pubis in sports activities. Physician Sportsmed 6:111, 1978.
Lombardo SJ, Benson DW. Stress fractures of the femur in runners. Am J Sports Med 10:219, 1982.
McBryde AM. Stress fractures in athletes. J Sports Med 3:212, 1973.
Skinner HB, Cook SD. Fatigue failure stress of the femoral neck: a case report. Am J Sports Med 10:245, 1982.
Stanitski CL, McMaster JH, Scranton PE. On the nature of stress fractures. Am J Sports Med 6:391, 1978.

Injuries to the Hip

Cooper DE, Warren RF, Barnes R. Traumatic subluxation of the hip resulting in aseptic necrosis and condrolysis in a professional football player. Am J Sports Med 19:322–324, 1991.

Frost A, Bauer M. Skier's hip: a new clinical entity? Proximal femur fractures sustained in cross-country skiing. J Orthop Trauma 5:57–50, 1991.

Kilgus DJ, Dorey FJ, Finerman GAM, Amstutz HC. Patient activity, sports participation, and impact loading on the durability of cemented total hip replacements. Clin Orthop 269:25–31, 1991.

Stenger A. Bo's hip dislocates stellar athletic career. Physician Sportsmed 19:17–18, 1991.

Stewart WJ. Aseptic necrosis of the head of the femur following traumatic dislocation of the hip joint. Case report and experimental studies. J Bone Joint Surg 15:413–438, 1933.

Vingard E, Alfredsson L, Goldi I, Hogstedt C. Sports and osteoarthrosis of the hip. An epidemiological study. Am J Sports Med 21:195–200, 1993.

Hip Arthroscopy

Dorfmann H, Boyer T, Henry P, DeBie B. A simple approach to hip arthroscopy. Arthroscopy 4:141–142, 1988.

Eriksson E, Arvidsson I, Arvidsson H. Diagnostic and operative arthroscopy of the hip. Orthopedics 9:169–178, 1986.

Glick JM. Hip arthroscopy using the lateral approach. Instr Course Lect 37:223–231, 1988.

Glick JM, Sampson TG, Gordon RB, et al. Hip arthroscopy by the lateral approach. Arthroscopy 3:4–12, 1987.

Okada Y, Awaya G, Ikeda T, et al. Arthroscopic surgery for synovial chondromatosis of the hip. J Bone Joint Surg 71B:198–199, 1989.

II

Upper Extremity

CHAPTER 4

Shoulder

I. Basic Sciences
  A. Anatomy
    1. Osteology—The shoulder is composed of three separate bones: the clavicle, the scapula, and the humerus.
      a. Clavicle—The *clavicle* is S shaped and is attached to the scapula through the acromioclavicular (AC) joint and the coracoclavicular ligaments (conoid and trapezoid) (Fig. 4–1). The clavicle articulates with the manubrium of the sternum through the sternoclavicular (SC) joint. The AC ligaments prevent anterior-posterior instability of this joint, and the coracoclavicular ligaments prevent inferior displacement of the acromion from the distal clavicle. The intra-articular disc in the AC joint tends to be incomplete, compared with the intra-articular disc in the SC joint, which is more consistently a complete structure. The clavicle is the first bone in the body to ossify and the last to fuse.
      b. Scapula—The *scapula* articulates with the chest wall (posterior ribs two to seven) (Fig. 4–2) and is the site of 17 muscle insertions (Fig. 4–3). The scapula has two important prominences: the coracoid process and the acromion. The coracoid process is the origin for the conjoined tendon (short head of the biceps and coracobrachialis), the insertion point of the pectoralis minor tendon, and is an attachment for the coracoacromial, coracohumeral, and transverse scapular ligaments (Fig. 4–4). The acromion is a broad, flat expansion of the scapular spine that projects over the humeral head and is the origin for most of the deltoid muscle. The acromion articulates with the distal clavicle at the AC joint.
      c. Humeral Head—The *humeral head* is normally retroverted 30° relative to the transepicondylar axis of the distal humerus, and the articular surface is inclined superiorly 130° relative to the shaft (Fig. 4–5). The greater and lesser tuberosities, located on opposite sides of the bicipital groove (Fig. 4–6) are the attachment sites for the four tendons of the rotator cuff (the supraspinatus, infraspinatus, and teres minor insert into the greater tuberosity, and the subscapularis inserts into the lesser tuberosity). The long head of the biceps tendon is constrained in the bicipital groove by the transverse humeral ligament as well as by the attachment of the subscapularis to the lesser tuberosity.
      d. Glenoid—The *glenoid* is the lateral thickening of the scapula that articulates with the humeral head. Although its articular surface is closely matched to that of the humeral head, the size mismatch renders this articulation minimally constrained. This anatomic arrangement is discussed in further detail later.
    2. Arthrology—The glenohumeral joint is the principal articulation of the shoulder; however, normal shoulder motion also requires coordinated scapulothoracic translation.
      a. Glenohumeral Joint–Although technically classified as a spheroidal (ball-and-socket) joint, the *glenohumeral joint* has little inherent stability provided by articular surface conformity. Contrary to the previously held opinion that the inherent instability of the glenohumeral joint was due to a mismatch in the radius of curvature between the glenoid and humeral head, it is now recognized that these articular surfaces are relatively well matched, with less than 2 mm of deviation in the radius of curvature between the two. It is actually the size mismatch between the humeral head and glenoid that contributes to a relative lack of intrinsic stability. In any position of rotation, only one third of the humeral head is covered by the glenoid. Stability is largely provided by static and dynamic soft tissue structures including the labrum, capsule (glenohumeral ligaments), and rotator cuff.

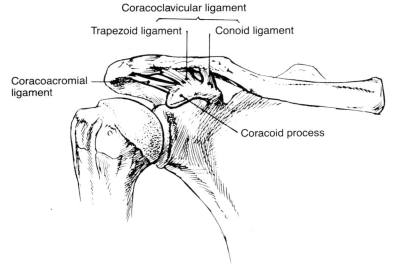

A

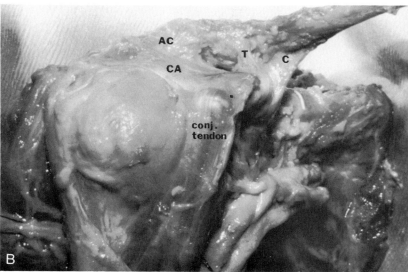

B

FIGURE 4–1. Anatomy of the acromioclavicular and coracoclavicular ligaments. *A*, Drawing demonstrating ligaments attached to the coracoid process. *B*, Dissection specimen showing the coracoclavicular ligament consisting of the conoid ligament (C) and trapezoid ligament (T). Also shown are the coracoacromial ligament (CA), acromioclavicular ligament/joint (AC), and conjoined (conj.) tendon.

(1) Glenohumeral Ligaments—The *glenohumeral ligaments* represent discrete thickenings in the capsule and serve as checkreins to abnormal motion (Fig. 4–7 and Color Figures 9 and 10). A significant variation in the size of these ligaments is noted among individuals. The glenohumeral ligaments limit excessive rotation and translation of the humeral head on the glenoid during arm motion. Additionally, complex interplay between these ligaments is dependent on arm position and direction of the applied force on the shoulder joint. Although the role of each ligament is controversial, the generally accepted function of each glenohumeral ligament is outlined below.

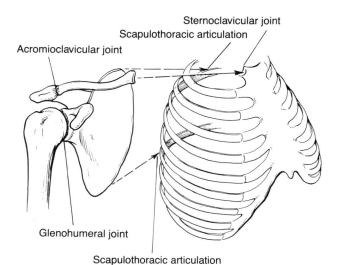

FIGURE 4–2. The shoulder girdle is attached to the thorax via the sternoclavicular and scapulothoracic articulations. (Reprinted with permission from Warner JJP, Caborn DN. Overview of shoulder instability. Crit Rev Phys Rehabil Med 4:145–198, 1992.)

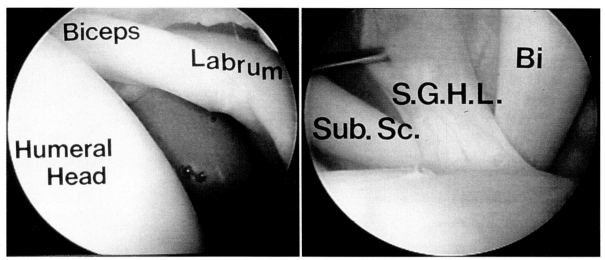

COLOR FIGURE 9. Arthroscopic views of the superior aspect of the glenohumeral joint. Note the normal relationship of the biceps tendon and labrum (*left*) and the position of the superior glenohumeral ligament (S.G.H.L.) between the biceps tendon (Bi) and the subscapularis tendon (Sub. Sc.) (*right*).

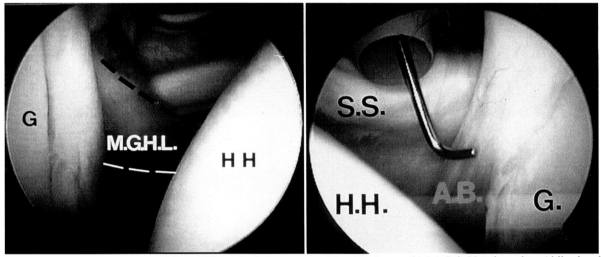

COLOR FIGURE 10. Arthroscopic views of the middle and inferior aspects of the glenohumeral joint. *Left,* Note how the middle glenohumeral ligament (M.G.H.L.) drapes over the subscapularis tendon (unlabeled) between the glenoid (G) and humeral head (HH). *Right,* The anterior band (A.B.) of the inferior glenohumeral ligament is intimately attached to the labrum, which in turn attaches to the glenoid (G.). The subscapularis (S.S.) and humeral head (H.H.) are also shown.

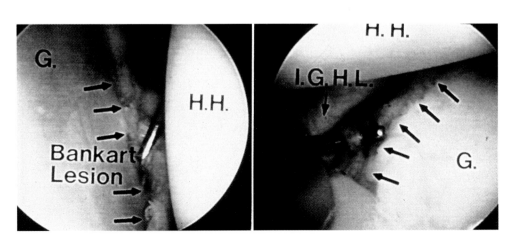

COLOR FIGURE 11. Bankart lesion (*arrows*) shown in relation to other structures. (G. = glenoid; H.H. = humeral head; I.G.H.L. = inferior glenohumeral ligament.)

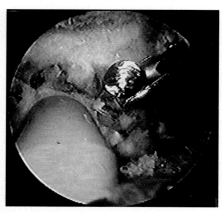

COLOR FIGURE 12. Arthroscopic acromioplasty requires adequate visualization and orientation. Note that a plastic cannula is located in the anterior portal.

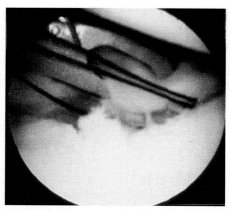

COLOR FIGURE 13. A suture punch is used to place sutures in the torn labrum for transglenoid techniques.

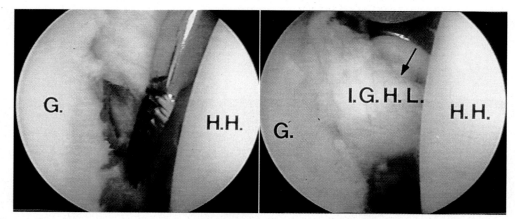

COLOR FIGURE 14. Arthroscopic Bankart repair using the Suretac device includes glenoid preparation (*left*) before inserting the tack through special cannulas (*right*). The first tack should be placed as inferiorly as possible after the torn labrum is lifted superiorly. Arrow indicates the direction of the tuck. (G. = glenoid; H.H. = humeral head; I.G.H.L. = inferior glenohumeral ligament.)

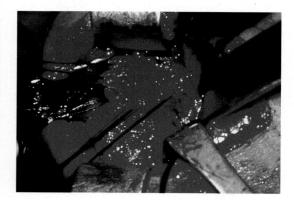

COLOR FIGURE 15. Open capsular shift.

COLOR FIGURE 16. Arthroscopically assisted rotator cuff repair as viewed arthroscopically (*left*) and from the exterior (*right*).

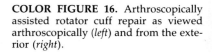
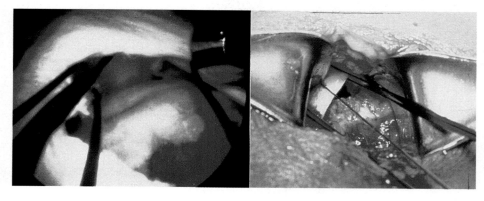

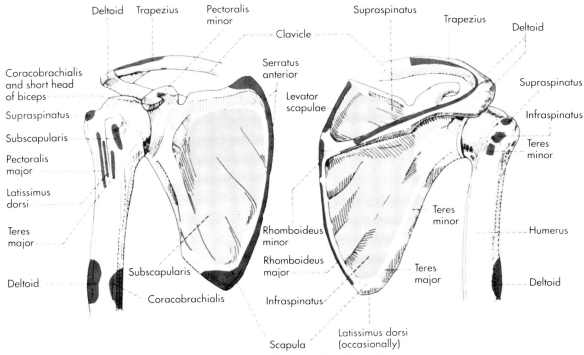

FIGURE 4–3. Origins and insertions of shoulder girdle muscles. (From Jenkins DB. *Hollinshead's Functional Anatomy of the Limbs and Back.* 6th ed. Philadelphia: WB Saunders, 1991, FIg. 5–3.)

Ligament	Function
Inferior glenohumeral ligament complex (IGHLC)	Primary stabilizer for anterior and inferior instability in abduction.
Middle glenohumeral ligament (MGHL)	Secondary stabilizer for inferior translation in adduction. May have a role in preventing anterior instability at 45° abduction.
Superior glenohumeral ligament (SGHL) and coracohumeral ligament (CHL)	Primary restraint to inferior translation in the adducted shoulder.

(a) Inferior Glenohumeral Ligament Complex (IGHLC)—This has traditionally been described as the major stabilizer of the glenohumeral joint. O'Brien and coworkers characterized this structure as a complex composed of two discrete bands (anterior and posterior) with an interposed axillary pouch. This arrangement simulates a hammock that supports the humeral head during abduction and rotation of the joint (Fig. 4–8). Through reciprocal tightening that occurs with both internal and external rotation, the IGHLC prevents inferior, anterior, and posterior instability in the abducted shoulder.

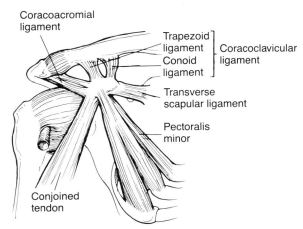

FIGURE 4–4. Attachments of muscles and ligaments to the coracoid process.

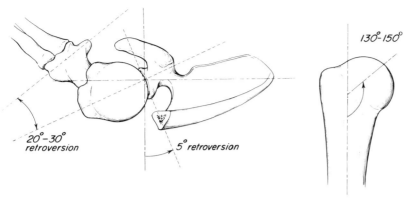

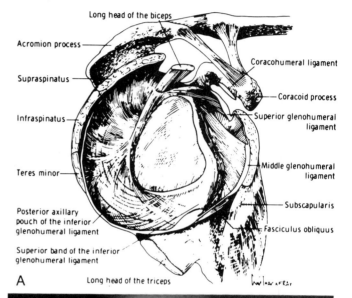

FIGURE 4–5. Normal articular orientations of the glenohumeral joint. (Reprinted with permission from Warner JJP, Caborn DN. Overview of shoulder instability. Crit Rev Phys Rehabil Med 4:145–198, 1992.)

(b) Middle Glenohumeral Ligament (MGHL)—This is present in approximately 80% of individuals and can be a discrete ligamentous band or a sheet-like thickening of the anterior capsule confluent with the IGHLC. It attaches slightly above and medial to the anterior band of the IGHLC on the glenoid (Fig. 4–7B and Color Figure 4–10). It has been shown to function principally to prevent anterior instability when the shoulder is abducted 45° and externally rotated.

(c) Superior Glenohumeral Ligament (SGHL)—This works in concert with the CHL to prevent inferior instability in the adducted arm. The SGHL courses from the supraglenoid tubercle into the rotator interval area and blends with the fibers of the CHL, which originates from the coracoid process. The two structures insert into the lesser tuberosity of the proximal humerus. Both structures have been described as constant and relatively well developed, being

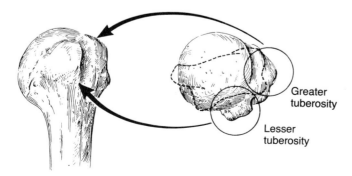

FIGURE 4–6. Relationship of greater and lesser tuberosities to the bicipital groove. (From Jobe CM. Gross anatomy of the shoulder. In Rockwood CA Jr, Matsen FA III [eds]. *The Shoulder*. Philadelphia: WB Saunders, 1990, p 47.)

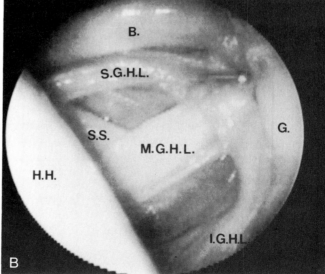

FIGURE 4–7. Glenohumeral ligaments. *A*, Anatomic identification. (From Turkel SJ, Panio MW, Marshall JL, Girgis FG. Stabilizing mechanisms preventing anterior dislocation of the gleno-humeral joint. J Bone Joint Surg 63A:1209, 1981.) *B*, Arthroscopic view. (B. = biceps; H.H. = humeral head; G. = glenoid; S.S. = subscapularis tendon; S.G.H.L. = superior gleno-humeral ligament; M.G.H.L. = middle glenohumeral ligament; I.G.H.L. = inferior glenohumeral ligament.)

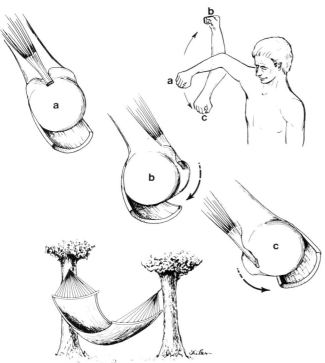

FIGURE 4–8. The inferior glenohumeral complex prevents anterior, posterior, and inferior dislocation by functioning like a hammock that supports the humeral head. With the arm in neutral, the ligament complex is relatively static (a). In external rotation (b) and internal rotation (c), the ligament complex rotates to the front and back of the shoulder, respectively, functioning as a checkrein against dislocation of the humeral head. (Reprinted with permission from Warner JJP, Caborn DN. Overview of shoulder instability. Crit Rev Phys Rehabil Med 4:145–198, 1992.)

(2) Glenoid Labrum—The *glenoid labrum* is a fibrocartilaginous thickening along the glenoid rim. Although its shape and attachment can vary significantly, the glenoid labrum has been shown to stabilize the humeral head in the glenoid via two mechanisms. First, it functionally deepens the glenoid cavity and provides a broader surface area for the humeral head (Fig. 4–9) and serves as a chock-block that prevents abnormal motion. Second, it serves as an anchoring point for the IGHLC along the glenoid rim.

b. Sternoclavicular Joint—The *sternoclavicular* (SC) *joint* is a gliding joint with a complete intra-articular disc. It rotates 30° during shoulder flexion. This joint has received little attention in the literature, although its importance as a connection of the shoulder girdle to the thoracic wall and its function in synergistic movement of the shoulder should not be overlooked. In general, the normal ratio of glenohumeral to scapulothoracic motion during shoulder abduction is approximately 2 : 1 although abnormal conditions such as rotator cuff pathology may alter this relationship.

c. Acromioclavicular Joint—The *acromioclavicular* (AC) *joint* has similar mor-

present in >90% of individuals. Biomechanical studies have suggested that the major stabilizing component of the two is the SGHL. Anatomic and histologic studies of the CHL support the belief that this ligament is unlikely to have a significant role as a suspensory structure in its physiologic state. In addition to their primary role in preventing inferior translation in adduction, the SGHL and CHL also have a secondary role in conjunction with the posterior capsule in preventing posterior instability of the flexed, adducted, and internally rotated shoulder.

(d) Posterior Capsule—The *posterior capsule* is that portion of the capsule that is superior to the posterior band of the IGHLC. It has been shown to be the thinnest portion of the shoulder capsule and is often blamed for the poor results associated with surgery for posterior instability.

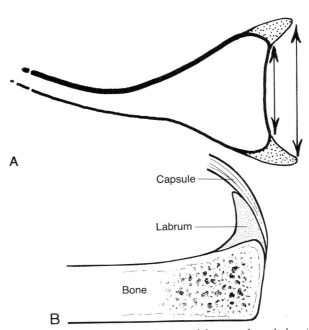

FIGURE 4–9. *A,* Superior (coronal) view of the scapula and glenoid. The glenoid labrum is a fibrocartilaginous extension of the edges of the glenoid that increases the surface area and depth of the glenoid fossa, thereby increasing stability of the joint. (Reprinted with permission from Warner JJP, Caborn DN. Overview of shoulder instability. Crit Rev Phys Rehabil Med 4:145–198, 1992.) *B,* Transverse section through the glenoid. Note that the capsule is intimately associated with the labrum.

phology to the SC joint but has an incomplete disc. This may be one of the reasons why degenerative changes affect this joint more frequently than they do the SC joint.

3. Surgical Approaches—Surgical approaches to the shoulder have been well described in several textbooks; however, a recent description of a layer concept has provided some additional insights into surgical anatomy of the shoulder (Fig. 4–10):

Layer	Components
I	Deltoid, pectoralis major
II	Clavipectoral fascia, conjoined tendon, pectoralis minor
III	Subdeltoid bursa, rotator cuff muscles
IV	Glenohumeral capsule, CHL

a. Anterior Approach—The *anterior approach* to the shoulder (Fig. 4–11) uses the interval between the deltoid (axillary nerve) and the pectoralis major (medial and lateral pectoral nerves). The subdeltoid interval is mobilized, and lateral retraction of the deltoid provides good exposure of the underlying structures. The conjoined tendon is identified at its attachment of the coracoid process, and the clavipectoral fascia is incised just lateral to the short head of the biceps muscle. The subscapularis tendon and muscle are exposed, and the anterior humeral circumflex vessels are identified along their inferior border and ligated. The subscapularis is dissected off the underlying capsule, into which its fibers blend laterally. Medially, a clear separation is noted between these two structures. Alternatively, the capsule can be exposed through a subscapularis muscle-splitting incision. A capsulotomy allows access to the glenohumeral joint.

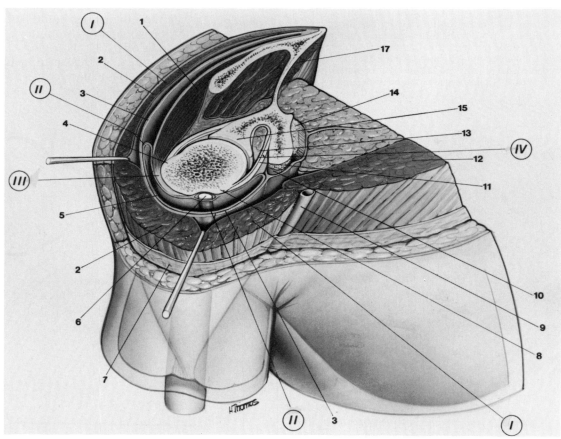

FIGURE 4–10. Cross-sectional view of the right shoulder at the level of the lesser tuberosity. Note the four layers of the shoulder:

Layer	Components
I	Deltoid (2), pectoralis major (12), fascia (7), cephalic vein (9).
II	Conjoined tendon (10), pectoralis minor (14).
III	Fascia (3), subdeltoid bursa (5), rotator cuff muscles (1, 17), suprascapular neurovascular bundle (not shown).
IV	Glenohumeral capsule (11), greater tuberosity (4), biceps long head (6), lesser tuberosity (8), synovium (13), glenoid (15).

(From Cooper DE, O'Brien SJ, Warren RF. Supporting layers of the glenohumeral joint: an anatomic study. Clin Orthop 289:144–155, 1993.)

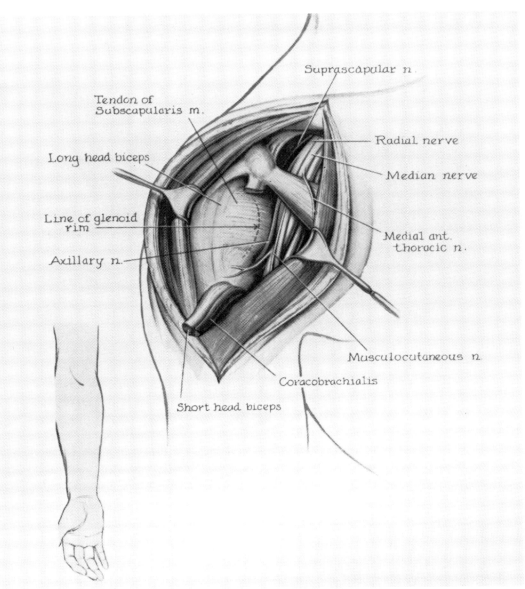

Suprascapular n.

Tendon of
Subscapularis m.

Radial nerve

Long head biceps

Median nerve

Line of glenoid
rim

Medial ant.
thoracic n.

Axillary n.

Musculocutaneous n.

Coracobrachialis

Short head biceps

FIGURE 4–11. Anterior approach to the shoulder through the deltopectoral interval. The conjoined tendon is reflected for demonstration purposes only. (m = muscle; n = nerve.) (From Kaplan EB. *Surgical Approaches to the Neck, Cervical Spine, and Upper Extremity.* Philadelphia: WB Saunders, 1966, p 57.)

The axillary and musculocutaneous nerves are the principal structures at risk with this exposure. The axillary nerve courses inferior to the anterior circumflex vessels, crossing over the subscapularis and running underneath the axillary portion of the joint capsule into the quadrilateral space. This nerve is at risk with dissections that are directed inferiorly or medially, such as an inferior capsular shift procedure. It should be palpated or visualized in these cases. The musculocutaneous nerve courses through the conjoined tendon about 1 to 5 cm distal to the coracoid process. It is principally at risk with procedures that transfer the coracoid process (i.e., the Bristow procedure) or with dissection underneath the conjoined tendon medially.

b. Posterior Approach—The *posterior approach* to the shoulder (Fig. 4–12) usually involves splitting the deltoid muscle through a longitudinal incision in the posterior axillary line. Traditional approaches, which were transverse and involved detachment of the deltoid off the posterior scapular spine and acromion, have been largely abandoned because of poor cosmesis. Splitting the deltoid muscle through this approach carries little risk for the axillary nerve

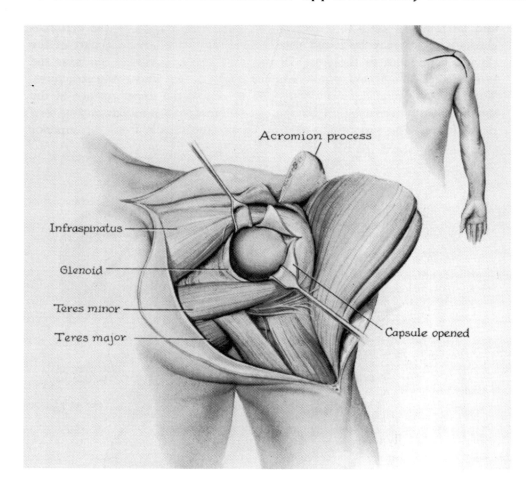

Infraspinatus

Acromion process

Glenoid

Teres minor

Teres major

Capsule opened

FIGURE 4–12. Posterior approach through the infraspinatus–teres minor interval. The deltoid is reflected and the acromion is split for demonstration purposes only. A deltoid-splitting approach is usually used. (From Kaplan EB. *Surgical Approaches to the Neck, Cervical Spine, and Upper Extremity*. Philadelphia: WB Saunders, 1966, p 61.)

as long as the dissection remains above the inferior border of the teres minor. The subdeltoid interval provides a good location for retraction to expose the underlying infraspinatus and teres minor tendons. The approach to the joint is in the interval between the infraspinatus (suprascapular nerve) and the teres minor (axillary nerve); however, in practice, the infraspinatus tendon is usually split longitudinally because determination of the internervous plane may be difficult.

The principal nerves at risk with this approach include the axillary nerve and the suprascapular nerve. The axillary nerve courses underneath the teres minor through the quadrilateral space and then extends on the undersurface of the deltoid around the humerus. It is at risk if the surgical dissection strays beneath the teres minor or if the posteroinferior capsule is not carefully visualized during the dissection. It can also be injured by excessive inferior retraction of the teres minor during surgery. The suprascapular nerve courses along the infraspinatus fossa about 3 cm medial to the

posterior glenoid margin. It is at risk with medial dissection along the scapula or excessive medial retraction during surgery.

   c. Traditional Approach—The traditional approach to open acromioplasty and *rotator cuff* repair (Fig. 4–13) is through an oblique anterosuperior incision from the midportion of the acromion toward the coracoid process. The deltoid is then detached from the anterior acromion edge and retracted inferiorly to allow for acromioplasty and cuff repair. If necessary, it may be split laterally between its anterior and medial portions for a distance of no more than 3 cm (to the level of the greater tuberosity). The axillary nerve is somewhat at risk if the deltoid split proceeds more inferiorly. The commonly referenced limit is said to be no more than 5 cm distal to the lateral acromion.

B. Biomechanics
   1. Introduction—Biomechanics of the glenohumeral joint is closely related to the anatomic architecture of this joint. Because it is a minimally constrained articulation, the soft tissue structures have a major role in

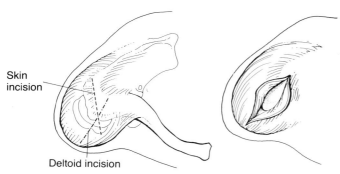

FIGURE 4–13. Approach for acromioplasty and rotator cuff repair (superior view). The skin incision is along Langer's lines.

stability. An understanding of both static and dynamic factors is important to appreciate the biomechanics of the shoulder:

Static Restraints	*Dynamic Restraints*
Articular anatomy	Rotator cuff
Glenoid labrum	muscles
Negative pressure	Biceps tendon
Capsule/ligaments	Scapulothoracic
	motion

2. Static Restraints
   a. Articular Anatomy—As previously noted, only one third of the articular surface of the humerus is covered by glenoid in any position of arm rotation. This anatomic arrangement, described by Saha as the glenohumeral index (ratio of the glenoid diameter to the humeral head diameter) (Fig. 4–14), describes the anatomic basis for relative instability of the glenohumeral joint. In the sagittal plane this ratio is 0.75, and in the transverse plane it is 0.6. Clinical conditions such as glenoid fractures, glenoid dysplasia, and labral detachment reduce this ratio and make the joint more susceptible to instability. In a normal shoulder, the combined retroversion of the humeral head and glenoid is 30° to 40°. Some surgeons have suggested that abnormal version of the glenoid or humerus may affect shoulder stability, but this is not universally accepted.
   b. Glenoid Labrum–As described earlier, the glenoid labrum functions through several mechanisms to stabilize the humeral head in the glenoid. It anchors the IGHLC and increases the glenoid depth, stabilizing the joint through a concavity-compression mechanism. This anatomic arrangement also acts in a fashion analogous to a chock-block, preventing the humeral head from translating with rotation.
   c. Negative Intra-articular Pressure (Fig. 4–15). Normally, the glenohumeral joint has a negative intra-articular pressure relative to the atmosphere. This is because of the closed space surrounded by an elastic sphere of ligaments and muscles. This negative intra-articular pressure is proportional to the force tending to displace the humeral head away from the glenoid, because a suction effect develops in this closed joint space surrounded by elastic soft tissue. Although this effect has a role in stabilizing the humeral head in the glenoid, it probably is clinically important only in an adducted shoulder resting at the side without any muscle activity.
   d. Glenohumeral Ligaments—These capsular thickenings reinforce the capsule and serve as static checkreins to extreme translations and rotations of the humeral head on the glenoid. These ligaments are named on the basis of their glenoid attachment. Material properties of the glenohumeral ligaments have recently been characterized (Bigliani and colleagues). The capsule (and ligaments) is normally a lax structure, with a surface area two times that of the hu-

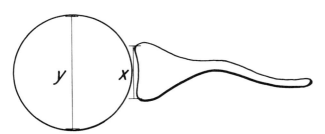

FIGURE 4–14. Glenohumeral index (GH_I = x/y). This illustrates the size mismatch between the glenoid diameter and humeral head diameter. (Reprinted with permission from Warner JJP, Caborn DN. Overview of shoulder instability. Crit Rev Phys Rehabil Med 4:145–198, 1992.)

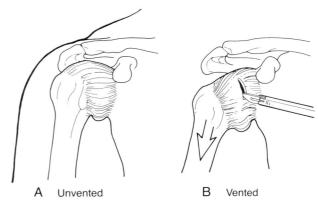

A   Unvented   B   Vented

FIGURE 4–15. Demonstration of normal negative intra-articular pressure. *A,* Unvented capsule. *B,* Vented capsule. (Note the inferior subluxation of the humerus.)

meral head. This is a necessary arrangement to permit the normal range of motion necessary for the joint. In addition, the capsule is prone to significant plastic deformation before complete failure; *therefore, it is likely that all traumatic injuries cause some laxity of the capsule even in the presence of a Bankart lesion.* Because of their different origins and insertions, each ligament has a different role depending on arm position and direction of applied force.

(1) SGHL and CHL—These structures parallel each other and are best considered together. The CHL was believed to be the more significant structure; however, investigations have now suggested otherwise. Together, these ligaments limit (1) external rotation with the arm in adduction, (2) inferior translation of the adducted humerus, and (3) posterior translation when the shoulder is adducted, flexed, and internally rotated.

(2) MGHL—This structure parallels the SGHL and has similar functions (Fig. 4–16). It is the most variable of the glenohumeral ligaments in terms of size and development, being well defined in approximately 60% of cases. Biomechanically, it

limits the following motions: (1) external rotation of the adducted shoulder, (2) inferior translation of the adducted and externally rotated humerus, and (3) anterior translation of the slightly abducted humerus (45°).

(3) IGHLC—This structure consists of an anterior and a posterior band and an intervening axillary pouch. The complex functions like a hammock or sling with the shoulder abducted (Fig. 4–17). Moreover, the anatomic arrangement allows for reciprocal tightening of the anterior and posterior bands during shoulder rotation, thus stabilizing the joint in both an anterior and a posterior direction. Biomechanically, this structure limits the following motions: (1) anterior translation of the abducted shoulder, (2) posterior translation of the abducted shoulder, and (3) inferior translation of the abducted shoulder.

3. Dynamic Restraints—In the past decade, a growing body of both experimental and clinical work has demonstrated that the most important stabilizing factor for the glenohumeral joint is the combined effect of the intrinsic muscles that cross it (i.e., the rotator cuff muscles and the long head of the biceps brachii). Stability may be afforded through several mechanisms. If one appreciates that the glenohumeral liga-

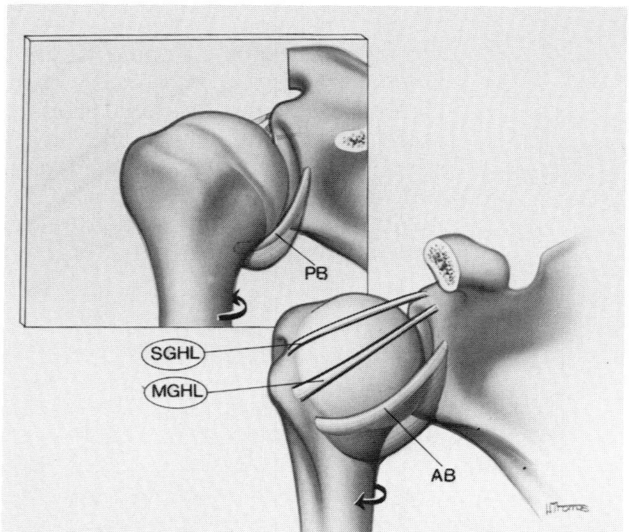

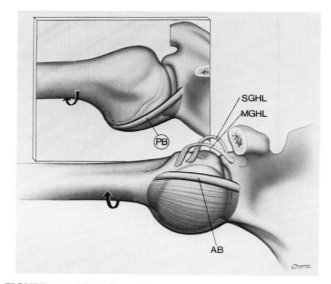

FIGURE 4–16. The superior and middle glenohumeral ligaments tighten with adduction and external rotation. (SGHL = superior glenohumeral ligament; MGHL = middle glenohumeral ligament; AB = anterior band [of the inferior glenohumeral ligament complex]; PB = posterior band [of the inferior glenohumeral ligament complex].) (From Warner JJP, Deng X-H, Warren RF, Tozilli AP. Static capsuloligamentous restraints to superior-inferior translation of the glenohumeral joint. Am J Sports Med 20:682–683, 1992.)

FIGURE 4–17. The inferior glenohumeral ligament complex tightens with abduction and external rotation. (SGHL = superior glenohumeral ligament; MGHL = middle glenohumeral ligament; AB = anterior band [of the inferior glenohumeral ligament complex]; PB = posterior band [of the inferior glenohumeral ligament complex].) (From Warner JJP, Deng X-H, Warren RF, Tozilli AP. Static capsuloligamentous restraints to superior-inferior translation of the glenohumeral joint. Am J Sports Med 20:682–683, 1992.)

ments function as passive checkreins only at the extremes of rotation and translation, then it is understandable why dynamic stabilization of the joint is essential, especially in the midranges of motion.

   a. Joint Compression—This enhances stability through a concavity-compression effect previously described. The magnitude of this effect is greater than that provided by capsular restraint.

   b. Barrier Effect—A contracting portion of the rotator cuff can function as an actual barrier to translation by becoming rigid with contraction.

   c. Secondary Dynamization—Secondary dynamization of the capsule can occur through direct attachments of rotator cuff tendons. Contraction of the rotator cuff may create tension in the capsule, thus stabilizing the joint.

   d. Steering Effect—A coordinated steering effect occurs through synergistic, sequential contractions of portions of the rotator cuff during arm motions.

C. Throwing—Significant forces, which may approach two to three times body weight, are generated in an athlete's shoulder with throwing. Repetitive throwing can result in overuse injuries that are manifested earlier in an athlete's shoulder than in the normal population. The five phases of throwing are described as follows (Fig. 4–18):

Phase	Maximum Stresses	Comments
Wind-up		Upper extremity flexion
Early cocking	Deltoid, cuff	Abduction, external rotation
Late cocking	Cuff, deltoid, inferior capsule	Begins with foot contact

Phase	Maximum Stresses	Comments
Acceleration	All tissues	Minimum activity
Follow-through	Posterior capsule	Maximum activity

In the cocking phase of throwing, a shear force tends to displace the humeral head anteriorly out of the glenoid. The magnitude of this shear force is close to body weight, and it must be resisted by the combined effect of muscle contraction, ligament tension, and labrum-glenoid concavity. As the arm is brought from the position of extreme extension-abduction-external rotation to maximum flexion-adduction-internal rotation during the acceleration phase of the throwing motion, the velocity of the hand approaches 7000°/sec; and in the follow-through phase of the throwing motion, the distraction force tending to pull the humeral head anteriorly again approaches body weight. In this situation, little stability is provided by either the glenoid or the labrum. Instead, all this kinetic energy must be absorbed by contracting rotator cuff and tension developed in the joint capsule. Because sports such as throwing, swimming, and tennis require repetitive overhead motions, it is easy to understand how the glenohumeral joint is at risk for overuse injury. Moreover, faulty mechanics of such overhead motions may occur as a result of either poor technique or fatigue and thus increase the risk for overuse injuries.

II. History and Physical Examination

  A. History—Two factors are particularly important in the initial evaluation of shoulder injuries—age and chief complaint. Instability, AC injuries, and other acute injuries are more common in the younger population. Older

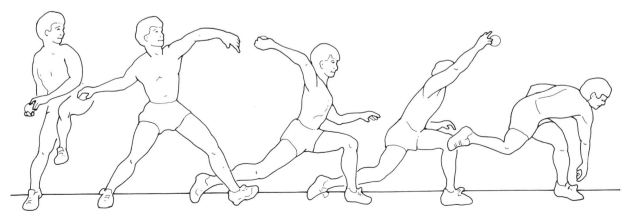

Wind-up   Early cocking   Late cocking   Acceleration   Follow-through

FIGURE 4–18. The five phases of throwing include wind-up, early cocking, late cocking, acceleration, and follow-through.

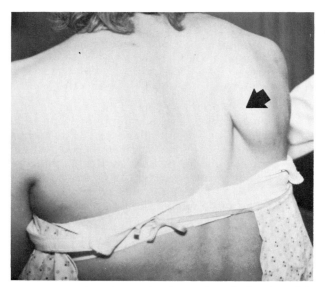

FIGURE 4–19. Clinical example of scapular winging (*arrow*) in a patient with long thoracic nerve palsy.

ing, neurovascular evaluation, and special testing is appropriate.

1. Observation—Patients should be evaluated while entering the room, while getting dressed, and throughout the examination for shoulder function and pain. Inspection for asymmetry, muscle wasting, deformities, swelling, and skin changes should be the first step in the examination. Muscle wasting commonly involves the rotator cuff muscles in patients with chronic rotator cuff tears. A rupture of the long head of the biceps classically presents with a bulge commonly referred to as a "Popeye" muscle. Scapular winging due to palsy of the serratus anterior may be observed as protrusion of the inferior angle of the scapula (Fig. 4–19). Dislocations and separations of the glenohumeral or AC joint may also be diagnosed merely by observing and inspecting a patient (Fig. 4–20).

2. Palpation—A thorough understanding of the underlying bony and soft tissue anatomy is essential in this portion of the examination. Bony landmarks including the SC joint, AC joint, acromion, greater tuberosity, and the area surrounding the bicipital groove should be palpated for tenderness, relationships to other structures, swelling, and deformity. The evaluation should also assess systemic laxity, including thumb-to-forearm flexibility; metacarpophalangeal, elbow, and knee hyperextension/recurvatum; and contralateral shoulder laxity. Findings of these examinations are important in classifying shoulder instability (Fig. 4–21).

3. Motion—Evaluation of shoulder range of motion typically includes forward flexion (elevation) (normal 150–180°), external rotation with the arm at the side (normal 30–60°) and with the arm 90° abducted (normal 70–90°), and internal rotation (graded on the basis of the highest verte-

patients are more likely to present with rotator cuff injuries and arthritis. It is important to establish the chronicity of the chief complaint and, for acute injuries, the mechanism of injury. Instability is usually associated with an injury to an abducted and externally rotated arm. AC injuries usually result from a fall directly onto the shoulder. Rotator cuff tears are usually associated with chronic pain with overhead activities and night pain. For instability, it is critical to obtain a thorough history of prior episodes of shoulder subluxation and dislocation, with particular emphasis on the amount of trauma involved in each injury and the direction of instability. For all shoulder problems, it is important to question a patient about associated symptoms and referred pain.

B. Physical Examination—As with any examination, an orderly sequence of observation, palpation, assessment of motion, strength test-

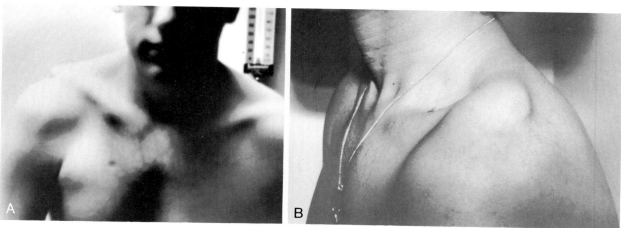

FIGURE 4–20. Clinical example of (*A*) grade III and (*B*) grade IV acromioclavicular separation.

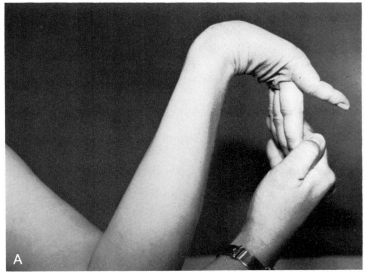

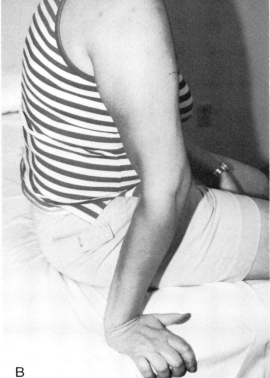

FIGURE 4–21. Congenital hyperlaxity associated with (*A*) metacarpophalangeal hyperextension and (*B*) excessive mobility.

bral body reached with the thumb midline behind the back) (normal T4–T8). Passive motion is also evaluated and recorded in patients with abnormal motion. It should be remembered that both age and sex can influence normal range of motion.

4. Strength Testing—Evaluation of muscle strength is often focused on the suspected pathology. Grading is based on a standardized scale (Table 4–1). Flexion, abduction, and external rotation strengths are commonly tested. Evaluation of the various muscles for specific problems is detailed in Table 4–2.

5. Neurovascular Examination—In addition to motor testing, sensory and reflex testing may be appropriate in the right clinical setting. Sensation over the lateral deltoid should be assessed in patients with shoulder instability to help verify the integrity of the axillary nerve. An understanding of the basic dermatomes is helpful: C5, lateral arm; C6, thumb; C7, middle finger; C8, small finger; and T1, medial arm. Reflex evaluation of the biceps (C5), brachioradialis (C6), and triceps (C7) may also be helpful in the right clinical setting. Palpation of pulses may also be indicated if vascular

TABLE 4–1. GRADING OF MUSCLE STRENGTH USING 0–5 SYSTEM

Grade	Degree of Muscle Strength	
0 = Zero	No palpable contraction.	(Nothing)
1 = Trace	Muscle contracts, but part normally motorized does not move, even without gravity.	(Trace)
2 = Poor	Muscle moves the part but not against gravity.	(With gravity eliminated)
3 = Fair	Muscle moves part through a range against gravity.	(Against gravity)
4 = Good	Muscle moves part even against added resistance; variations in resistance are graded plus or minus.	(Near normal)
5 = Excellent	Normal strength against full resistance is present.	(Normal)

(From Rockwood CA Jr, Matsen EA III [eds]. *The Shoulder.* Philadelphia: WB Saunders, 1990, p 165.)

TABLE 4–2. SHOULDER MUSCLE TESTING CHART

Muscle	Innervation	Myotomes	Technique for Testing
Trapezius	Spinal accessory	C2–C4	Patient shrugs shoulders against resistance.
Sternomastoid	Spinal accessory	C2–C4	Patient turns head to one side with resistance over opposite temporal area.
Serratus anterior	Long thoracic	C5–C7	Patient pushes against wall with outstretched arm. Scapular winging is observed.
Latissimus dorsi	Thoracodorsal	C7–C8	Downward/backward pressure of arm against resistance. Muscle palpable at inferior angle of scapula during cough.
Rhomboids Levator scapulae	Dorsal Scapular	(C4) C5*	Hands on hips pushing elbows backward against resistance.
Subclavius	Nerve to subclavius	C5–C6	None.
Teres major	Subscapular (lower)	C5–C6	Similar to latissimus dorsi; muscle palpable at lower border of scapula.
Deltoid	Axillary	C5–C6 (C7)	With arm abducted 90°, downward pressure is applied. Anterior and posterior fibers may be tested in slight flexion and extension.
Subscapularis	Subscapular (upper)	C5	Arm at side with elbow flexed to 90°. Examiner resists internal rotation.
Supraspinatus	Suprascapular	C5 (C6)	Arm abducted against resistance (not isolated). With arm pronated and elevated 90° in plane of scapula, downward pressure is applied.
Infraspinatus	Suprascapular	C5 (C6)	Arm at side with elbow flexed 90°. Examiner resists external rotation.
Teres minor	Axillary	C5–C6 (C7)	Same as for infraspinatus.
Pectoralis major	Medial and lateral pectoral	C5–T1	With arm flexed 30° in front of body, patient adducts against resistance.
Pectoralis minor	Medial pectoral	C8, T1	None.
Coracobrachialis	Musculocutaneous	(C4) C5–C6 (C7)	None.
Biceps brachii	Musculocutaneous	(C4) C5–C6 (C7)	Flexion of the supinated forearm against resistance.
Triceps	Radial	(C5) C6–C8	Resistance to extension of elbow from varying position of flexion.

* Numbers in parentheses indicate a variable but not rare contribution.
(From Rockwood CA Jr, Matsen FA III [eds]. *The Shoulder*. Philadelphia: WB Saunders, 1990, p 166.)

injury is suspected. A modified Adson or Wright test, which consists of arm extension abduction and external rotation, neck extension, and rotation to the opposite shoulder with or without patients' holding their breath, may cause the radial pulse in the affected arm to be obliterated and symptoms to develop in patients with thoracic outlet syndrome (Fig. 4–22). Elevation of both arms and rapid opening and closing of the hands may also cause fatigue, cramping, or hand and finger blanching and tingling in patients with thoracic outlet syndrome.

6. Special Testing—Certain provocative maneuvers and tests are useful for increasing the specificity of the diagnosis.

 a. Instability—Glenohumeral translation is tested with the arm in various positions of abduction. This is particularly useful for examination under anesthesia. The amount of translation is graded on the basis of the final position of the humerus in relation to the glenoid (Fig. 4–23). Inferior stress is applied to determine if a patient has a *sulcus sign* (Fig. 4–24). Widening of the subacromial space with inferior traction is associated

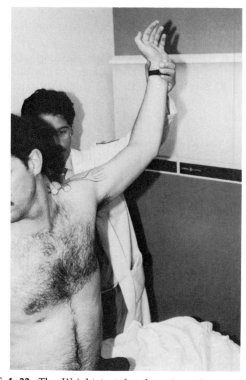

FIGURE 4–22. The Wright test for thoracic outlet syndrome is a modification of the classic Adson test. The arm is extended, abducted, and externally rotated, and the neck is extended and rotated to the opposite shoulder. Loss of pulse and reproduction of symptoms is consistent with thoracic outlet syndrome.

GRADE   GLENOHUMERAL   CLINICAL
        TRANSLATION

Trace

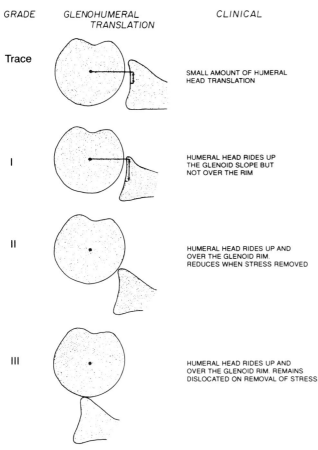

SMALL AMOUNT OF HUMERAL
HEAD TRANSLATION

I

HUMERAL HEAD RIDES UP
THE GLENOID SLOPE BUT
NOT OVER THE RIM

II

HUMERAL HEAD RIDES UP AND
OVER THE GLENOID RIM.
REDUCES WHEN STRESS REMOVED

III

HUMERAL HEAD RIDES UP AND
OVER THE GLENOID RIM. REMAINS
DISLOCATED ON REMOVAL OF STRESS.

FIGURE 4–23. Translation of the shoulder has been classified by many schemes, including the one shown here. All schemes quantify the amount of translation in relation to the glenoid. (From Hawkins RJ, Bokor DJ. Clinical evaluation of shoulder problems. In Rockwood CA Jr, Matsen FA III [eds]. *The Shoulder.* Philadelphia: WB Saunders, 1990, p 168.)

with an inferior (and usually multidirectional) component to instability. The *apprehension test* consists of abduction and external rotation of the shoulder, which reproduces pain and the sensation of instability in patients with anterior instability (Fig. 4–25*A*). A companion test, the *relocation test*, involves application of posterior stress on the proximal arm after supine apprehension testing (Fig. 4–25*B*). This usually relieves the apprehension and allows increased external rotation in patients with anterior instability. These tests are, however, more sensitive than specific.

b. Impingement Syndrome—Three examination features are usually described for evaluating shoulder impingement (Fig. 4–26). The *impingement sign* basically involves passive forward elevation of the arm beyond 90°, causing painful pinching of the rotator cuff under the coracoacromial arch. This pain is re-

lieved with a subacromial injection of lidocaine in patients with true impingement syndrome (*impingement test*). One additional test for impingement is forcible internal rotation of the shoulder with the arm forward-flexed 90° and adducted (impingement-reinforcement or *Hawkins test*). This also causes impingement of the cuff under the anterior acromion. The impingement *test* is the most sensitive and specific maneuver for detection of impingement.

c. Acromioclavicular Pain—In addition to direct tenderness over the AC joint, patients with arthritis or osteolysis of this joint often have pain with forceful horizontal adduction of the shoulder. As in the impingement test, injection of the AC joint with lidocaine resolves this pain.

d. Biceps Tendinitis—Tenderness directly over the area of the bicipital groove is usually present in patients with bicipital tendinitis. Two additional tests are also commonly used to assist in the diagnosis: the Yergason and Speed tests. The *Yergason test* involves resisted supination of the hand with the elbow flexed. The *Speed test* involves resisted forward elevation of the arm with the elbow extended and the forearm supinated (Fig. 4–27). Both of these maneuvers may create pain felt in the biceps region in

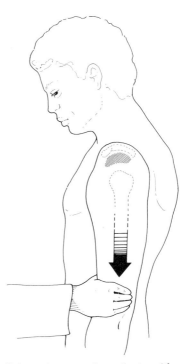

FIGURE 4–24. Sulcus sign seen in patients with multidirectional instability. Traction on the arm results in inferior displacement of the humerus.

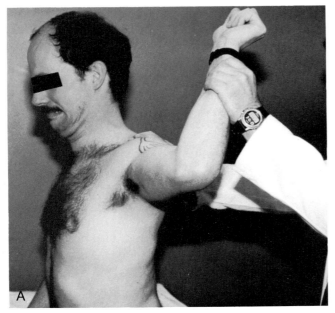

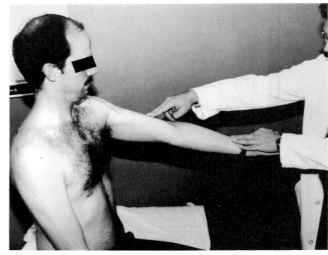

FIGURE 4–27. Speed test. Resisted forward elevation of the supinated arm elicits pain in patients with tendinitis of the long head of the biceps.

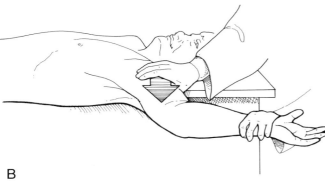

FIGURE 4–25. *A*, Apprehension test. The patient notes pain and becomes apprehensive about his shoulder dislocating in this position. *B*, Relocation test. Anterior pressure on the proximal arm relocates the humerus and causes relief of the apprehension.

patients with tendinitis of the long head of the biceps.

e. Cervical Spine—Evaluation of the cervical spine, including assessment of range of motion and a thorough neurologic evaluation, is helpful in distinguishing cervical from shoulder pathology. This is a common differential diagnosis to make in patients with shoulder pain. The *Spurling test*, lateral flexion and rotation of the neck with compression, elicits pain on the side to which the head is tilted (Fig. 4–28). Another useful observation is that patients who have shoulder pain due to cervical spine disease localize their pain to the

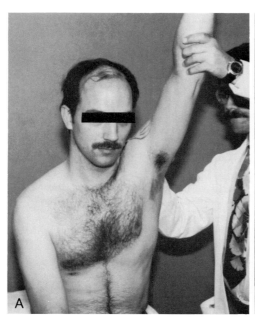

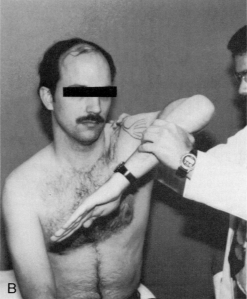

FIGURE 4–26. *A*, Impingement sign/test. Passive forward flexion of the arm causes pain as the rotator cuff muscles are impinged by the coracoacromial arch and the undersurface of the acromion. This pain is relieved by a subacromial injection of anesthetic. *B*, Hawkins sign/test. Placing the arm in this position also produces pain in patients with impingement syndrome.

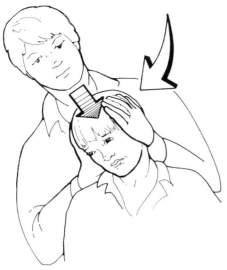

FIGURE 4–28. Spurling test. Lateral flexion and rotation with some compression causes nerve root encroachment and pain on the ipsilateral side.

trapezius area. Patients with shoulder pain due to impingement localize their pain over the deltoid area.

III. Radiography of the Shoulder
  A. Standard Radiographs—The trauma series of shoulder radiographs includes a true anteroposterior (AP) and an axillary lateral of the shoulder. The true AP view is angulated 45° from the plane of the thorax. The advantage of this view over the standard AP view of the shoulder is that the glenohumeral joint can

be seen in true profile without any overlap of the humeral head on the glenoid (Fig. 4–29). The *axillary lateral* is taken with the arm abducted 70° to 90° with the radiographic beam directed cranially (Fig. 4–30). Although this view can be obtained in almost any patient, an occasional patient may be unable to abduct his or her arm enough for this view. Several techniques can be used in this setting. The arm usually can be carefully passively abducted to allow this film to be taken. In other cases, a curved cassette can be placed in the axilla and the beam can be directed inferiorly onto the cassette. Alternatively, the arm can be forward flexed rather than abducted (Fig. 4–31A). The Velpeau axillary lateral can be obtained without even removing the injured extremity from its immobilized position. The patient is simply asked to lean backward over the edge of the radiography table, and the beam is directed from superior to inferior (Fig. 4–31B). If none of these techniques are possible, a scapulolateral view should be obtained. This view, also known as the transscapular or *scapular Y* view, is taken from posteromedial to anterolateral parallel to the spine of the scapula. This view is a true lateral of the scapula and forms the letter Y, which is composed of the coracoid anteriorly and the scapular spine/acromion posteriorly. The glenoid fossa is located at the intersection of the three arms of the Y (Fig. 4–32).
  B. Special Radiographs––Various special views have been developed to visualize specific abnormalities of the shoulder.
    1. Anterior Instability—In addition to the true AP and axillary lateral views, the *West*

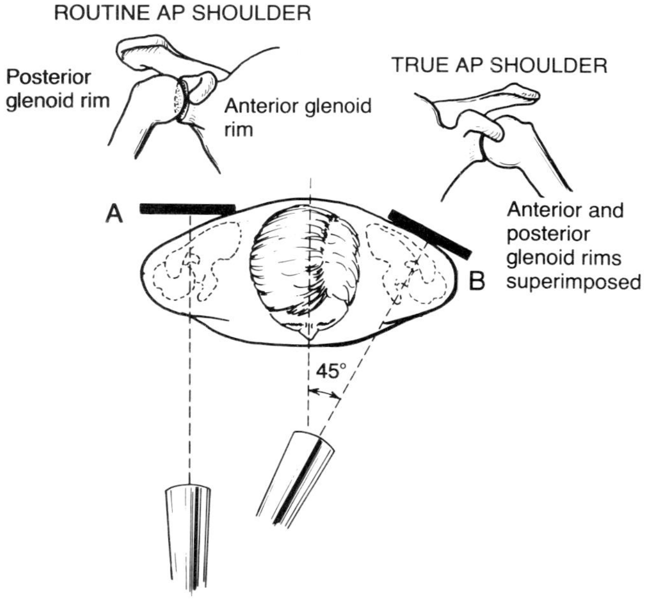

ROUTINE AP SHOULDER

Posterior glenoid rim

Anterior glenoid rim

TRUE AP SHOULDER

A

B

Anterior and posterior glenoid rims superimposed

45°

FIGURE 4–29. The true AP of the shoulder allows clear visualization of the joint space without overlap. A, Routine AP. B, True AP. (Reprinted with permission from Warner JJP, Caborn DN. Overview of shoulder instability. Crit Rev Phys Rehabil 4:145–198, 1992.)

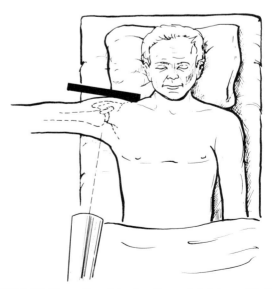

FIGURE 4–30. The axillary lateral radiograph is taken with the arm abducted 70° to 90°. (Reprinted with permission from Warner JJP, Caborn DN. Overview of shoulder instability. Crit Rev Phys Rehabil Med 4:145–198, 1992.)

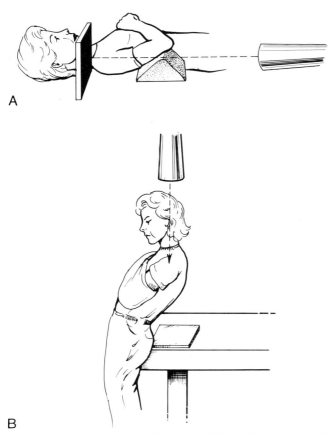

A

B

FIGURE 4–31. Techniques to obtain a modified axillary lateral without abducting the arm include (*A*) placing the arm on a foam block in forward flexion (trauma axillary lateral) and (*B*) a Velpeau view. (Reprinted with permission from Warner JJP, Caborn DN. Overview of shoulder instability. Crit Rev Phys Rehabil Med 4:145–198, 1992.)

Point and *Stryker notch* views are commonly recommended to evaluate the anteroinferior glenoid rim and the presence of an impression fracture of the humeral head (Hill-Sachs lesion), respectively. The West Point view is essentially an axillary lateral taken with a patient prone and the beam angled 25° in two planes (Fig. 4–33). The Stryker notch view is a 10° cephalic tilt radiograph

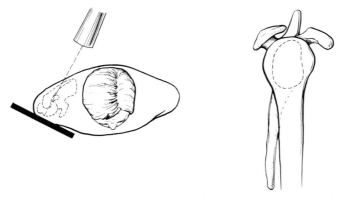

FIGURE 4–32. Positioning for the scapular Y view. (Reprinted with permission from Warner JJP, Caborn DN. Overview of shoulder instability. Crit Rev Phys Rehabil Med 4:145–198, 1992.)

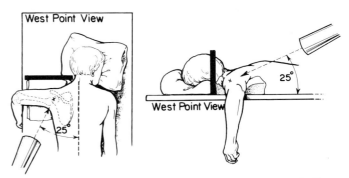

FIGURE 4–33. The West Point modified axillary radiograph allows visualization of the anteroinferior glenoid rim. (Reprinted with permission from Warner JJP, Caborn DN. Overview of shoulder instability. Crit Rev Phys Rehabil Med 4:145–198, 1992.)

taken with a patient supine with his or her affected hand on the head (Fig. 4–34). This view allows the presence and size of a Hill-Sachs impression fracture to be ascertained. Another view sometimes helpful in evaluating recurrent anterior instability is the apical oblique or Garth view. This view, which is a true AP with a 45° caudal tilt, allows evaluation of the anterior inferior glenoid (like the West Point view). Finally, an AP radiograph with the arm in internal rotation is also helpful in identifying a Hill-Sachs lesion (Fig. 4–35).

2. Acromioclavicular Pain—In addition to standard views, a 10° cephalic tilt (*Zanca*) view is helpful to evaluate AC arthritis or distal clavicle osteolysis (Fig. 4–36). This view is taken with approximately half the voltage of a standard AP shoulder radiograph. With AC separations, an AP radiograph is taken of both shoulders on a wide cassette, and the coracoclavicular distance is measured and compared. For more subtle injuries, a stress view can be obtained with 10 to 20 pounds of weight suspended from the patient's wrists.

3. Sternoclavicular Injuries—Two special views have been described for evaluation of this joint—the Hobbs view and the serendipity view. The *Hobbs view* is a posteroanterior (PA) of the joint taken with the patient slumped over the cassette and resting on the elbows. The *serendipity view*, named for its method of discovery by Dr. Rockwood, is a 40° cephalic tilt view with the patient supine. Interpretation of the film is based on evaluation of the longitudinal axis of the clavicle compared with the opposite side. Anterior dislocation of the clavicle is suggested by superior displacement of the clavicle from the longitudinal axis and posterior dislocation by inferior displacement. Computed tomography (CT) is often a helpful adjunct to

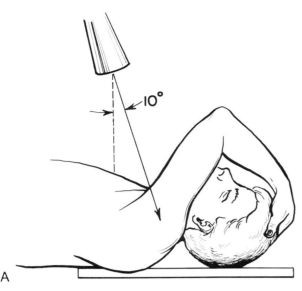

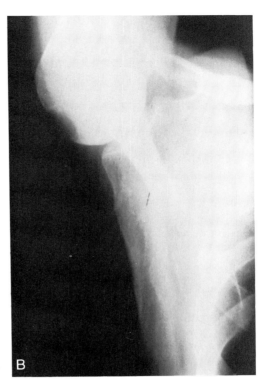

FIGURE 4–34. The Stryker notch radiograph allows visualization of a Hill-Sachs impression fracture of the posterior humeral head. *A,* Positioning the arm for the view. (Reprinted with permission from Warner JJP, Caborn DN. Overview of shoulder instability. Crit Rev Phys Rehabil Med 4:145–198, 1992.) *B,* Example of Hill-Sachs defect using this view.

the evaluation of SC dislocation, especially with posterior displacement.

4. Impingement Syndrome—AP views may show superior migration of the humerus and cystic or sclerotic changes in the greater tuberosity in patients with chronic massive rotator cuff tears. Two specific views are helpful in assessing associated acromial morphology—the supraspinatus outlet view and the 30° caudal tilt. The *supraspinatus outlet view* is similar to the

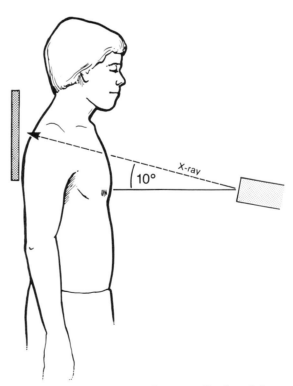

FIGURE 4–36. AC (Zanca) view allows visualization of the acromioclavicular joint. It is important to use soft tissue techniques in obtaining this radiograph. (From Rockwood CA Jr, Szalay EA, Curtis RJ Jr, et al. X-ray evaluation of shoulder problems. In Rockwood CA Jr, Matsen FA III [eds]. *The Shoulder.* Philadelphia: WB Saunders, 1990, p 192.)

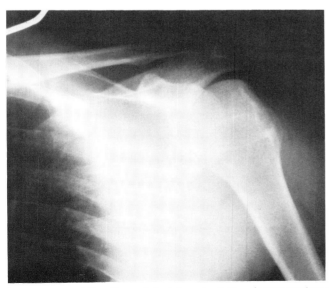

FIGURE 4–35. AP radiograph in internal rotation demonstrating a Hill-Sachs defect.

scapulolateral radiograph, except that the tube is angled 5° to 10° caudally. Bigliani and associates characterized three shapes of the acromion on the basis of this view: flat (I), curved (II), and hooked (III) (Fig. 4–37). Investigators at the Southern California Orthopaedic Institute further classified the acromion on the basis of its thickness: A, <8 mm; B, 8 to 12 mm; and C, >12 mm (Fig. 4–38). Another view that is helpful in identifying subacromial spurring is the *30° caudal tilt*, as described by Rockwood (Fig. 4–39). Subacromial spurs can be well characterized with a combination of the two views (Fig. 4–40).

C. Arthrography—Standard arthrography is still frequently used in evaluating rotator cuff tears. Dye that is injected into the glenohumeral joint and escapes into the subacromial space is diagnostic of a full-thickness rotator cuff tear. This study does not allow the tear to be quantified, however. Arthrography can also be used in conjunction with CT to evaluate intra-articular pathology such as Bankart tears.

D. Magnetic Resonance Imaging (MRI)—As in the knee, MRI of the shoulder has rapidly

emerged as the preferred imaging technique for various shoulder conditions (Fig. 4–41). Advances in technology, surface coils, and imaging techniques will likely further improve the diagnostic sensitivity and specificity of this imagining modality for shoulder pathology.

IV. Shoulder Arthroscopy
   A. Introduction—Shoulder arthroscopy has dramatically increased in popularity during the past decade and has evolved from a diagnostic to a therapeutic tool. Advantages of arthroscopic over open procedures include less invasiveness, muscle preservation, smaller incisions, improved visualization and access, and easier rehabilitation. Arthroscopic acromioplasty has evolved into a widely accepted procedure. Arthroscopic treatment of anterior instability has also been described, and its short-term efficacy established. Recognition and treatment of superior labral tears have rapidly evolved. Other possibilities for arthroscopic shoulder surgery are on the horizon.
   B. Positioning and Setup—Two methods of positioning are routinely used for shoulder

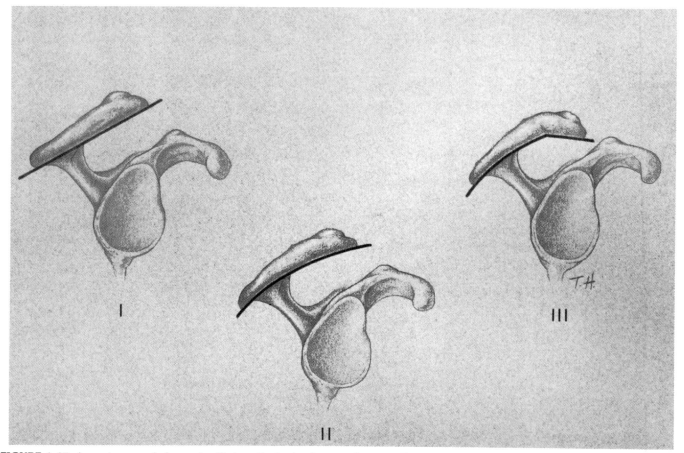

FIGURE 4–37. Acromion morphology, classified on the basis of supraspinatus outlet view, as described originally by Bigliani. (From Esch JC. Shoulder arthroscopy in the older age group. Op Techn Orthop 1:200, 1991.)

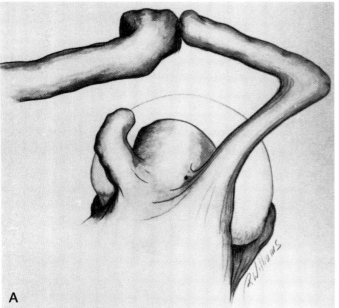

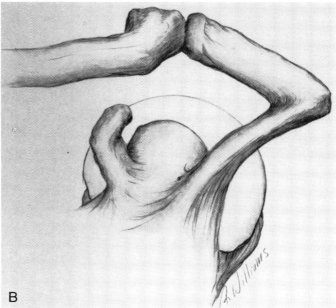

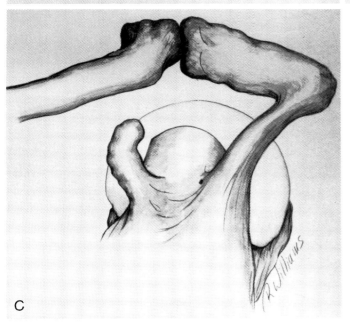

FIGURE 4–38. The acromion can also be subclassified on the basis of its thickness: *A*, <8 mm thick; *B*, 8 to 12 mm thick; *C*, >12 mm thick. (From Snyder SJ, Wuh HCK. Arthroscopic evaluation and treatment of the rotator cuff superior labrum anterior-posterior lesion. Op Tech Orthop 1:212–213, 1991.)

arthroscopy. The lateral decubitus position is the traditional method. More recently, the beach chair position has been successfully used for shoulder arthroscopy. The advantages of the beach chair position include normal vertical orientation of glenohumeral anatomy, free movement of the arm, avoidance of the use of traction, and easy conversion to an open procedure. Equipment used for shoulder arthroscopy is similar to that used in the knee. Commercially available cannulas with rubber diaphragms are helpful to maintain portals and allow easy insertion of arthroscopic instruments. Routine use of epinephrine in the arthroscopic solution is help-

ful to reduce the amount of bleeding with arthroscopic procedures about the shoulder. Anesthesia can be accomplished with regional (interscalene block) or general anesthesia. Examination of the shoulder before final positioning is helpful to confirm clinical suspicions of instability.

C. Diagnostic Arthroscopy
   1. Portals—Routine arthroscopy is usually carried out using two portals. Other portals are reserved for special applications (Fig. 4–42).
      a. Posterior Portal—The posterior portal is established 2 cm distal and 2 cm medial to the posterolateral corner of the

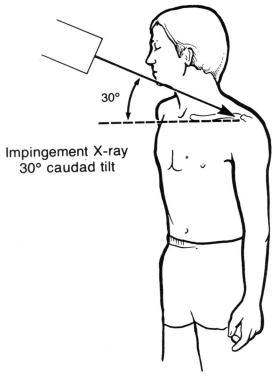

30°

Impingement X-ray
30° caudad tilt

FIGURE 4–39. Thirty-degree caudal tilt view for assessing acromial spurs. (From Rockwood CA Jr, Szalay EA, Curtis RJ Jr, et al. X-ray evaluation of shoulder problems. In Rockwood CA Jr, Matsen FA III [eds]. *The Shoulder*. Philadelphia: WB Saunders, 1990, p 197.)

acromion. Local anesthetic with epinephrine typically is injected around this and the anterior portal, and a spinal needle is introduced from the posterior portal into the glenohumeral joint. Ster-

ile saline is injected into the joint to distend the joint capsule, confirm the proper orientation for the portal, and introduce the arthroscope with a reduced chance of scope trauma to the articular cartilage. Saline should flow freely into the joint. After 10 to 20 mL of fluid is instilled, the syringe should be disconnected, and fluid should freely flow back through the needle, confirming proper placement. The remaining 40 to 50 mL of saline is then introduced into the joint. The posterior portal is then established, and the arthroscope is introduced into the glenohumeral joint. The biceps and superior labrum are visualized to establish orientation, and systematic examination of the joint is then carried out. Diagnostic arthroscopy can usually be successfully carried out through this portal alone.

b. Anterior Portal—The anterior portal is used for instrumentation. Some surgeons prefer to establish this portal from inside out using a Wissinger rod. Alternatively, a spinal needle can be used from outside in, and its location confirmed by direct arthroscopic visualization before creating the anterior portal. The portal should be located lateral to the coracoid and just distal to the acromion. Placing the arm in adduction reduces the chance of musculocutaneous nerve injury. It is often helpful to locate the portal with a spinal needle and then introduce the cannula just un-

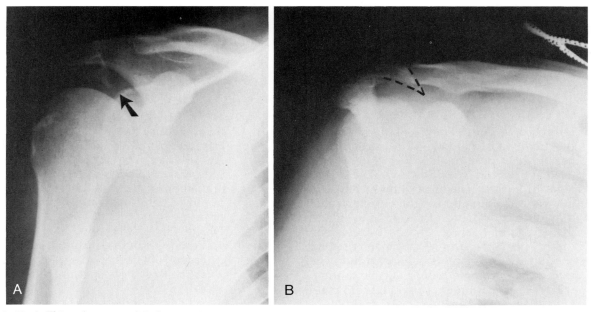

FIGURE 4–40. *A*, Thirty-degree caudal tilt view demonstrating large subacromial spur and spike. *B*, Supraspinatus outlet view showing a hooked (type III) acromion.

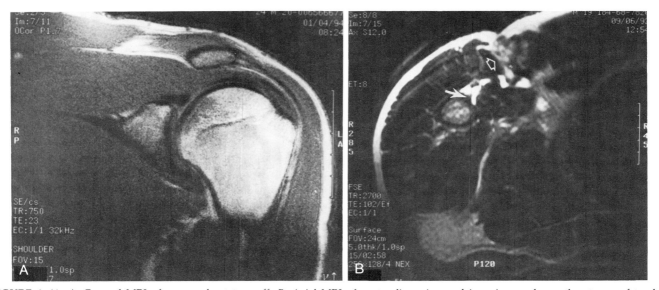

FIGURE 4–41. *A,* Coronal MRI of a normal rotator cuff. *B,* Axial MRI of pectoralis major avulsion. Arrow shows the stump of tendon remaining on the proximal humerus; open arrow shows accordioning of ruptured muscle. (From Miller MD, Johnson DA, Theate LA, et al. Rupture of the pectoralis major tendon in a football player. Am J Sports Med 21:475–477, 1993.)

der the biceps tendon. An arthroscopic cannula allows insertion of various instruments through this portal.

  c. Additional Portals—Other portals that can be useful for specific applications include the anteroinferior portal, the lateral portal, and the supraspinatus (Neviaser) portal. The anteroinferior portal is used for arthroscopic Bankart repair. It is located approximately 2 cm distal to the anterior portal and again is established from outside in with a spinal needle. When locating the portal,

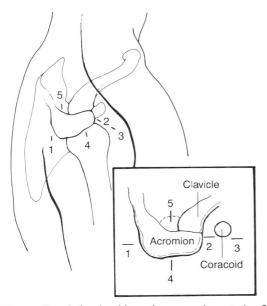

FIGURE 4–42. Portals for shoulder arthroscopy: 1, posterior; 2, anterior superior; 3, anterior inferior; 4, lateral; 5, supraspinatus (Neviaser) portal.

the spinal needle should enter the joint just superior to the subscapularis tendon. Because this portal is usually used for arthroscopic Bankart repair, it should be placed as low as possible so that it enters the joint just superior to the subscapularis tendon. The lateral portal is used for subacromial decompression and is located at the lateral margin of the acromion. Again, a spinal needle and cannula are helpful in establishing and maintaining this portal. The supraspinatus (Neviaser) portal is preferred by some surgeons for inflow or for visualization of the anterior glenoid. This portal is placed in the corner of the supraspinatus fossa and oriented slightly anteriorly and laterally. Studies have shown that the portal is well lateral to the suprascapular nerve and artery. This portal should also be placed with the arm adducted and with the trochar angled posteriorly to avoid injury to the tendinous portion of the rotator cuff.

 2. Examination Sequence—An orderly sequence for arthroscopic evaluation of the shoulder begins with visualization of the biceps tendon and superior labrum (see Color Figure 9). The arthroscope is then swept inferiorly, and the anteroinferior labrum and axillary pouch are visualized. Next, the articular surface of the glenoid is carefully examined for defects. The arthroscope is then swept superiorly, and the arm is externally rotated to examine the rotator cuff near its insertion at the greater tuberosity. Positioning the arm in external

rotation also allows visualization of the posterior labrum and posterior aspect of the humeral head. The arm is rotated to evaluate the articular surface of the humeral head (Fig. 4–43). Next, the glenohumeral ligaments are visualized and probed to assess capsular integrity (see Color Figures 9 and 10). The labrum is examined and probed for the presence of a Bankart lesion (Color Figure 11).

3. Subacromial Bursoscopy—This can be accomplished through the posterior portal as well. The arthroscope is removed and reintroduced with a blunt obturator placed through the same portal and directed superiorly. The undersurface of the acromion is contacted by the obturator to ensure introduction into the correct space and then gently pushed out the anterior portal. A cannula is then placed over the arthroscope into the subacromial bursa. The scope is then slowly backed out, into the bursa, so that just the end of the cannula can be visualized. A lateral portal can then be established using a spinal needle. A shaver is introduced through the lateral portal, and a window is made in the bursal tissue to allow visualization of the inferior surface of the acromion and the coracoacromial ligament. Both electrocautery and the shaver are used alternately to allow hemostasis and improved visualization. If subacromial decompression is planned, the acromion is exposed and a bony acromioplasty is accomplished with a motorized bur (Fig. 4–44 and Color Figure 12).

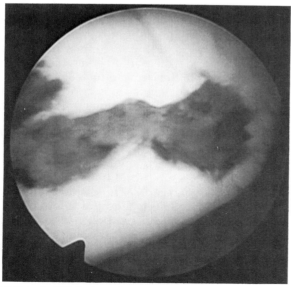

FIGURE 4–43. Hill-Sachs defect (posterior humeral head impression fracture) as seen arthroscopically.

V. Shoulder Instability
  A. Introduction—Anterior shoulder subluxation or dislocation accounts for the majority of shoulder instability. Patients typically report a history of trauma to the arm while it was in a position of abduction and external rotation. They may describe a period when their arm loses sensation and strength (dead-arm syndrome). Matsen describes two different categories of anterior shoulder instability: *t*ramatic *u*nilateral dislocation with a *B*ankart lesion and usually requiring *s*urgery (TUBS) and *a*traumatic *m*ultidirectional instability that is *bi*lateral and responds to *r*ehabilitation and rarely requires an *i*nferior capsular shift (AMBRI). Although this distinction may be helpful, in practice there may often be a degree of clinical overlap. Nevertheless, all patients who present with shoulder instability should be carefully questioned about previous episodes and the extent of the trauma involved and should be examined for generalized ligamentous laxity.
  B. Diagnosis—As alluded to earlier, the history and physical examination usually allow determination of the proper diagnosis. Important physical examination tests include the apprehension maneuver and the relocation test. Radiographs should be carefully reviewed for signs of a bony Bankart lesion (best seen on a West Point or Garth view) and a Hill-Sachs lesion (best seen on the Stryker notch and AP in internal rotation views). MRI is rapidly replacing CT arthrography in the imaging of labral lesions, although this appears to be more sensitive than specific. The use of gadolinium for MRI arthrography may further improve specificity of this test.
  C. Treatment of Anterior Instability
    1. Initial Treatment—Early treatment includes reduction of the dislocation, usually with some variation of the traction-countertraction technique. Results of postreduction radiographs and neurovascular examination should be carefully documented. In older patients, it is important to evaluate the rotator cuff to ensure that it is not torn.
    2. Nonoperative Treatment—The consensus is that a conservative approach is most appropriate after a first episode of traumatic anterior dislocation. Some investigators have suggested that arthroscopic stabilization may be appropriate in this setting. Numerous reports have documented a high recurrence rate with anterior instability, ranging from 50% to 90%. The recurrence rate appears to be directly related to the age of the patient, with younger patients more likely to have recurrent instability. One study from the U.S. Naval Academy, however, demonstrated a recurrence of

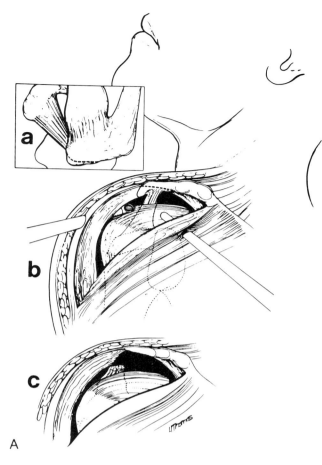

FIGURE 4–44. *A*, Technique for subacromial bursoscopy and acromioplasty. *a*, Coracoacromial ligament. *b*, Arthroscopic placement of instruments for acromioplasty. *Dotted lines* indicate the amount of intended resection. *c*, Following coracoacromial ligament resection. (From Altchek DW, Warren RF, Skyhar MJ. Shoulder arthroscopy. In Rockwood CA Jr, Matsen FA III [eds]. *The Shoulder*. WB Saunders, 1990, p 269.) *B*, Conversion from a type III to a type I acromion using arthroscopic techniques.

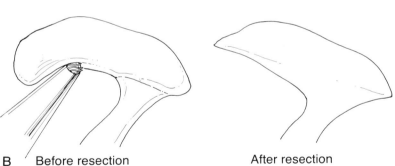

B   Before resection   After resection

only 25%, suggesting that a rehabilitation program with a high compliance rate can be successful, even in young adults. Most surgeons favor a 2- to 4-week period of immobilization based on a patient's age (longer for younger patients). This is followed by a period of intense rehabilitation including rotator cuff and scapular stabilizer strengthening. The length of this program is highly variable, from several months to years. A prolonged trial of therapy is most critical in patients with AMBRI. Success rates for rehabilitation of shoulder instability of atraumatic etiology (80%) were significantly better than in those patients with traumatic instability (16%) in one study.

3. Surgical Treatment—Many patients with TUBS ultimately have recurrences and symptoms that lead to surgical consideration. Some patients with AMBRI also need surgery. Because capsular laxity is an important consideration in the AMBRI group, open Bankart repair with some form of capsular shift is the procedure of choice for these patients. In the TUBS group, open procedures have also been the standard. Nevertheless, as previously described, arthroscopic treatment has many advantages. Early reports of arthroscopic

repair techniques have been discouraging because of high recurrence rates; however, much of this appears to be related to technical errors and poor patient selection. Some surgeons are reporting success rates that approach those of open Bankart repairs. At present, however, open capsular repair techniques are the most reliable approach.

a. Examination Under Anesthesia—Regardless of whether an arthroscopic or an open procedure has been selected, an examination under anesthesia can contribute helpful information before surgery. As in the knee, the examination under anesthesia can help quantify the degree and direction of instability (Fig. 4–45). One study demonstrated the utility of this examination, with a sensitivity of 100% and a specificity and predictive value of 93%. Various schemes have been used to quantify this instability, based on the amount of translation of the humeral head (see Fig. 4–23). It is also helpful to compare findings with those in the contralateral shoulder.

b. Diagnostic Arthroscopy—Although the debate over the essential lesion continues, arthroscopy has contributed greatly to our understanding of normal and pathologic anatomy of the shoulder (see Fig. 4–31 and Color Figures 9 and 11). One study reported arthroscopic findings in acute dislocations to fall into one of three groups (Fig. 4–46):

Group	Frequency	Pathology
1	13%	Capsular tear only
2	24%	Capsule and partial labral tear
3	63%	Capsular tear with labral detachment

Although labral tears were identified in the majority of the cases and all of the cases that were grossly unstable, the appropriateness of a simple Bankart repair without simultaneous correction of capsular laxity is still controversial. In vitro studies have demonstrated that the capsule must plastically deform before failure of its labral attachment, suggesting that some degree of capsular shift is necessary in addition to the Bankart repair.

c. Arthroscopic Treatment—Several techniques for arthroscopic Bankart repair have been developed. Simple debridement of labral injuries has not proved to be effective. Repair using a metal staple, first described by Johnson, has been associated with complications, mainly related to hardware adjacent to the joint. The initial high failure rate of 20% declined to 8% once it was recognized that the shoulder should be immobilized after a repair with this approach. Arthroscopic transglenoid Bankart suture repair (Fig. 4–47 and Color Figure 13), as described by Morgan and popularized by Caspari and others, has become widely used by arthroscopic surgeons. Unfortunately, results have been variable, with failure rates approaching 40% in some long-term follow-up studies. Additionally, the risk of articular cartilage injury, injury to the suprascapular nerve with drilling, and muscle problems with tying of sutures over the infraspinatus muscle make this procedure undesirable. Maki has modified this technique using an intra-articular knot-tying technique to avoid entrapment of adjacent soft tissues (Fig. 4–48). He reported a 93% success rate with this procedure, but transglenoid drilling, with its attendant risk, is still required. Because of these concerns, Warren developed a cannulated, biodegradable fixation device that allows secure soft tissue fixation without some of the risks described earlier. This Suretac device (Acufex Co., Mansfield, MA) can be placed arthroscopically under direct visualization. This device has been adopted for use in cases of TUBS with discrete Bankart lesions and intact capsular tissue. The technique is described next.

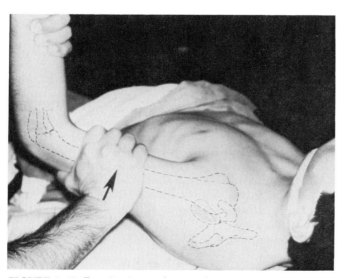

FIGURE 4–45. Examination under anesthesia. Anterior drawer test demonstrating anterior instability with the arm in a neutral position.

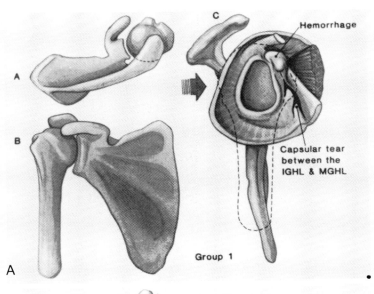

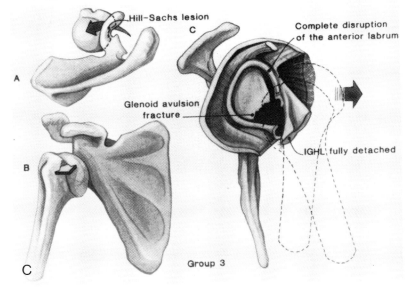

FIGURE 4-46. Classification of shoulder pathology associated with acute dislocations. *A,* In group 1, note capsular tearing without associated labral tear. *B,* Group 2 includes capsular and partial labral tears. *C,* Group 3, capsular and complete labral tear (Bankart), is most common. *A,* Superior view. *B,* AP view. *C,* Sagittal view. (From Baker CL, Uribe JW, Whitman C. Arthroscopic evaluation of acute initial anterior shoulder dislocation. Am J Sports Med 18:25–28, 1990.)

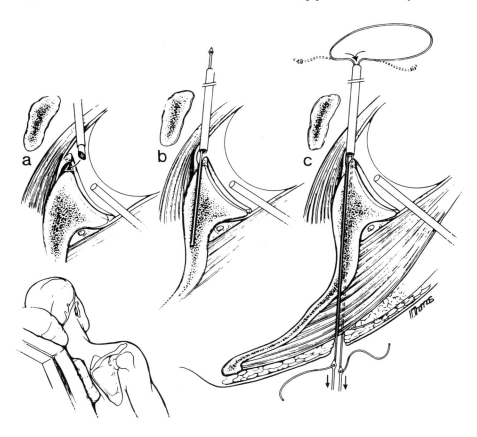

FIGURE 4–47. Transglenoid suture technique of arthroscopic Bankart repair. *a*, Glenoid rim preparation. *b*, Transglenoid drilling. *c*, Suture passage. (From Altchek DW, Warren RF, Skyhar MJ. Shoulder arthroscopy. In Rockwood CA Jr, Matsen FA III [eds]. *The Shoulder*. Philadelphia: WB Saunders, 1990, p 275.)

(1) Suretac Technique (Fig. 4–49 and Color Figure 14)—After examination is conducted under anesthesia and the patient is placed in a modified beach chair position, diagnostic arthroscopy is carried out through a standard posterior portal. The quality and laxity of the glenohumeral ligaments are recorded, and the labrum is examined. If a discrete Bankart lesion is identified and the labral and capsular tissue is of good quality, then arthroscopic stabilization is carried out. Electrocautery, a special sharp-tipped rasp, and a motorized bur are used to extend the Bankart lesion down to the 6 o'clock position (right shoulder) and to prepare a bleeding cancellous bed on the anterior scapular neck. The detached labrum and inferior glenohumeral ligament are pierced with the cannulated drill and guide wire. The drill is advanced into the anterior scapula approximately 1 cm and then carefully removed, leaving the guide wire in place. The tack is then placed over the guide wire and impacted against the bony surface, effectively restoring the labrum and inferior glenohumeral ligament. As with all arthroscopic procedures, one must be willing to convert to open procedures if the capsule is friable, excessively lax, or contracted. Additionally, all patients with multidirectional instability are best treated with an open procedure.

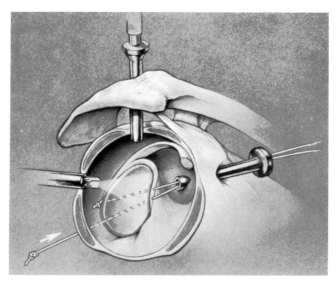

FIGURE 4–48. Modified technique for arthroscopic transglenoid Bankart repair with sutures tied into a knot and then secured to the posterior glenoid rim. (From Maki NJ. Arthroscopic stabilization: suture technique. Op Tech Orthop 1:180–183, 1991.)

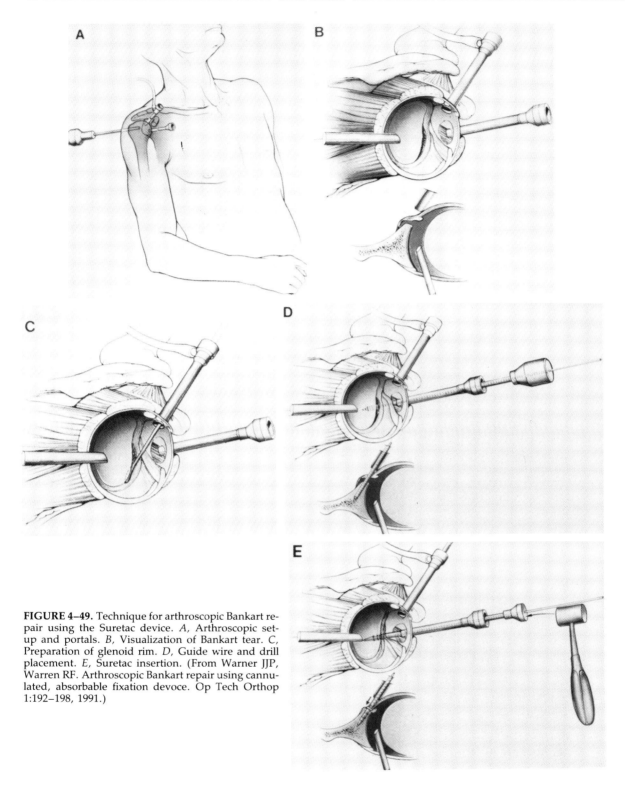

FIGURE 4–49. Technique for arthroscopic Bankart repair using the Suretac device. *A,* Arthroscopic set-up and portals. *B,* Visualization of Bankart tear. *C,* Preparation of glenoid rim. *D,* Guide wire and drill placement. *E,* Suretac insertion. (From Warner JJP, Warren RF. Arthroscopic Bankart repair using cannulated, absorbable fixation devoce. Op Tech Orthop 1:192–198, 1991.)

d. Open Bankart Repair and Capsular Shift—This procedure remains the standard against which arthroscopic procedures are compared, and it is the procedure of choice for patients with multidirectional instability. The Bankart lesion is repaired through drill holes, resulting in an anatomic repair (Fig. 4–50). Modifications of this repair, including the use of suture anchors, are often used because they are technically less difficult. The inferior capsular shift, as described by Neer (Fig. 4–51 and Color Figure 15), is usually performed

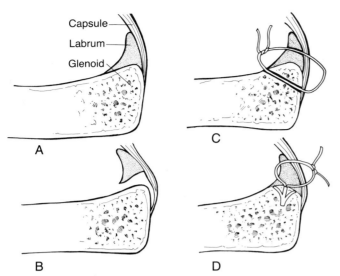

Capsule
Labrum
Glenoid

A
B
C
D

FIGURE 4–50. *A,* Normal relationships of the glenoid and capsulolabral complex. *B,* Bankart injury with stripping of the labrum and capsule. *C,* Bankart repair using the traditional method of placing sutures through drill holes. *D,* Bankart repair with suture anchors.

in conjunction with the Bankart repair to address associated capsular pathology.
D. Posterior Shoulder Instability
1. Introduction—Posterior shoulder dislocation is uncommon but not rare in the athletic population. Posterior subluxation, however, can occur with repeated overuse or after a traumatic episode. Physical examination may reveal pain with forward flexion to 90° along with internal rotation. The shoulder may actually be subluxated in this position. This examination can also be accomplished with the patient supine with a posteriorly directed force applied (posterior apprehension test) (Fig. 4–52). Voluntary instability and associated psychologic disturbance must always be ruled out in patients with this type of instability.
2. Treatment—Initial management includes extensive physical therapy with emphasis on strengthening the external rotators and posterior deltoid. Modifications to throwing including emphasizing the lower extremity during follow-through can also be helpful. Surgical results have traditionally been disappointing, although recent reports are more optimistic. The approach is through a vertically oriented incision and deltoid split. Deep dissection is in the interval between the infraspinatus and teres minor tendon (Fig. 4–53). The association of posterior instability and glenoid retroversion remains unclear, although preoperative CT evaluation may be appropriate in cases in which abnormal version is suspected. Postoperative management con-

sists of 6 weeks of immobilization with the arm 15° abducted and in neutral rotation and 0° flexion (gunslinger brace). Active-assisted range of motion is then initiated, and strengthening commences at 12 weeks. As with anterior procedures, competitive throwing and contact sports are usually delayed 6 to 9 months.

VI. Subacromial Impingement/Rotator Cuff Disease
A. Introduction—Although rotator cuff tears are more common in the older population, impingement and rotator cuff disease are increasingly common in athletes who engage in overhead throwing. Increased forces and repetitive throwing motions can affect the supraspinatus tendon insertion, which is already at risk for attritional injury by virtue of its relatively poor blood supply. Neer identified three stages of subacromial impingement syndrome (Table 4–3). The only difference in athletes who throw is that the age ranges described by Neer are often younger in these athletes. Advances in arthroscopic evaluation and treatment of rotator cuff problems have been applied with some success to athletes who engage in throwing.
B. Presentation—Patients typically present with insidious onset of shoulder pain exacerbated by overhead activities/throwing. The pain may be referred to the deltoid insertion or the midarm. Inspection of the shoulder may demonstrate atrophy of the rotator cuff muscles, but usually only in chronic cases. Pain with forward flexion (impingement sign) that resolves with subacromial lidocaine injection (impingement test) and pain with forward flexion and internal rotation (Hawkins sign) help confirm the diagnosis. Plain radiographs may demonstrate subacromial sclerosis on the AP view. The axillary lateral view is helpful in identifying an unfused os acromionale (Fig. 4–54). The supraspinatus outlet view and 30° caudal tilt view are also helpful in characterizing acromion morphology (see the earlier section on radiology). In young athletes, it is critical to exclude glenohumeral instability in the differential diagnosis. In these cases, the impingement is functional and secondary to the instability. Careful physical examination often resolves this diagnostic dilemma.
C. Treatment
1. Nonoperative Treatment—This is the mainstay of management, particularly in athletes. Activity modification, avoiding repeated motions of the shoulder in which the humerus makes a >10° angle above the scapular spine, and an aggressive rotator cuff strengthening program are initiated. Modification to throwing motions (tilting the thorax to the opposite side) or swimming strokes (emphasizing body roll), as

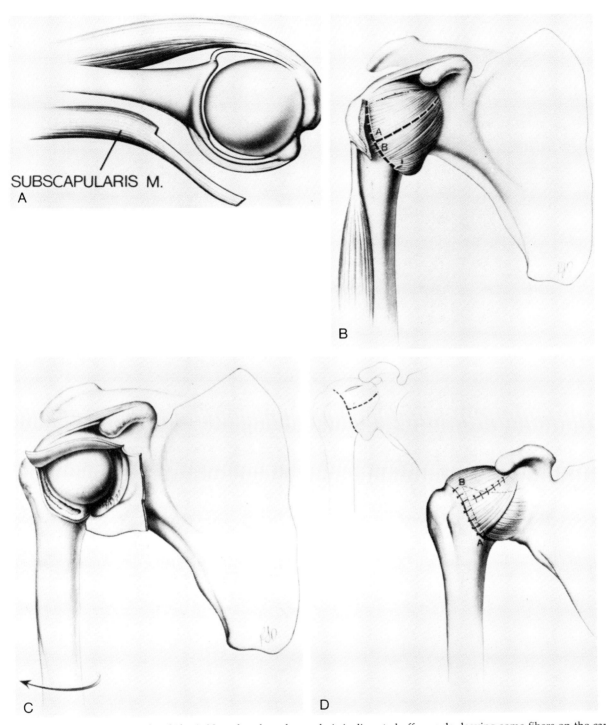

FIGURE 4–51. Anterior-inferior capsular shift. *A*, Note that the subscapularis is dissected off capsule, leaving some fibers on the capsule to make it more amenable to repair. *B*, T incision used in the capsule can be based on the humerus, as shown here, or on the glenoid. *C*, Exposure of the joint is facilitated by external rotation. A Fukuda retractor is placed into the joint to inspect (and repair if necessary) the labrum. *D*, Location of flaps following shift. (Reprinted with permission from Neer CS II, Foster CR. Inferior capsular shift for involuntary inferior and multidirectional instability of the shoulder. A preliminary report. J Bone Joint Surg 62A:897–908, 1980.)

well as pre- and postparticipation stretching, can be helpful in athletes. Various therapeutic modalities such as ultrasound or iontophoresis are sometimes helpful in some patients. Subacromial injection of corticosteroids is often helpful; how-

ever, relief is only temporary. Repetitive injections should be avoided because of the possibility of weakening the tendons.
2. Open Subacromial Decompression— Open subacromial decompression is recommended for patients with persistent im-

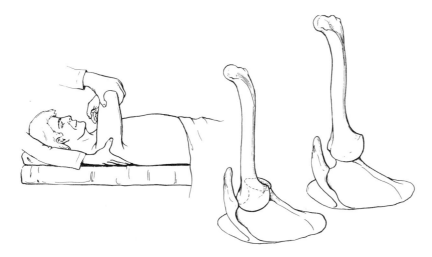

FIGURE 4–52. Posterior apprehension test for posterior instability. (Reprinted with permission from Warner JJP, Caborn DN. Overview of shoulder instability. Crit Rev Phys Rehabil Med 4:145–198, 1992.)

pingement syndrome refractory to 6 months to a year of nonoperative treatment and in conjunction with rotator cuff repair in patients with rotator cuff tears. This procedure involves subperiosteal dissection of the deltoid off of the acromion, excision of

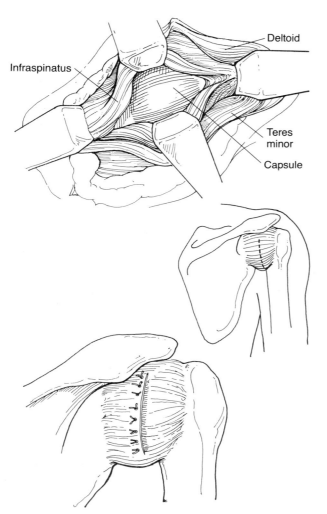

FIGURE 4–53. Posterior capsular shift.

the coracoacromial ligament, and removal of the anterior and inferior portion of the acromion (Fig. 4–55). After completion of the acromioplasty, the rotator cuff is carefully inspected at various degrees of shoulder rotation to ensure that there is no tear. After the rotator cuff tear is addressed (discussed later), the deltoid is repaired back to bone through drill holes, and the subcutaneous tissue and skin are closed in the standard fashion.

3. Arthroscopic Subacromial Decompression—Subacromial bursoscopy is accomplished as described earlier. A bur is introduced through the lateral portal, and systematic resection of the anterior-inferior acromion is accomplished. The goal is to convert a thick (type C) or hooked (type 3) acromion into a thin, flat acromion (Fig. 4–56; see Color Figure 12). After completion of the acromioplasty, the arthroscope can be inserted through the lateral portal and the subacromial space can be directly evaluated with the arms in various degrees of forward flexion.

4. Open Rotator Cuff Repair—After open acromioplasty, the rotator cuff tear is visualized. The torn tendon is mobilized by a combination of blunt and sharp dissection including the bursa, deltoid attachments, coracohumeral ligament, and if necessary, attachments around the periphery of the glenoid (Fig. 4–57). The edge of the torn tendon(s) is debrided with a sharp blade, and sutures are placed into the edge of the mobilized cuff. A bony trough is made at the junction of the articular surface and the greater tuberosity (Fig. 4–58A). Drill holes are placed at least 2 cm distal to the bony trough on the lateral cortex of the proximal humerus, spaced at approximately 1-cm intervals. Sutures are passed from the edge of the cuff into the bony trough using a suture passer (Fig. 4–58B). The sutures are

TABLE 4–3. STAGES OF SUBACROMIAL IMPINGEMENT SYNDROME

Stage	Age	Pathology	Clinical Course	Treatment
I	<25	Edema and hemorrhage	Reversible	Conservative
II	25–40	Fibrosis and tendinitis	Activity-related pain	Therapy/operative
III	>40	AC spur and cuff tear	Progressive disability	Acromioplasty/repair

(From Miller MD. *Review of Orthopaedics*. Philadelphia: WB Saunders, 1992, p 98.)

tied together over the lateral cortex of the humerus. Wound closure is then similar to that described earlier for open subacromial decompression. Revision rotator cuff surgery is more difficult and less successful, especially with poor rotator cuff tissue and a previously detached deltoid.

5. Arthroscopically Assisted Rotator Cuff Repair—This technique, which is possible in relatively acute tears that are easily mobilized, avoids detachment of the deltoid from the acromion and the morbidity associated with the open approach. After arthroscopic acromioplasty, the cuff tear is identified and, using a grasper placed through the lateral portal, assessed for mobility and repairability. PDS sutures are placed in the edge of the tendon using a suture punch (Fig. 4–59 and Color Figure 16) and brought out through the lateral

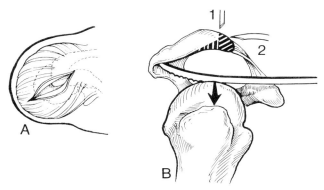

FIGURE 4–55. Technique for open acromioplasty. *A*, Exposure. *B*, Anterior (1) and inferior (2) acromioplasty.

portal. A trough is fashioned at the junction of the humeral head and greater tuberosity using a bur. A longitudinal incision is then made, incorporating the arthroscopic portal, and the deltoid muscle is split longitudinally, staying well proximal to the axillary nerve (usually located 5 cm distal to the lateral acromion) (Fig. 4–60). Sutures are then placed through the bony trough and tied over the lateral cortex of the humerus, as described earlier for the open technique.

D. Subcoracoid Impingement—Patients with excessively long or laterally placed coracoid processes may have impingement of this process on the proximal humerus with forward flexion (120–130°) and internal rotation of the arm. This condition is usually iatrogenic following surgery that causes posterior capsular tightness and loss of internal rotation. Local anesthetic injection should relieve these symptoms. CT with the arms crossed on the chest is helpful in evaluating this unusual disorder. Treatment for chronic symptoms involves resection of the lateral aspect of the coracoid process.

VII. Biceps Tendon Injuries
A. Introduction—The biceps serves as a dynamic and static humeral head depressor. Biceps tendinitis is usually secondary to impingement syndrome; however, isolated biceps tendinitis occasionally occurs without any known precipitating cause. Subluxation of the biceps tendon can occur with disruption of the trans-

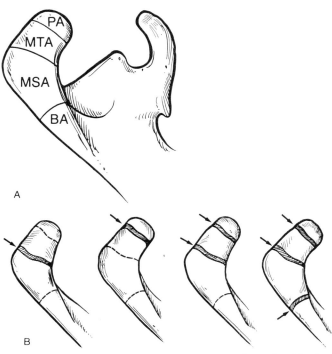

FIGURE 4–54. Acromion ossification centers. Failure of ossification most commonly occurs between the mesoacromion and the metaacromion. It is important to identify os acromiale before acromioplasty. (PA = pre-acromion; MTA = meta-acromion; MSA = mesoacromion; BA = basiacromion.) (From Rockwood CA Jr, Matsen FA III [eds]. *The Shoulder*. Philadelphia: WB Saunders, 1990, p 343.)

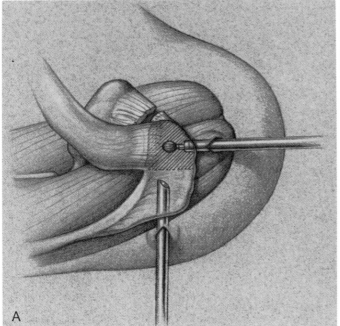

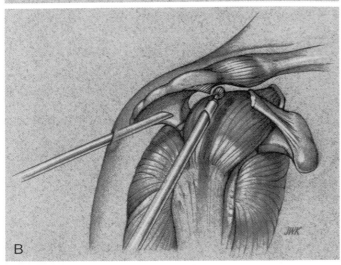

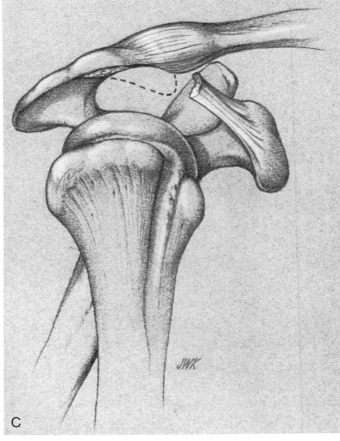

FIGURE 4–56. Technique for arthroscopic acromioplasty. *A,* Superior view. Shaded area represents extent of resection. *B,* Lateral view demonstrating decompression. *C,* Completion of decompressions results in conversion to a type I acromion. (From Harner CD. Arthroscopic subacromial decompression. Op Tech Orthop 1:229–234, 1991.)

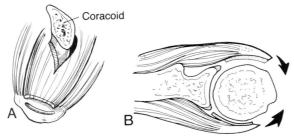

FIGURE 4–57. Techniques for mobilization of the rotator cuff. *A,* Mobilization from the coracoid. *B,* Mobilization from the glenoid labrum. Additional mobilization requires disinsertion-advancement of the affected rotator cuff muscles.

verse humeral ligament, the coracohumeral ligament, or the subscapularis. Rupture of the biceps tendon is unusual in young athletes but can occur in older individuals. Proximal rupture usually gives a characteristic appear-

ance on physical examination ("Popeye" muscle) and rarely requires surgery in and of itself. Distal ruptures do require surgical reattachment and are addressed in Chapter 5. Superior labral injuries, which can disrupt the biceps anchor, have only recently been characterized.

B. Biceps Tendinitis—This is usually caused by concomitant impingement syndrome and rotator cuff tears (especially anterior tears). Additionally, stenosis of the bicipital groove can lead to an attrition tendinitis of the tendon. Physical examination is usually notable for tenderness in the bicipital groove, best identified with the arm internally rotated approximately 10°. The tenderness classically changes with rotation of the arm. The Speed test and Yergason sign (described earlier) can help confirm the diagnosis. Local anesthetic injec-

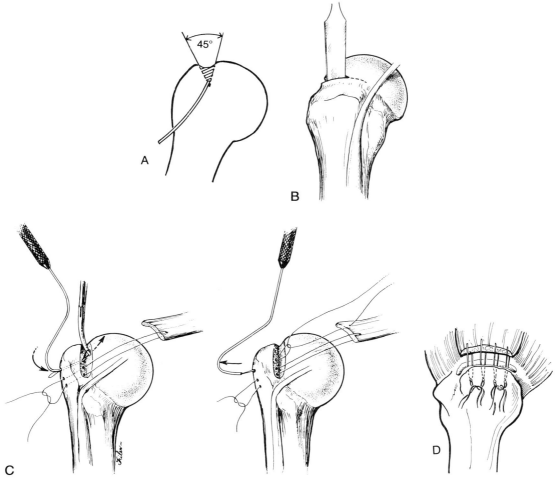

FIGURE 4–58. Technique for open rotator cuff repair. *A,* A bony trough is planned adjacent to the articular surface of the humerus. *B,* An osteotome is used to create a 1-cm-wide trough. *C,* Sutures are passed into the trough. This is facilitated by the use of a suture passer. *D,* Sutures are secured on the lateral cortex of the humerus.

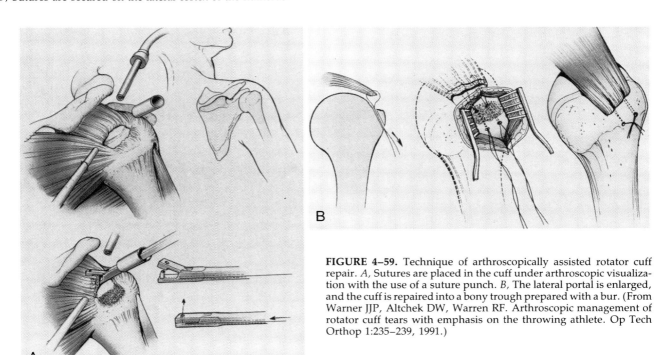

FIGURE 4–59. Technique of arthroscopically assisted rotator cuff repair. *A,* Sutures are placed in the cuff under arthroscopic visualization with the use of a suture punch. *B,* The lateral portal is enlarged, and the cuff is repaired into a bony trough prepared with a bur. (From Warner JJP, Altchek DW, Warren RF. Arthroscopic management of rotator cuff tears with emphasis on the throwing athlete. Op Tech Orthop 1:235–239, 1991.)

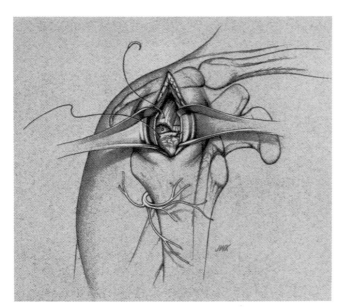

FIGURE 4–60. Longitudinal incision used for rotator cuff repair that avoids detachment of the deltoid. Note the position of the axillary nerve. (From Harner CD. Arthroscopic subacromial decompression. Op Tech Orthop 1:229–234, 1991.)

tion in the area around the tendon should relieve the pain. Radiographs are helpful to evaluate associated impingement. Additionally, a bicipital groove view taken 15° medial to the AP axis, with the patient supine with the arm externally rotated, can help characterize the groove. Initial treatment is nonoperative, including strengthening, various modalities, and local injection (around, not into, the tendon).

Operative treatment almost always involves subacromial decompression. Tenodesis of the biceps tendon into the proximal humerus using the keyhole technique is reserved

for patients with tendinitis that has not responded to prolonged nonoperative management (Fig. 4–61). Younger patients and those whose work requires repetitive forceful supination are more likely to benefit from this procedure. Subacromial decompression is usually performed at the same time because of reports of associated or later development of impingement.

C. Subluxation of the Biceps Tendon—A tear in the medial portion of the coracohumeral ligament or the subscapularis attachment can result in subluxation and medial displacement of the tendon from the bicipital groove. Instability can sometimes be identified by moving the arm from abduction and external rotation to internal rotation while palpating the bicipital groove. The tendon may sublux or dislocate from the groove with a palpable or audible click. Nonoperative treatment is similar to that for tendinitis (described earlier). Operative treatment includes evaluation and treatment of associated impingement and rotator cuff tears. The tendon is reduced into the groove, which is deepened if necessary, and the fibrous roof reconstructed with local tissue.

D. Superior Labral Lesions—Superior labrum anterior posterior (SLAP) lesions have been described by investigators at the Southern California Orthopaedic Institute. These surgeons have identified four varieties of SLAP lesions (Fig. 4–62):

Type	Description	Treatment
I	Fraying with intact anchor	Arthroscopic debridement
II	Detachment of biceps anchor	Arthroscopic/open stabilization

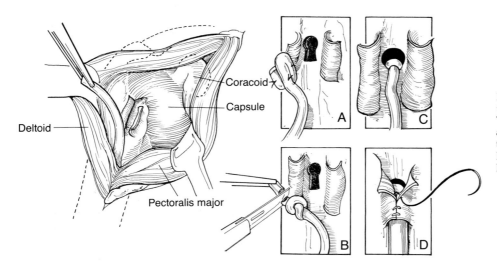

FIGURE 4–61. Reattachment of the biceps tendon using the keyhole technique. *A,* The free edge of the tendon is mobilized, and a keyhole is made with a bur. *B,* The tendon is prepared for placement into the keyhole (*C*). *D,* Repair of the transverse humeral ligament.

Type I

Type II

Type III

Type IV

FIGURE 4–62. Superior labral anterior posterior (SLAP) lesion classification:

I   Fraying with intact anchor
II Detachment of biceps anchor
III Bucket-handle tear of superior labrum, biceps intact
IV Bucket-handle tear of superior labrum into biceps

(From Snyder SJ, Wuh HCK. Arthroscopic evaluation and treatment of the rotator cuff superior labrum anterior posterior lesion. Op Tech Orthop 1:212–213, 1991.)

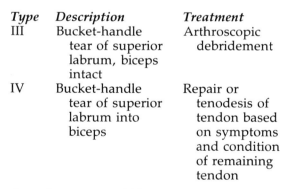

Type	Description	Treatment
III	Bucket-handle tear of superior labrum, biceps intact	Arthroscopic debridement
IV	Bucket-handle tear of superior labrum into biceps	Repair or tenodesis of tendon based on symptoms and condition of remaining tendon

Complex tears, a fifth category, are a result of a combination of one or more of the other four varieties of SLAP lesions. Diagnosis of SLAP lesions is sometimes difficult. Patients often report a history of a compression injury to the shoulder. Acute hyperflexion (as occurs in gymnastics) can sometimes result in a SLAP lesion. Physical examination may demonstrate tenderness with resisted biceps motion, clicking with motion, and a positive Speed test. MRI of SLAP lesions is improving, and gadolinium enhancement may improve its diagnostic accuracy. These lesions are most often identified arthroscopically with inspection and probing (Fig. 4–63).

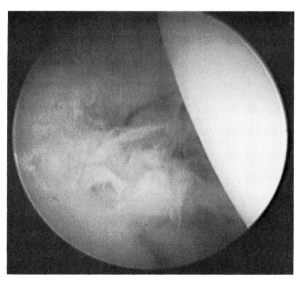

FIGURE 4–63. Arthroscopic view of a type I SLAP lesion before debridement.

VIII. Fractures
  A. Introduction—Although a comprehensive discussion of fractures about the shoulder is beyond the scope of this text, certain fractures are common in athletics and merit some discussion. Greater tuberosity fractures are commonly associated with anterior shoulder dislocation, especially in patients older than 40 years. Humeral shaft fractures can occur with arm wrestling. Clavicle fractures are common in bicyclists. Coracoid fractures can occur in association with AC separations, usually secondary to direct trauma.
  B. Proximal Humeral Fractures—Although these fractures commonly occur in older sedentary individuals, proximal humeral fractures can occur in athletes. The four-part classification scheme of Neer applies in the classification and treatment of these injuries (Fig. 4–64). Displacement of 1 cm or angulation of >45° results in classification as a "part" in this scheme. Treatment includes open reduction and internal fixation of type III and IV fractures in younger individuals and hemiarthroplasty for older patients. Percutaneous stabilization of unstable proximal humeral fractures is also an attractive option. Additionally, it is usually necessary to fix displaced greater tuberosity fractures in younger patients. Lesser tuberosity fractures, which may be associated with posterior dislocations, usually heal without surgical intervention, although one must be aware of the possibility of an associated subscapularis tendon tear (Fig. 4–65).
  C. Scapular Fractures—Fractures of the body of the scapula usually do not require surgical treatment. Treatment of associated injuries (usually pulmonary) should take priority.
  D. Coracoid Fractures—Although these fractures are unusual, they can occur. If they are associated with complete AC injuries, most surgeons favor surgical intervention. These combined injuries can be associated with suprascapular nerve injury, which may require exploration. The fracture can be visualized on Stryker notch or 35° cephalic tilt radiographs. Three-dimensional CT can provide excellent visualization of the fracture (Fig. 4–66).
  E. Clavicle Fractures—As noted, fractures of the clavicle are very common. The vast majority of these fractures can be successfully treated nonoperatively. Some authorities recommend primary open reduction and internal fixation of displaced distal clavicle fractures (Fig. 4–67), but as with grade III AC separations, many surgeons now advocate initial nonoperative management. Indications for primary open repair and fixation include progressive neurovascular compromise, compromised skin integrity after unsuccessful closed reduction, open fractures, floating shoulder, and inability to tolerate closed immobilization. Clavicle nonunion is unusual but can occur. Failure of the fracture to heal within 4 to 6 months may require open reduction and internal fixation with bone grafting. Intercalary iliac crest grafting may be necessary in cases with segmental defects (Fig. 4–68).

IX. Acromioclavicular and Sternoclavicular Injuries
  A. Acromioclavicular Separation—This is a common athletic injury, usually resulting from a fall directly onto the shoulder. The classification scheme described by Rockwood is well accepted (Fig. 4–69). It may sometimes be necessary to obtain stress radiographs with hanging weights in order to demonstrate downward displacement of the affected arm (Fig. 4–70). Treatment of grades I and II injuries includes the use of a sling followed by physical therapy.
  Treatment of grade III injuries remains controversial. Some authorities recommend open reduction and temporary stabilization of the coracoclavicular joint with a screw, pins, suture, or various other techniques, particularly for laborers and noncontact athletes. Most surgeons, however, recommend closed treatment of these injuries. Almost all authorities agree that open treatment is appropriate for types IV, V, and VI injuries. Treatment of chronic symptomatic separations is best accomplished via a modified Weaver-Dunn procedure. This technique basically involves resection of the distal clavicle and transfer of the coracoacromial ligament to the resected end (Fig. 4–71). As in primary repairs, various fixation devices have been proposed to stabilize the repair temporarily. Unfortunately, most of these devices require later removal, usually in the operating room. The use of braided absorbable suture (PDS) as originally

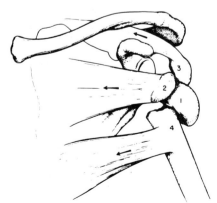

FIGURE 4–64. Neer's four-part classification scheme of proximal humeral fractures: 1 = humeral head; 2 = lesser tuberosity; 3 = greater tuberosity; 4 = shaft. (From Neer CS, Rockwood CA Jr. Fractures and dislocations of the shoulder. In Rockwood CA Jr, Green DP [eds]. *Fractures in Adults.* Philadelphia: JB Lippincott, 1984, p 696.)

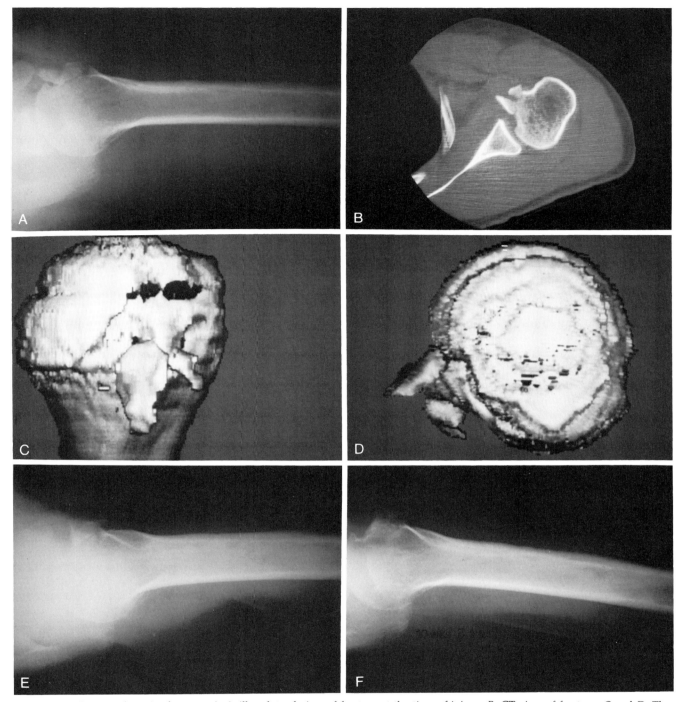

FIGURE 4–65. Lesser tuberosity fracture. *A,* Axillary lateral view of fracture at the time of injury. *B,* CT view of fracture. *C* and *D,* Three-dimensional CT reconstruction of fracture at the time of injury. *E,* Fracture 4 weeks after injury. *F,* Fracture 10 weeks after injury.

described by Hawkins, Warren, and others is favored. This is passed under the coracoid and secured on the superior aspect of the clavicle. This fixation gradually absorbs and provides adequate temporary stability until the reconstructed ligament heals.

B. Distal Clavicle Osteolysis—This condition is common in weight lifters and can follow traumatic injuries. Patients complain of localized pain, aching, and weakness exacerbated by weight lifting. Examination may demonstrate pain with flexion and adduction across the chest. Local injections into the AC joint may at least temporarily relieve the pain. Typical radiographic changes in the distal clavicle include osteopenia, osteolysis, tapering, and cystic changes (Fig. 4–72). Treatment involves activity modification, rest, and nonsteroidal

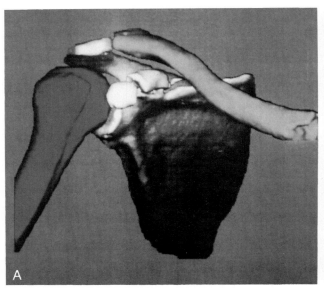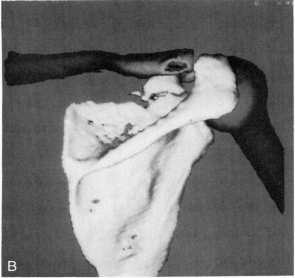

FIGURE 4–66. Three-dimensional CT reconstruction of a coracoid fracture. *A,* Anterior view. *B,* Posterior/superior view.

anti-inflammatory medications. Distal clavicle excision may occasionally be required.

C. Acromioclavicular Degenerative Joint Disease—Arthritis of this joint can be isolated or may occur in conjunction with subacromial impingement syndrome. Examination most often reveals pain with crossed-chest adduction. Injection of the joint with local anesthetic often relieves this pain, and bone scan confirms the diagnosis. Distal clavicle resection is often curative. Reports of arthroscopic distal clavicle resection are encouraging. If an open approach is used, subperiosteal dissection of the deltoid off the clavicle causes less morbid-

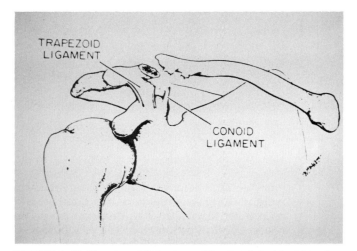

FIGURE 4–67. Neer type IIB fracture of the distal clavicle. Note that the fracture is interligamentous and is associated with displacement of the proximal fragment. (From Neer CS. Fracture of the distal clavicle with detachment of the coracoclavicular ligaments in adults. J Trauma 3:101, 1963.)

ity than dissection off the acromion, because the distal clavicle is removed and the deltoid does not need to be reattached.

D. Sternoclavicular Subluxation/Dislocation—Injuries of the SC joint are unusual but can be serious. These injuries are most commonly caused by motor vehicle accidents but can occur in athletes as a result of direct trauma. Localized tenderness, prominence, or other findings are important. Radiographs should include Hobbs and serendipity views, but a CT should be obtained if there is any question of dislocation. Anterior dislocation is more common than posterior dislocation. Treatment involves closed reduction, which is usually successful. If this fails, open reduction using a sterile towel clip should be attempted. Vascular surgery consultation is important in posterior dislocations because of the risk of vascular injury/entrapment. The use of hardware in and around the SC joint should be avoided because of the significant risk of migration. Patients with spontaneous subluxation of the SC joint should be treated nonoperatively because this is a self-limited condition.

X. Muscle Ruptures
   A. Pectoralis Major Muscle Rupture—Although this is an uncommon injury that usually occurs in weight lifters, numerous cases of this injury have been reported in the literature. As with all tendon ruptures in young athletes, the individual should be questioned about anabolic steroid use. The mechanism of injury is related to excessive tension on a maximally eccentrically contracted muscle. High forces applied to an arm that is extended can result

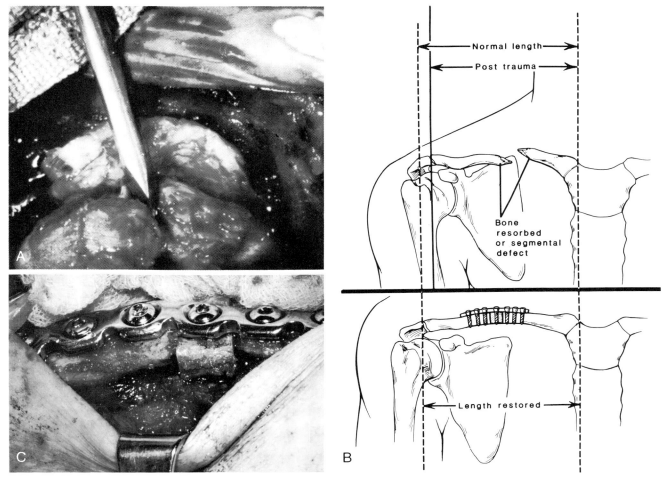

FIGURE 4–68. Technique for open reduction, bone grafting, and internal fixation of a clavicle nonunion. *A*, Surgical exposure. *B*, Measurement of the defect and plan for open reduction and external fixation and segmental bone grafting. *C*, Clinical example of this technique. (*B* from Craig EV. Fractures of the clavicle. In Rockwood CA Jr, Matsen FA III [eds]. *The Shoulder*. Philadelphia: WB Saunders, 1990, p 406.)

in injury. Swelling, a palpable defect, ecchymosis, and weak adduction/internal rotation may be present. Although radiographs may demonstrate the loss of a soft tissue shadow, MRI is the most reliable method to confirm the injury. Surgical repair of complete ruptures to bone through drill holes or suture anchors (Fig. 4–73) is usually necessary.

B. Deltoid Ruptures—Most injuries to the deltoid muscle are strains and partial injuries that occur with repetitive throwing in athletes. These usually respond to ice, mobilization, and therapy. Complete ruptures of the deltoid are unusual, but when they occur, they are usually a result of inadequate repair after rotator cuff surgery. Reconstruction of defects of the deltoid is challenging. These are some of the most debilitating injuries to the shoulder. A deltoidplasty consisting of mobilization and transfer of the middle third of the deltoid anteriorly may improve function in selected cases, but the deltoid should be carefully repaired back to bone after any procedure in which it is dissected.

C. Triceps Rupture—This injury is also unusual and may be associated with systemic illness (e.g., renal osteodystrophy). Repair of the avulsion back to bone has been successful in the limited cases reported.

D. Subscapularis Rupture—This injury has been described in connection with recurrent dislocations; however, isolated tears can occur without instability. These ruptures usually result from trauma in patients who are younger than those typically developing degenerative rotator cuff tears. Several physical examination findings are diagnostic: increased passive external rotation, weak internal rotation (Fig. 4–74), and a "lift-off" sign (Fig. 4–75). MRI or ultrasonography may be helpful to confirm the diagnosis. In most cases, surgical treatment is appropriate, although this can be technically difficult owing to the need to mobilize the axillary nerve.

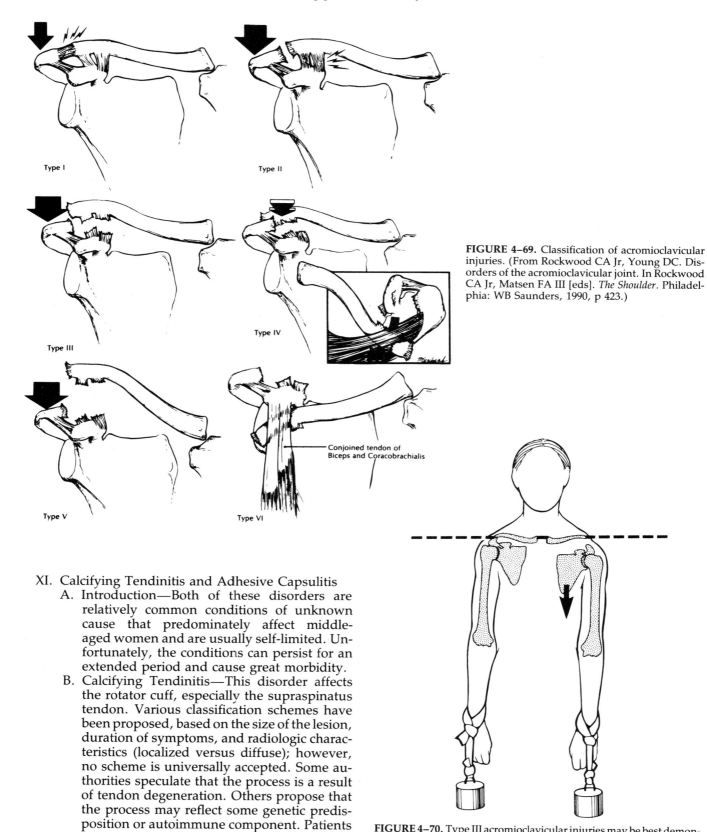

FIGURE 4–69. Classification of acromioclavicular injuries. (From Rockwood CA Jr, Young DC. Disorders of the acromioclavicular joint. In Rockwood CA Jr, Matsen FA III [eds]. *The Shoulder*. Philadelphia: WB Saunders, 1990, p 423.)

Type I

Type II

Type III

Type IV

Type V

Type VI

Conjoined tendon of Biceps and Coracobrachialis

XI. Calcifying Tendinitis and Adhesive Capsulitis
   A. Introduction—Both of these disorders are relatively common conditions of unknown cause that predominately affect middle-aged women and are usually self-limited. Unfortunately, the conditions can persist for an extended period and cause great morbidity.
   B. Calcifying Tendinitis—This disorder affects the rotator cuff, especially the supraspinatus tendon. Various classification schemes have been proposed, based on the size of the lesion, duration of symptoms, and radiologic characteristics (localized versus diffuse); however, no scheme is universally accepted. Some authorities speculate that the process is a result of tendon degeneration. Others propose that the process may reflect some genetic predisposition or autoimmune component. Patients complain of pain late in the process, during the so-called resorptive phase. Radiographs typically demonstrate calcification within the soft tissue of the rotator cuff (Fig. 4–76). Nonoperative treatment is usually successful.

FIGURE 4–70. Type III acromioclavicular injuries may be best demonstrated by measuring the distance between the coracoid and clavicle on bilateral AP radiographs of the shoulder with 10 to 15 pounds of weights hanging from both arms. (From Rockwood CA Jr, Young DC. Disorders of the acromioclavicular joint. In Rockwood CA Jr, Matsen FA III [eds]. *The Shoulder*. Philadelphia: WB Saunders, 1990, p 421.)

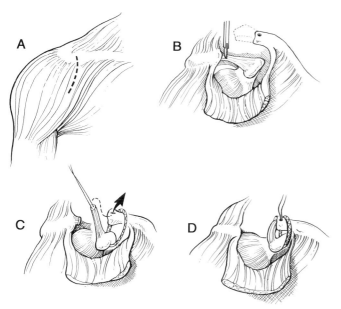

FIGURE 4–71. Weaver-Dunn procedure for symptomatic chronic acromioclavicular separations. *A,* Skin incision. *B,* Distal clavicle resection. *C,* Mobilization of the coracoacromial ligament and fixation of the clavicle to the coracoid. *D,* Transfer and fixation of the coarcoacromial ligament to the clavicle.

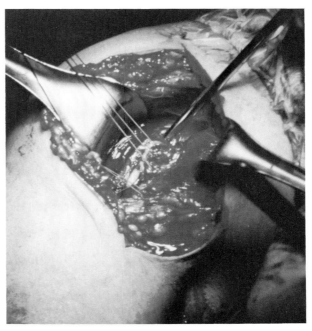

FIGURE 4–73. Repair of pectoralis major avulsion using suture anchors. (From Miller MD, Johnson DA, Theate LA, et al. Rupture of the pectoralis major tendon in a football player. Am J Sports Med 21:475–477, 1993.)

Physical therapy is important, and modalities such as ultrasound and iontophoresis can be helpful. Some authorities have recommended needling and local anesthetic injection. The efficacy of local steroid injection is controversial. Radiotherapy has also been reported to have mixed results. Surgery, consisting of removal of the calcific deposit, usually through a deltoid-splitting approach, has been reported to have a high success rate. Bursoscopy has also been advocated to remove the depos-

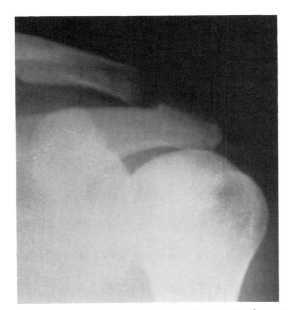

FIGURE 4–72. Distal clavicle osteolysis. Note cystic changes and osteopenia of distal clavicle.

its. All authors describe the deposits as being chalky or like toothpaste. Early mobilization after surgery is important to success.

C. Adhesive Capsulitis
  1. Introduction—Commonly referred to by the inaccurate term *frozen shoulder,* adhesive capsulitis is also a disorder of unknown cause and is characterized clinically by pain and a restricted range of active and passive glenohumeral motion. The diagnosis can be confirmed after other conditions that mimic adhesive capsulitis are ruled out, including posterior dislocation of the shoulder, ruptured rotator cuff, severe impingement, cervical arthritis, Pancoast tumor, and neuromuscular disease. Adhesive capsulitis is the end result of an inflammatory reaction of the shoulder joint and capsule, leading to a stiff and painful shoulder. Factors associated with the development of adhesive capsulitis include trauma following chest or breast surgery, diabetes, prolonged immobilization, thyroid disease, and various medical problems (e.g., pulmonary disease, myocardial infarction, cerebrovascular accident). Much like calcific tendinitis, the disease may have a genetic focus or autoimmune component. The pathology of adhesive capsulitis has been characterized as chronic inflammation, fibrosis, and perivascular inflammation of the subsynovial layer of the capsule, suggesting an overreactive reparative inflammatory process.

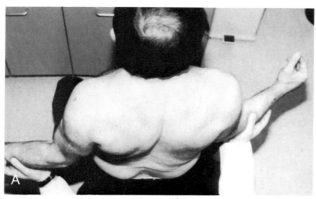
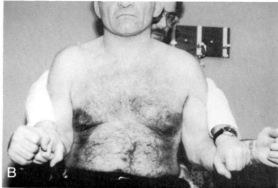

FIGURE 4–74. Patient with a subscapularis tendon rupture demonstrating (A) increased external rotation and (B) internal rotation weakness.

2. Disease Stages
   a. Clinical Stages—Three stages of idiopathic adhesive capsulitis are generally recognized: (1) a painful phase characterized by gradual onset of diffuse shoulder pain, (2) a stiffening phase with a gradual decrease in range of motion, affecting activities of daily living, and (3) a thawing phase characterized by a gradual return of motion. These stages can often be prolonged, lasting for years.
   b. Arthroscopic Stages—Neviaser has arthroscopically evaluated many patients with adhesive capsulitis and has

characterized the process as having four stages:

Stage 1 is characterized by a patchy fibrinous synovitis, existing primarily in the dependent fold area without capsular contracture.

Stage 2 is associated with capsular contraction, fibrinous adhesions, and synovitis.

Stage 3 is typified by increased capsular contraction but resolving synovitis.

Stage 4 is identified as severe capsular contraction without any other intra-articular process.

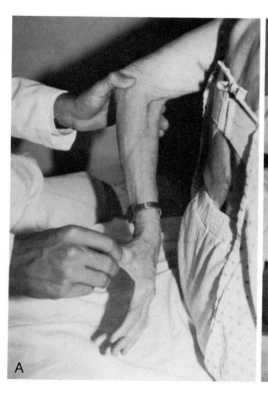
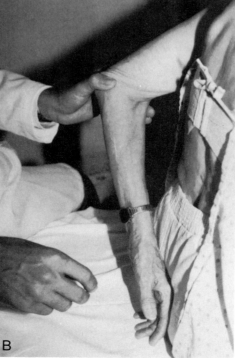

FIGURE 4–75. Positive lift-off sign. *A*, Patient with a subscapularis tendon tear is positioned. *B*, Patient is unable to hold the arm in the prior position or to lift it away from the back.

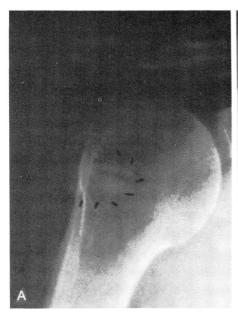
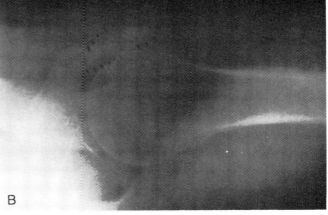

FIGURE 4–76. *A,* AP and *B,* Axillary lateral radiographs demonstrating calcific tendinitis near the subscapularis insertion on the lesser tuberosity. (From Re P, Karzel RP. Management of rotator cuff calcificatons. Orthop Clin North Am 24:128, 1993.)

3. Imaging—Radiographic findings in frozen shoulder are often minimal. Osteopenia and mild arthritic changes are sometimes noted, but early radiographs may appear normal. Nevertheless, it is important to obtain AP and axillary lateral views of the affected shoulder to rule out other shoulder disorders. The axillary view may help preclude unrecognized dislocations, fractures, and locking osteophytes. Technetium bone scan results are often diffusely positive but are nonspecific and are of little use in a clinical setting. Shoulder arthrography demonstrates a significant reduction in the capsular volume and loss of the normal axillary recess (Fig. 4–77).

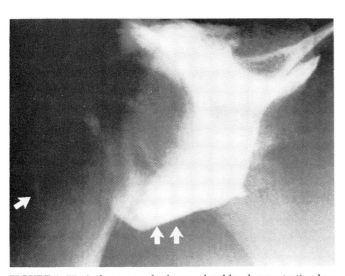

FIGURE 4–77. Arthrogram of a frozen shoulder demonstrating loss of axillary fold (*double arrows*). (From Rockwood CA, Matsen FA III [eds]. *The Shoulder.* Philadelphia: WB Saunders, 1990, p 819.)

4. Treatment—Treatment options that have been reported for adhesive capsulitis include local steroids, oral steroids, physical therapy, nerve stimulation, manipulations, ultrasound, acupuncture, infiltration brisement, arthroscopy, and open surgery. Treatment of adhesive capsulitis continues to be a matter of debate; however, many authorities suggest that this disease is self-limited. Manipulation under anesthesia may be required for severe cases of adhesive capsulitis, when motion is limited to <90° of flexion or 0° of external rotation despite 3 to 6 months of physical therapy. The role of arthroscopy in frozen shoulder has not yet been established.

XII. Nerve Disorders
    A. Brachial Plexus Injury—Brachial plexus injuries are unfortunately an all too common occurrence in sports, especially football. The mechanism of injury usually is related to tackling or falling on shoulder and neck (Fig. 4–78). One study, however, suggests that the mechanism of injury more commonly involves compression of the fixed brachial plexus between the shoulder pad and the superior medial scapula when the pad is compressed into the area of Erb's point (just superior to the clavicle). These injuries, commonly called "burners" or "stingers," are usually transient, lasting only a few seconds. Evaluation of affected players should include a complete neurologic examination and cervical spine radiographs (including flexion and extension views). Complete resolution of symptoms is required before returning to play. Recurrent episodes of burners can be a difficult problem, and cervical MRI and electrodiag-

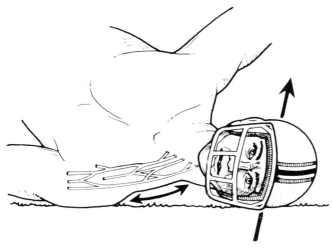

FIGURE 4–78. Mechanism of injury for brachial plexus traction injury. Contact force with the ground (*single-headed arrow*) causing traction on the plexus (*double-headed arrow*). (From Rowe CR [ed]. *The Shoulder.* New York: Churchill Livingstone, 1988, p 419.)

nostic studies may be appropriate. More serious injuries of the brachial plexus are uncommon in sports, with the exception of motorcycle riding. Root avulsions (loss of serratus anterior, rhomboids, deltoid, and rotator cuff muscles) are associated with a poor prognosis. Distal ruptures of the upper trunk may be amenable to nerve grafting or tendon transfers.

B. Thoracic Outlet Syndrome—This disorder is caused by compression of the nerves and vessels to the upper limb where they pass through the scalene muscles and first rib. This condition can be associated with a cervical rib, scapular ptosis, and scalene muscle abnormalities. Patients often complain of pain and paresthesias, usually in an ulnar distribution. The Adson/Wright test and the abduction stress test (described previously) may be helpful in making the diagnosis. Muscle strengthening and postural training can be helpful. Surgical treatment is occasionally indicated for refractory cases and involves scalene muscle release and first rib resection. First rib resection does have some risks, including pneumothorax, vascular injury, and severe causalgia.

C. Long Thoracic Nerve Palsy—Injury to this nerve results in scapular winging due to serratus anterior dysfunction. This condition is relatively common in competitive swimmers. Simple observation is usually called for, because many of these injuries spontaneously resolve. Treatment with a modified thoracolumbar brace with a scapular pad may be effective because it allows the nerve to regenerate by avoiding scapular winging and recurrent traction. For chronic palsies that do not recover and that are significantly bothersome to patients, pectoralis major transfer has had some success.

D. Suprascapular Nerve Compression—The suprascapular nerve can be compressed by various structures including a ganglion or fracture callus in the area of the transverse suprascapular ligament. Weakness and atrophy of the supraspinatus and infraspinatus result, along with pain over the shoulder (Fig. 4–79). Electrodiagnostic studies can confirm the clinical diagnosis. MRI can also be helpful in certain circumstances. Surgical release of the ligament and removal of any other impinging lesions can be performed through a transverse incision with splitting of the trapezius. The suprascapular nerve can also be injured with mobilization of chronic retracted tears of the rotator cuff.

E. Other Nerve Injuries—Other injuries, including those of the axillary nerve, the spinal accessory nerve, and the musculocutaneous nerves, are usually the result of a surgical insult to these structures. Several months of observation is appropriate before considering exploration and repair of the affected nerve. Tendon transfers for permanent trapezius palsy include the Eden-Lange procedure, which transfers the levator scapulae and rhomboids.

XIII. Other Shoulder Disorders
A. Glenohumeral Degenerative Joint Disease—Although degenerative joint disease is more common in older patients, athletes who engage in throwing may develop arthritis at a younger age than usual. Arthritis may also be associated with other shoulder disorders, including instability and rotator cuff disease. Certain iatrogenic factors may also contribute to the development of osteoarthritis of the shoulder, including the use of hardware in

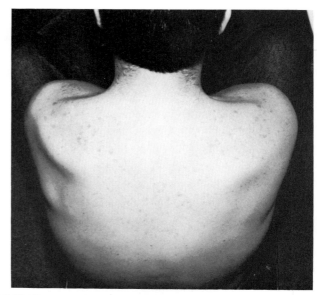

FIGURE 4–79. Infraspinatus atrophy demonstrated in a patient with left suprascapular nerve entrapment.

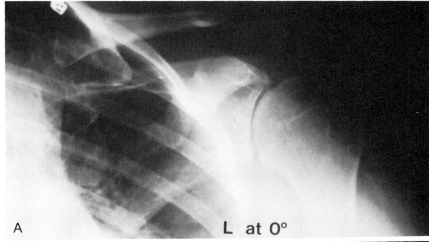

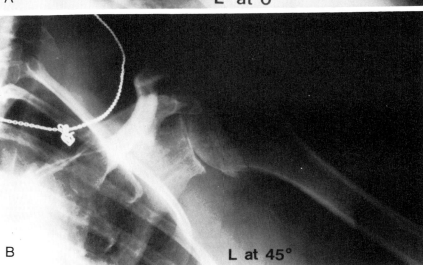

FIGURE 4–80. Neutral (*A*) and 45° abduction (*B*) AP radiograph of a shoulder demonstrating glenohumeral arthritis.

and around the shoulder and overtightening of the shoulder capsule during shoulder reconstruction. Radiographs, including a true AP film taken in abduction, can be helpful in characterizing the amount of arthritis (Fig. 4–80). In some cases, arthroscopic debridement of the shoulder may be a temporizing measure before considering other more invasive forms of surgery. Because the shoulder is not considered a weight-bearing joint, this form of treatment may have more success than in the knee.

B. Snapping Scapula—This unusual disorder can be caused by abnormalities of the scapula itself or by inflammation of the bursa between the scapula and the thoracic rib cage. Patients occasionally reproduce this snapping voluntarily, and treatment of these individuals simply involves encouraging them not to do this. Other patients may respond to scapular strengthening exercises, local injections, or other forms of treatment. Reports of resection of the medial border of the scapula, usually done in conjunction with bursal debridement, are encouraging.

C. Reflex Sympathetic Dystrophy—As in the knee, this condition can be difficult for the patient and physician alike.

Selected References

Basic Sciences

Bigliani LU, Pollock RG, Soslowsky LJ, et al. Tensile properties of the inferior glenohumeral ligament. J Orthop Res 10:187–197, 1992.

Blasier RB, Guldberg RE, Rothman ED. Anterior shoulder stability: contributions of rotator cuff forces and the capsular ligaments in a cadaver model. J Shoulder Elbow Surg 1:140–150, 1992.

Clark JM, Harryman DT II. Tendons, ligaments, and capsule of the rotator cuff. Gross and microscopic anatomy. J Bone Joint Surg 74A:713–725, 1992.

Cooper DE, Arnoczsky SP, O'Brien SJ, et al. Anatomy, histology, and vascularity of the glenoid labrum. J Bone Joint Surg 74A:46–52, 1992.

Cooper DE, O'Brien SJ, Arnoczky SP, Warren RF. The structure and function of the coracohumeral ligament. An anatomic and microscopic study. J Shoulder Elbow Surg 2:70–77, 1993.

Cooper DE, O'Brien SJ, Warren RF. Supporting layers of the glenohumeral joint: an anatomic study. Clin Orthop 289:144–155, 1993.

Cooper DE, Warner JJP, Deng X, et al. Anatomy and function of the coracohumeral ligament. J Bone Joint Surg 74B(suppl 1):90, 1992.

Ferrari DA. Capsular ligaments of the shoulder. Anatomical and functional study of the anterior superior capsule. Am J Sports Med 18:20–24, 1990.

Flatow EL. The biomechanics of the acromioclavicular, sternoclavicular, and scapulothoracic joints. Instr Course Lect 42:237–245, 1993.

Gibb TD, Sidler JA, Thompson DJ II, et al. An effect of capsular venting on glenohumeral laxity. Clin Orthop 268:120, 1991.

Harryman DT II. Common surgical approaches to the shoulder. Instr Course Lect 41:3–11, 1992.

Howell SM, Galinat BJ. The glenoid-labral socket. A constrained articular surface. Clin Orthop 243:122, 1989.

Iannotti JP, Gabriel JP, Schneck SL, et al. The normal glenohumeral relationships. An anatomical study of one hundred and forty shoulders. J Bone Joint Surg 74A:491–500, 1992.

Jobe CM. Gross anatomy of the shoulder. In Rockwood CA Jr, Matsen FA III (eds). The Shoulder. Philadelphia: WB Saunders, 1990, pp 34–97.

Jobe FW, Tibone JE, Perry J, Moynes D. An EMG analysis of the shoulder in throwing and pitching. Am J Sports Med 11:3–5, 1983.

Kumar VP, Balasubramaniam P. The role of atmospheric pressure in stabilizing the shoulder: an experimental study. J Bone Joint Surg 67B:719, 1985.

Morrey BF, An K-N. Biomechanics of the shoulder. In Rockwood CA Jr, Matsen FA III (eds). The Shoulder. Philadelphia: WB Saunders, 1990, pp 209–245.

O'Brien SJ, Neves MC, Rozbruch, SR, et al. The anatomy and histology of the inferior glenohumeral ligament complex of the shoulder. Am J Sports Med 18:449, 1990.

O'Connell PW, Nuber GW, Mileski RA, Lautenschlager E. The contribution of the glenohumeral ligaments to anterior stability of the shoulder joint. Am J Sports Med 18:579–584, 1990.

Saha AK. Dynamic stability of the glenohumeral joint. Acta Orthop Scand 42:491, 1971.

Sarrafian SK. Gross and functional anatomy of the shoulder. Clin Orthop 173:11, 1983.

Shaffer BS, Conway J, Jobe FW, et al. Infraspinatus muscle-splitting incision in posterior shoulder surgery. An anatomic and electromyographic study. Am J Sports Med 22:113–120, 1994.

Soslowsky LJ, Flatow EL, Bigliani LU, Mow VC. Articular geometry of the glenohumeral joint. Clin Orthop 285:181–190, 1992.

Warner JJP. The gross anatomy of the joint surfaces, ligaments labrum, and capsule. In Matsen FA III, Fu FH, Hawking RJ (eds). The Shoulder: A Balance of Mobility and Stability. Rosemont, IL: American Academy of Orthopaedic Surgeons, 1993, pp 7–28.

Warner JJP, Caborn DN. Overview of shoulder instability. Crit Phys Rehabil Med 4:145–198, 1992.

Warner JJP, Caborn DNM, Berger R, et al. Dynamic capsuloligamentous anatomy of the glenohumeral joint. J Shoulder Elbow Surg 2:115–133, 1993.

Warner JJP, Deng XH, Warren RF, Torzilli PA. Static capsuloligamentous restraints to superior-inferior translation of the glenohumeral joint. Am J Sports Med 20:675–685, 1992.

Warner JJP, Deng X, Warren RF, Torzilli PA. Superior-inferior translation in the intact and vented glenohumeral joint. J Shoulder Elbow Surg 2:99–105, 1993.

Warner JJP, Micheli LJ, Arslanian LE, et al. Scapulothoracic motion in normal shoulders and shoulders with glenohumeral instability and impingement syndrome: a study using Moire topographic analysis. Clin Orthop 285:191–199, 1992.

History and Physical Examination

Gerber C, Ganz R. Clinical assessment of instability of the shoulder with special reference to anterior and posterior drawer tests. J Bone Joint Surg 66B:551–556, 1984.

Hawkins R, Bokor DJ. Clinical evaluation of shoulder problems. In Rockwood CA Jr, Matsen FA III (eds). The Shoulder. Philadelphia: WB Saunders, 1990, pp 149–177.

Hawkins RJ, Hobeika P. Physical examination of the shoulder. Orthopedics 6:1270–1278, 1983.

Hawkins RJ, Mohtadi NGH. Clinical evaluation of shoulder instability. Clin J Sports Med 1:59–64, 1991.

Hoppenfeld S. Physical Examination of the Spine and Extremities. Norwalk, CT: Appleton-Century-Crofts, 1976.

Neer CS, Welsh RP. The shoulder in sports. Orthop Clin North Am 8:583–591, 1977.

Poppen NK, Walker PS. Normal and abnormal motion of the shoulder. J Bone Joint Surg 58A:195–201, 1976.

Yergason RM. Supination sign. J Bone Joint Surg 13A:160, 1931.

Radiography of the Shoulder

Beltran J. The use of magnetic resonance imaging about the shoulder. J Shoulder Elbow Surg 1:287–295, 1992.

Bigliani LU, Morrison D, April EW. The morphology of the acromion and its relationship to rotator cuff tears. Orthop Trans 10:228, 1986.

Engebretsen L, Craig EV. Radiologic features of shoulder instability. Clin Orthop 291:29–44, 1993.

Garth WP Jr, Slappey CE, Ochs CW. Roentgenographic demonstration of instability of the shoulder: the apical oblique projection—a technical note. J Bone Joint Surg 66A: 1450–1453, 1984.

Hall RH, Isaac F, Booth CR. Dislocations of the shoulder with special reference to accompanying small fractures. J Bone Joint Surg 41A:489–494, 1959.

Hill HA, Sachs MD. The grooved defect of the humeral head: a frequently unrecognized complication of dislocations of the shoulder joint. Radiology 35:690–700, 1940.

Hobbs DW. Sternoclavicular joint: a new axial radiographic view. Radiology 90:801–802, 1968.

Jahnke AH, Petersen SA, Neumann C, et al: A prospective comparison of computerized arthrotomography and magnetic resonance imaging of the glenohumeral joint. Am J Sports Med 20:695–701, 1992.

Kozo O, Yamamuro T, Rockwood CA. Use of a thirty-degree caudal tilt radiograph in the shoulder impingement syndrome. J Shoulder Elbow Surg 1:246–252, 1992.
Recht MP, Resnick D. Instructional Course Lectures: magnetic resonance imaging studies of the shoulder. Diagnosis of lesions of the rotator cuff. J Bone Joint Surg 75A:1244–1253, 1993.
Rockwood CA Jr, Green DP, Bucholz RW. Rockwood and Green's Fractures in Adults. 3rd ed. Philadelphia: JB Lippincott, 1991.
Rockwood CA Jr, Szalay EA, Curtis RJ, et al. X-ray evaluation of shoulder problems. In Rockwood Ca Jr, Matsen FA III (eds). The Shoulder. Philadelphia: WB Saunders, 1990, pp 178–207.
Rokous JR, Feagin JA, Abbott HG. Modified axillary roentgenogram. Clin Orthop 82:84–86, 1972.
Zanca P. Shoulder pain: involvement of the acromioclavicular joint. Analysis of 1000 cases. AJR 112:493–506, 1971.

Shoulder Arthroscopy

Altchek DW, Warren RF, Skyhar MJ. Shoulder arthroscopy. In Rockwood CA Jr, Matsen FA III (eds). The Shoulder. Philadelphia: WB Saunders, 1990, pp 258–277.
Caborn DM, Fu FH. Arthroscopic approach and anatomy of the shoulder. Op Tech Orthop 1:126–133, 1991.
Fu FH, Harner CD. Overview of shoulder arthroscopy: procedure selection. Op Tech Orthop 1:123–125, 1991.
Nisbet JK, Paulos LE. Subacromial bursoscopy. Op Tech Orthop 1:221–228, 1991.
Skyhar MJ, Altchek DW, Warren RF, et al. Shoulder arthroscopy with the patient in the beach chair position. Arthroscopy 4:256–259, 1988.
Souryal TO, Baker CL. Anatomy of the supraclavicular portal in shoulder arthroscopy. Arthroscopy 6:297–300, 1990.
Warner JJP. Shoulder arthroscopy in the beach-chair position: basic setup. Op Tech Orthop 1:147–154, 1991.
Wolf EM. Anterior portals in shoulder arthroscopy. Arthroscopy 5:201–208, 1989.

Shoulder Instability

Altchek DW, Warren RF, Skyhar MJ. Shoulder arthroscopy. In Rockwood CA Jr, Matsen FA III (eds). The Shoulder. Philadelphia: WB Saunders, 1990, pp 258–277.
Altchek DW, Warren RF, Skyhar MJ, Ortiz G. T-plasty modification of the Bankhart procedure for multidirectional instability of the anterior and inferior types. J Bone Joint Surg 73A:105–112, 1991.
Altchek DW, Warren RD, Wickiewicz TL, Ortiz G. Arthroscopic labral debridement. A three-year follow-up study. Am J Sports Med 20:702–706, 1992.
Arciero RA, Wheeler JH III, Ryan JB, McBride JT. Arthroscopic Bankart repair for acute, initial anterior shoulder dislocations (paper 308). American Academy of Orthopaedic Surgeons, 60th Annual Meeting, San Francisco, CA, February 1993.
Baker CL, Uribe JW, Whitman C. Arthroscopic evaluation of acute initial anterior shoulder dislocations. Am J Sports Med 18:25–28, 1990.
Bankart ASB. The pathology and treatment of recurrent dislocation of the shoulder joint. Br J Surg 26:23–29, 1939.
Burkhead WZ, Rockwood CA Jr. Treatment of instability of the shoulder with an exercise program. J Bone Joint Surg 74A:890–896, 1992.
Caspari RB. Arthroscopic stabilization for shoulder instability. Operative Techniques in Shoulder Surgery. Gaithersburg, MD: Aspen, 1991, pp 57–63.
Cofield RH, Nessler JP, Weinstable R. Diagnosis of shoulder instability by examination under anesthesia. Clin Orthop 291:45–53, 1993.
Cooper RA, Brems JJ. The inferior capsular shift procedure for multi-directional instability of the shoulder. J Bone Joint Surg 74A:1516–1521, 1992.
Detrisac DA. Arthroscopic shoulder staple capsulorrhaphy for traumatic anterior instability. In McGinty JB (ed). Operative Arthroscopy. New York: Raven Press, 1991.
Fronich J, Warren RF, Bowen MK. Posterior subluxation of the glenohumeral joint. J Bone Joint Surg 71A:205–211, 1989.
Glasgow SG, Bruce RA, Yacobucci JN, Torg JS. Arthroscopic resection of glenoid labral tears in the athlete: A report of 29 cases. Arthroscopy 8:23–30, 1992.
Grana WA, Buckley PD, Yates CK. Arthroscopic Bankart suture repair. Am J Sports Med 21:348–353, 1993.
Harryman DT II, Sidles JA, Harris SL, Matsen FA III. Laxity of the normal glenohumeral joint: a quantitative in-vivo assessment. J Shoulder Elbow Surg 1:66–76, 1992.
Hawkins RB. Arthroscopic stapling repair for shoulder instability: a retrospective study of 50 cases. Arthroscopy 5:122–128, 1989.
Hovelius L. Anterior dislocation of the shoulder in teenagers and young adults: five-year prognosis. J Bone Joint Surg 69A:393–399, 1987.
Hovelius L, Thorling J, Fredin H. Recurrent anterior dislocation of the shoulder. Results after the Bankart and Putti-Platt operations. J Bone Joint Surg 61A:566–569, 1979.
Hurley JA, Anderson TE, Dear W, et al. Posterior shoulder instability. Surgical versus conservative results with evaluation of glenoid version. Am J Sports Med 20:396–400, 1992.
Ioti E, Motzkin NE, Morrey BF, An KN. Scapular inclination and inferior stability of the shoulder. J Shoulder Elbow Surg 1:131–139, 1992.
Lippit S, Matsen FA III. Mechanisms of glenohumeral joint stability. Clin Orthop 291:20–28, 1993.
Lyons FA, Rockwood CA Jr. Current concepts review. Migration of pins used in operations on the shoulder. J Bone Joint Surg 72A:1262–1267, 1990.
Maki NJ. Arthroscopic stabilization: suture technique. Op Tech Orthop 1:180–183, 1991.
Mallon WJ. Shoulder instability. In Frymoyer JW (ed). Orthopaedic Knowledge Update 4: Home Study Syllabus. 1993, pp 297–302. Rosemont IL: American Academy of Orthopaedic Surgeons.
Matthews LS, Vetter WL, Oweida SJ, et al. Arthroscopic staple capsulorrhaphy for recurrent anterior shoulder instability. Arthroscopy 4:106–111, 1988.
Morgan CD, Bodenstab AB. Arthroscopic Bankart suture repair; techniques and early results. Arthroscopy 3:111–112, 1982.

Neer CS II, Foster CR. Inferior capsular shift for involuntary inferior and multidirectional instability of the shoulder. A preliminary report. J Bone Joint Surg 62A:897–908, 1980.

Paulos LE, Evans IK, Pinkowski JL. Anterior and anterior-inferior shoulder instability. Treatment by glenoid labrum reconstruction and a modified capsular shift procedure. J Shoulder Elbow Surg 2:275–285, 1993.

Perthes G. Uber Operationen bei Habitueller Schulterluxation. Dtsch Z Chir 85:199–227, 1906.

Protzman RR. Anterior instability of the shoulder. J Bone Joint Surg 62A:909–918.

Rowe CR, Patel D, Southmayd WW. The Bankart procedure—a long-term end-result study. J Bone Joint Surg 55A:445–460, 1973.

Rowe CR, Sakellarides HT. Factors related to recurrences of anterior dislocation of the shoulder. Clin Orthop 20:40–47, 1961.

Rubenstein DL, Jobe FW, Glousman RE, et al. Anterior capsulolabral reconstruction of the shoulder in athletes. J Shoulder Elbow Surg 1:229–237, 1992.

Simonet WT, Cofield RH. Prognosis in anterior shoulder dislocation. Am J Sports Med 12:19–24, 1984.

Small NC. Complications in arthroscopic surgery performed by experienced arthroscopists. Arthroscopy 4:215–221, 1988.

Turkel SJ, Panio MW, Marshall JL, et al. Stabilizing mechanisms preventing anterior dislocation of the glenohumeral joint. J Bone Joint Surg 63A:1208–1217, 1981.

Warner JJP, Marks PH. Management of complications of surgery for anterior shoulder instability. Sports Med Arthrosc Rev 1:272–292, 1993.

Warner JJP, Marks PH. Reconstruction of the antero-superior shoulder capsule with the subscapularis tendon. A case report. J Shoulder Elbow Surg 2:260–263, 1993.

Warner JJP, Warren RF. Arthroscopic Bankart repair using a cannulated, absorbable fixation device. Op Tech Orthop 1:192–198, 1991.

Zuckerman JD, Matsen FA III. Complications about the glenohumeral joint related to the use of screws and staples. J Bone Joint Surg 66A:175–180, 1984.

Impingement Syndrome/Rotator Cuff

Adamson GJ, Tibone JE. Ten year assessment of primary rotator cuff repairs. J Shoulder Elbow Surg 2:57–63, 1993.

Bigliani LU, Cordasco FA, McIlveen SJ, Musso ES. Operative treatment of failed repairs of the rotator cuff. J Bone Joint Surg 74A:1505–1515, 1992.

Bigliani LU, Cordasco FA, McIlveen SJ, Musso ES. Operative repair of massive rotator cuff tears. Long term results. J Shoulder Elbow Surg 1:66–76, 1992.

Caspari RB, Thal R. A technique for arthroscopic subacromial decompression. Arthroscopy 8:23–30, 1992.

Ellman H, Kay SP, Worth M. Arthroscopic treatment of full thickness rotator cuff tears: two to seven year follow-up study. Arthroscopy 9:301–314, 1993.

Etoi E, Tabata S. Conservative treatment of rotator cuff tears. Clin Orthop 275:152–160, 1992.

Gerber C. Latissmus dorsi transfer for the treatment of irreparable tears of the rotator cuff. Clin Orthop 275:152–160, 1992.

Gerber C, Terrier F, Ganz R. The role of the coracoid process in the chronic impingement syndrome. J Bone Joint Surg 67B:703–708, 1985.

Hawkins RJ, Kennedy JC. Impingement syndrome in athletes. Am J Sports Med 8:151–158, 1980.

Holsbeeck E. Subacromial impingement: open versus arthroscopic decompression. Arthroscopy 8:173–178, 1992.

Itoi E, Tabatta S. Incomplete rotator cuff tears. Results of operative treatment. Clin Orthop 284:156–160, 1992.

Kimio N, Ozaki J, Tomito Y, Tamai S. Magnetic resonance imaging of rotator cuff tearing and degenerative changes: correlation with histologic pathology. J Shoulder Elbow Surg 2:156–164, 1993.

Lazarus MD, Chansky HA, Misra S, et al. Comparison of open and arthroscopic subacromial decompression. J Shoulder Elbow Surg 3:1–11, 1994.

Matsen FA III, Arntz CT. Subacromial impingement. In Rockwood CA Jr, Matsen FA III (eds). The Shoulder. Philadelphia: WB Saunders, 1990, pp 623–646.

Matsen FA III, Arntz CT. Rotator cuff tendon failure. In Rockwood CA Jr, Matsen FA III (eds). The Shoulder. Philadelphia: WB Saunders, 1990, pp 647–677.

Neer CS II: Anterior acromioplasty for the chronic impingement syndrome in the shoulder. J Bone Joint Surg 54A:41–50, 1972.

Neviaser RJ, Neviaser TJ. Reoperation for failed rotator cuff repair: analysis of fitty cases. J Shoulder Elbow Surg 1:283–286, 1992.

Rockwood CA Jr, Lyons FR. Shoulder impingement syndrome: diagnosis, radiographic evaluation, and treatment with a modified Neer acromioplasty. J Bone Joint Surg 75A:409–424, 1993.

Ryu RKN. Arthroscopic subacromial decompression: a clinical review. Arthroscopy 8:141–147, 1992.

Speer KP, Lohnes J, Garrett WC. Arthroscopic subacromial decompression: results in advanced impingement syndrome. Arthroscopy 7:291–296, 1991.

Walch G, Boileau P, Noel E, Donell ST. Impingement of the deep surface of the supraspinatus tendon on the posterosuperior glenoid rim. An anatomic study. J Shoulder Elbow Surg 1:238–245, 1992.

Warner JJP, Altchek DW, Warren RF. Arthroscopic management of rotator cuff tears with emphasis on the throwing athlete. Op Tech Orthop 1:235–239, 1991.

Zuckerman JD, Kummer FJ, Cuomo F, et al. The influence of coracoacromial arch anatomy on rotator cuff tears. J Shoulder Elbow Surg 1:4–14, 1992.

Biceps Injuries

Andrews J, Carson W, McLeod W. Glenoid labrum tears related to the long head of the biceps. Am J Sports Med 13:337–341, 1985.

Burkhead WZ Jr. The biceps tendon. In Rockwood CA Jr, Matsen FA III (eds). The Shoulder. Philadelphia: WB Saunders, 1990, pp 791–836.

Froimson AI, Oh I. Keyhole tenodesis of biceps origin at the shoulder. Clin Orthop 112:245–249, 1974.

Resch H, Golser K, Thoeni H, Sperner G. Arthroscopic repair of superior glenoid labral detachment (the SLAP lesion). J Shoulder Elbow Surg 2:147–155, 1993.
Synder SJ, Wuh HCK. Arthroscopic evaluation and treatment of the rotator cuff and superior labrum anterior posterior lesion. Op Tech Orthop 1:207–220, 1991.
Warren RF. Lesions of the long head of the biceps tendon. Instr Course Lect 34:204–209, 1985.

Fractures

Bigliani LU, Craig EV, Butters KP. Fractures of the proximal humerus. In Rockwood CA Jr, Green DP, Bucholz RW (eds). *Rockwood and Green's Fractures in Adults.* 3rd ed. Philadelphia: JB Lippincott, 1991, pp 871–927.
Butters KP. Fractures and dislocations of the scapula. In Rockwood CA Jr, Green DP, Bucholz RW (eds). *Rockwood and Green's Fractures in Adults.* 3rd ed. Philadelphia: JB Lippincott, 1991, pp 928–990.
Craig EV. Fractures of the clavicle. In Rockwood CA Jr, Green DP, Bucholz RW (eds). *Rockwood and Green's Fractures in Adults.* 3rd ed. Philadelphia: JB Lippincott, 1991, pp 928–990.
Cuomo F, Flatow EL, Maday MG, et al. Open reduction and internal fixation of two- and three-part displaced surgical neck fractures of the proximal humerus. J Shoulder Elbow Surg 1:287–295, 1992.
Goss TP. Fractures of the glenoid neck. J Shoulder Elbow Surg 3:42–52, 1994.
Jaberg H, Warner JJP, Jakob RP. Percutaneous stabilization of unstable fractures of the humerus. J Bone Joint Surg 74A:508, 1992.
Koval KJ, Sanders R, Zuckerman JD, et al. Modified tension band wiring of displaced surgical neck fractures of the humerus. J Shoulder Elbow Surg 2:99–105, 1993.
Sidor ML, Zuckerman JD, Lyon T, et al. Classification of proximal humerus fractures. The contribution of the scapular lateral and axillary radiographs. J Shoulder Elbow Surg 3:24–27, 1994.
Zuckerman JD, Koval KJ, Cuomo F. Fractures of the scapula. Instr Course Lect 42:271–281, 1983.

Acromioclavicular and Sternoclavicular Injuries

Cahill BR. Osteolysis of the distal part of the clavicle in male athletes. J Bone Joint Surg 64A:1053–1058, 1982.
Gartsman GM. Arthroscopic resection of the acromioclavicular joint. Am J Sports Med 21:71–77, 1993.
Lewonowski K, Basset GS. Complete posterior sternoclavicular epiphyseal separation: a case report and review of the literature. Clin Orthop 281:84–88, 1992.
Richards RR. Acromioclavicular joint injuries. Instr Course Lect 42:259–269, 1993.
Rockwood CA Jr. Injuries to the acromioclavicular joint. In Rockwood CA Jr, Green DP (eds). *Fractures in Adults.* Vol 1. 2nd ed. Philadelphia: JB Lippincott, 1984, pp 860–910.
Rockwood CA Jr. Disorders of the sternoclavicular joint. In Rockwood CA Jr, Matsen FA III (eds). *The Shoulder.* Philadelphia: WB Saunders, 1990, pp 477–525.
Rockwood CA Jr, Young DC. Disorders of the acromioclavicular joint. In Rockwood CA Jr, Matsen FA III (eds). *The Shoulder.* Philadelphia: WB Saunders, 1990, pp 413–476.
Scavenius M, Iverson BF. Nontraumatic clavicular osteolysis in weight lifters. Am J Sports Med 20:463–467, 1992.

Muscle Ruptures

Berson BL. Surgical repair of the pectoralis major rupture in an athlete. Am J Sports Med 7:348–351, 1979.
Caughey MA, Welsh P. Muscle ruptures affecting the shoulder girdle. In Rockwood CA Jr, Matsen FA III (eds). *The Shoulder.* Philadelphia: WB Saunders, 1991, pp 863–873.
Gerber C, Krushell RJ. Isolated rupture of the tendon of the subscapularis muscle. J Bone Joint Surg 73B:389–394, 1991.
Kretzler HH Jr, Richardson AB. Rupture of the pectoralis major muscle. Am J Sports Med 17:453–458, 1989.
Liu J, Chang C, Chou Y, et al: Avulsion of the pectoralis major tendon. Am J Sports Med 20:366–368, 1992.
McAuliffe TB, Dowd GS. Avulsion of the subscapularis tendon: a case report. J Bone Joint Surg 69A:1454, 1987.
Miller MD, Johnson DL, Fu FH, et al. Rupture of the pectoralis major muscle in a collegiate football player. Am J Sports Med 21:475–477, 1993.
Symeonides PP. The significance of the subscapularis muscle in the pathogenesis of recurrent anterior dislocation of the shoulder. J Bone Joint Surg 54B:476–483, 1972.
Wolfe SW, Wickiewics TL, Cananaugh JT. Ruptures of the pectoralis major muscle. An anatomic and clinical analysis. Am J Sports Med 20:587–593, 1992.

Calcific Tendinitis and Adhesive Capsulitis

Ark JW, Flock TJ, Flatow EL, Bigliani LU. Arthroscopic treatment of calcific tendinitis of the shoulder 8:183–188, 1992.
Bulgen DY, Binder AI, Hazleman BL, et al. Frozen shoulder: prospective clinical study with an evaluation of three treatment regimens. Ann Rheum Dis 43:353–360, 1984.
Bulgen DY, Binder A, Hazleman BL, Park JP. Immunological studies in frozen shoulder. J Rheumatol 9:893, 1982.
Coventry MB. Problem of the painful shoulder. JAMA 151: 177–185, 1953.
Fareed DU, Gallivan WR. Office management of frozen shoulder syndrome. Clin Orthop 242:177–183, 1989.
Faure G, Daculsi G. Calcified tendinitis: a review. Ann Rheum Dis 42(suppl):49–53, 1983.
Grey RG. The natural history of "idiopathic" frozen shoulder. J Bone Joint Surg 60A:564, 1978.
Harmon HP. Methods and results in the treatment of 2580 painful shoulders. With special reference to calcific tendinitis and the frozen shoulder. Am J Surg 95:527–544, 1958.
Harryman DT II. Shoulders: frozen and stiff. Instr Course Lect 42:247–257, 1993.
Lapidus PW. Infiltration therapy of acute tendinitis with calcification. Surg Gyencol Obstet 76:715–725, 1943.
Leffert RE. The frozen shoulder. Instr Course Lect 34:199–203, 1985.
Lippmann RK. Observations concerning the calcific cuff deposits. Clin Orthop 20:49–60, 1961.
McLaughlin HL. On the frozen shoulder. Bull Hosp J Dis Orthop Inst 12:383, 1951.

McLaughlin HL. Selection of calcium deposits for operation—the technique and results of operation. Surg Clin North Am 43:1501–1504, 1963.

Miller MD, Wirth MA, Rockwood CA Jr. Thawing the frozen shoulder: the "patient" patient. Orthopedics (in press).

Moseley HF. The results of nonoperative and operative treatment of calcified deposits. Surg Clin North Am 43:1505–1506, 1963.

Murnaghan JS. Adhesive capsulitis of the shoulder: current concepts and treatment. Orthopaedics II:153–158, 1988.

Murnaghan JP. Frozen shoulder. In Rockwood CA Jr, Matsen FA III. *The Shoulder.* Philadelphia: WB Saunders, 1990.

Neviaser JG. Adhesive capsulitis and the stiff and painful shoulder. Orthop Clin North Am II:327–331, 1980.

Neviaser RJ, Neviaser TJ. The frozen shoulder. Diagnosis and management. Clin Orthop 223:59–64, 1987.

Neviaser TJ. Adhesive capsulitis. In McGinty JB (ed). *Operative Arthroscopy.* New York: Raven Press, 1991, pp 561–566.

Shaffer B, Tibone JE, Kerlan RK. Frozen shoulder. A long-term follow-up. J Bone Joint Surg 74A:738–746, 1992.

Simon WH. Soft tissue disorders of the shoulder. Frozen shoulder, calcific tendinitis, and bicipital tendinitis. Ortho Clin North Am 6:521–539, 1949.

Uthoff HK, Sarkar K, Maynard JA. Calcifying tendinitis. Clin Orthop 118:164–168, 1976.

Wiley AM, Older MWJ. Shoulder arthroscopy, investigations with a fiberoptic instrument. Am J Sports Med 17:31–37, 1989.

Nerve Disorders

Bigliani L, Perez-Sanz JR, Wolfe IN. Treatment of the trapezius paralysis. J Bone Joint Surg 67A:871–877, 1985.

Black KP, Lombardo JA. Suprascapular nerve injuries with isolated paralysis of the infraspinatus. Am J Sports Med 18:225, 1990.

Burkhead WZ, Scheinberg RR, Box G. Surgical anatomy of the axillary nerve. J Shoulder Elbow Surg 1:31–36, 1992.

Drez D. Suprascapular neuropathy in the differential diagnosis of rotator cuff injuries. Am J Sports Med 4:443, 1976.

Fechter JD, Kuschner SH. The thoracic outlet syndrome. Orthopedics 16:1243–1254, 1993.

Kauppila LI. The long thoracic nerve. Possible mechanisms of injury based on autopsy study. J Shoulder Elbow Surg 2:244–248, 1993.

Leffert RD. Neurological problems. In Rockwood CA Jr, Matsen FA III (eds). *The Shoulder.* Philadelphia: WB Saunders, 1990, pp 750–773.

Markey KL, DiBeneditto M, Curl WW. Upper trunk brachial plexopathy. The stinger syndrome. Am J Sports Med 23:650–655, 1993.

Marmor L, Bechtal CO. Paralysis of the serratus anterior due to electric shock relieved by transplantation of the pectoralis major muscle. J Bone Joint Surg 45A:156–160, 1983.

Narakas A. Brachial plexus injury. Orthop Clin North Am 12:303, 1981.

Post M, Grinblat E. Suprascapular nerve entrapment: diagnosis and results of treatment. J Shoulder Elbow Surg 2:190–197, 1993.

Post M, Mayer J. Suprascapular nerve entrapment: diagnosis and treatment. Clin Orthop 223:126, 1987.

Sedel L. Results of surgical repair of brachial plexus injuries. J Bone Joint Surg 64B:54, 1982.

Vastamaki M, Kauppila LI. Etiologic factors in isolated paralysis of the serratus anterior muscle. A report of 197 cases. J Shoulder Elbow Surg 2:244–248, 1993.

Warner JJP, Krushell RJ, Masquelet A, Gerber C. Anatomy and relationships of the suprascapular nerve. Anatomical constraints to mobilization of the supraspinatus and infraspinatus muscles in the management of massive rotator cuff tears. J Bone Joint Surg 74A:36–45, 1992.

Other Shoulder Disorders

Matthews LS, Wolock BS, Martin DF. Arthroscopic management of degenerative arthritis of the shoulder. In McGinty JB (ed). *Operative Arthroscopy* New York: Raven Press, 1991, pp 567–572.

Miller MD, Warner JJP. The abduction (weight bearing) radiograph of the shoulder (poster). American Academy of Orthopaedic Surgeons, 61st Annual Meeting, New Orleans, 1994.

CHAPTER 5

Elbow

I. Anatomy and Biomechanics
  A. Anatomy—The elbow consists of a compound ginglymus (hinge) joint (humeroulnar) and a trochoid (pivot) joint (humeroradial). The distal humerus is composed of two condyles forming the articular surfaces of the trochlea (which articulates with the ulna) and the capitellum (which articulates with the radial head) (Figure 5–1). The medial epicondyle serves as the attachment of the important ulnar (medial) collateral ligament and the flexor-pronator muscles of the forearm. The lateral epicondyle, which is less prominent, serves as the attachment for the lateral collateral ligament and the extensor muscles of the forearm. The proximal radius is composed of a head with a central fovea that articulates with the capitellum, a neck, and a proximal tuberosity for the insertion of the biceps tendon (Fig. 5–2). The proximal ulna is made up of two curved processes, the olecranon and the coronoid, with an intervening trochlear notch. The elbow contains a relatively thin capsule and the following ligaments (Fig. 5–3):

Ligament	Components	Comments
Ulnar collateral	Anterior, posterior, and transverse	Anterior bundle most important
Radial collateral	Radial collateral Lateral ulnar collateral Accessory collateral	
Annular ligament	Osseofibrous ring	Functions in rotatory movements

In addition to these ligaments, the quadrate ligament (inferior to the annular ligament) and the oblique cord (ulnar to the radial tuberosity) also contribute to the elbow joint. Numerous vessels and nerves of clinical significance surround the elbow (Fig. 5–4). The location of these structures is a major determinant of surgical incisions and arthroscopic portal placement. Important approaches to the elbow include the anterolateral, posterior, and posterolateral approaches. The anterolateral approach (Henry) is between the pronator teres (median nerve) and brachioradialis (radial nerve) (Fig. 5–5). The posterior approach usually includes an olecranon osteotomy (Fig. 5–6); however, Bryan and Morrey have described a more extensive exposure that spares the triceps. The posterolateral, or Kocher, approach to the elbow uses the interval between the anconeus (radial nerve) and the main extensor origin (posterior interosseous nerve) (Fig. 5–7).

  B. Functional Anatomy—Several studies have provided more details about the cubital tunnel and the medial collateral ligament.
    1. Cubital Tunnel—The cubital tunnel, through which the ulnar nerve courses, begins at the cubital tunnel retinaculum (Fig. 5–8). This structure and the aponeurosis of the flexor carpi ulnaris form the roof of the cubital tunnel. The floor of the cubital tunnel is formed by the joint capsule and the posterior and transverse components of the medial collateral ligament (MCL). The anterior component of the MCL is anterior to the ulnar nerve. The retinaculum, which is normally tight in full flexion, can be tight in lesser degrees of flexion if additional pathology is affecting the area or an accessory muscle, the anconeus epitrochlearis, is present.
    2. Medial Collateral Ligament—The anterior portion of the MCL is the primary constraint to valgus instability. Studies of this band indicate that only 20% of the width of the medial epicondyle can be safely removed without affecting the origin of the anterior portion of the MCL (Fig. 5–9).
  C. Biomechanics—The elbow is a loose hinge with slight varus/valgus and rotational laxity (3–5°) throughout flexion and extension. The elbow serves three functions—(1) as a component joint of the lever arm in positioning the hand, (2) as a fulcrum for the forearm lever, and (3) as a weight-bearing joint for patients using crutches. Motion of the elbow includes

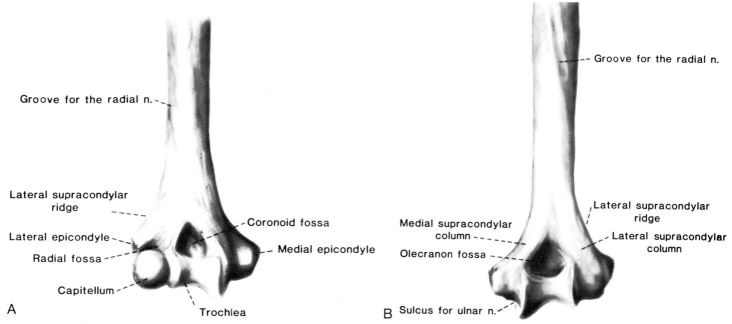

Groove for the radial n.

Groove for the radial n.

Lateral supracondylar ridge

Lateral epicondyle

Radial fossa

Capitellum

Coronoid fossa

Medial epicondyle

A

Trochlea

Medial supracondylar column

Olecranon fossa

Lateral supracondylar ridge

Lateral supracondylar column

B Sulcus for ulnar n.

FIGURE 5–1. Anterior (*A*) and posterior (*B*) aspects of the distal humerus demonstrating important bony landmarks. (From Morrey BF [ed]. *The Elbow and Its Disorders.* 2nd ed. Philadelphia: WB Saunders, 1993, pp 20, 21.)

flexion and extension (0–150° normal, 30–130° functional) and pronation and supination (80–90° normal, 50° functional). The normal carrying angle (valgus angle at the elbow) is about 10° to 15° (slightly higher in females than males).

The elbow is one of the most stable joints in the body. Both bony and soft tissue restraints contribute to the stability of this joint. The bony architecture resists varus and valgus forces (especially the former) and has increased stability in extension. The collateral ligaments and capsule are also important stabilizing forces, especially in flexion. Several muscles cross the elbow and serve as dynamic stabilizers. Flexion of the elbow is primarily accomplished by the biceps, brachialis (the workhorse of flexion), and brachioradialis; extension, by the triceps (especially the medial head); pronation, by the pronator teres; and supination, by the supinator muscle. The anconeus muscle provides additional stability to the elbow, because it is active with almost all motions. The greatest forces in the elbow occur with the joint in extension owing to the relatively poor mechanical advantage of the flexors and extensors (insertions very near the center of axis of the joint). The force across the radiohumeral joint is maximal with the elbow extended and the forearm pronated.

II. History and Physical Examination
 A. History—Patients frequently present with elbow pain. A precise history includes a patient's description of the onset of pain, the location, analgesics used, and aggravating motions. Careful investigation into whether any other symptoms exist may help preclude cervical, shoulder, wrist, and other problems. In athletes who engage in throwing, repetitive overhand throwing with medial pain during late cocking or acceleration may suggest instability of the ulnar collateral ligament.
 B. Physical Examination—Like most areas of orthopaedics, evaluation of the elbow joint should progress through an orderly sequence of inspection, palpation, assessment of motion, strength testing, and instability evaluation.

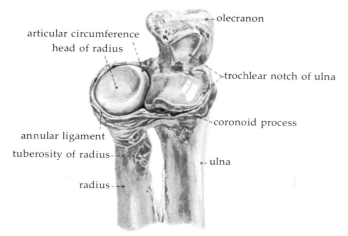

olecranon

articular circumference head of radius

trochlear notch of ulna

coronoid process

annular ligament

tuberosity of radius

ulna

radius

FIGURE 5–2. Proximal radius and ulna. (From Langman J, Woerdeman MW. *Atlas of Medical Anatomy.* Philadelphia: WB Saunders, 1976.)

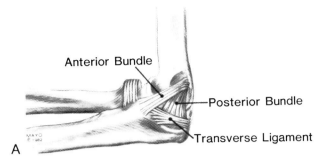

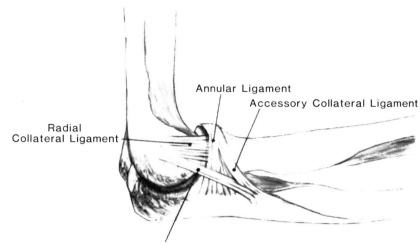

FIGURE 5–3. Orientation of the medial (ulnar) collateral ligament (*A*) and the lateral (radial) collateral ligament complex (*B*). (From Morrey BF [ed]. *The Elbow and Its Disorders.* 2nd ed. Philadelphia: WB Saunders, 1993, pp 29, 30.)

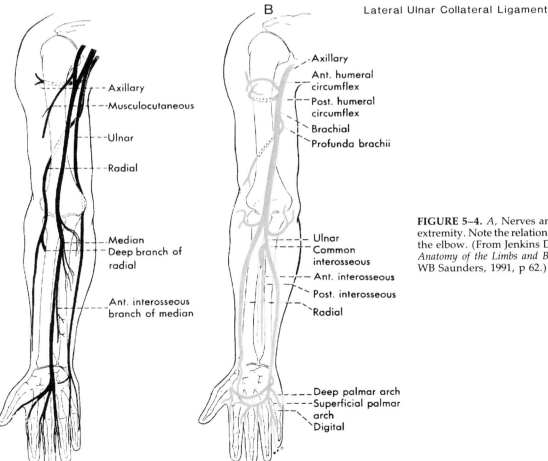

FIGURE 5–4. *A,* Nerves and *B,* vessels of the upper extremity. Note the relationships of these structures to the elbow. (From Jenkins DB. *Hollinshead's Functional Anatomy of the Limbs and Back.* 6th ed. Philadelphia: WB Saunders, 1991, p 62.)

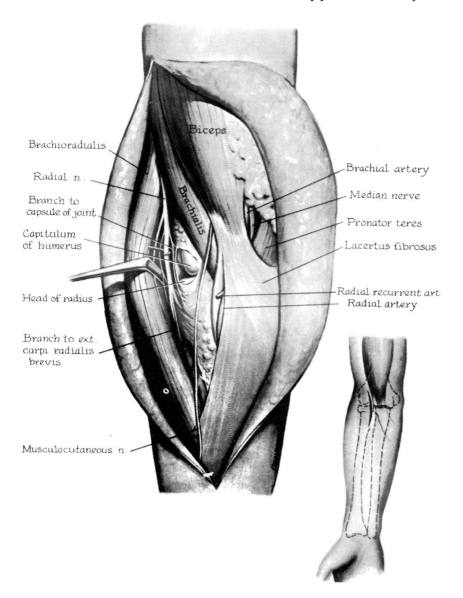

FIGURE 5–5. Anterior approach to the elbow. (From Kaplan EB. *Surgical Approaches to the Neck, Cervical Spine and Upper Extremity.* Philadelphia: WB Saunders, 1966, p 77.)

1. Inspection—Patients should first be assessed for any gross deformities, swelling, or muscle atrophy. The axial alignment can be checked by evaluating the carrying angle, although this is difficult to assess in patients with flexion contractures. The lateral infracondylar recess can be obliterated with swelling. The posterior elbow may be swollen with olecranon bursitis, and a defect may be present with a triceps tendon rupture. Proximal and distal joints of the upper extremity should also be evaluated.
2. Palpation—The bony landmarks, including the epicondyles and the radial head, should be palpated for tenderness. The collateral ligaments should be palpated with the elbow flexed 30° or more. The muscle groups' origins should be palpated with

resisted wrist extension or flexion to evaluate for the possibility of epicondylitis. The cubital fossa and olecranon fossa should be palpated for tenderness or deformity. Additionally, the cubital tunnel can be palpated, and localized tenderness or the Tinel sign may be present in patients with ulnar nerve impingement (Fig. 5–10).
3. Range of Motion—Assessment of elbow flexion-extension and pronation-supination is one of the most important aspects of the physical examination. Normal flexion-extension is 0° to 140° (+/− 10°), pronation 70°, and supination 85°. Functional range of motion for most activities of daily living is 30° to 130° flexion-extension with 50° each of pronation and supination (Fig. 5–11). Differences in active and passive motion are usually caused

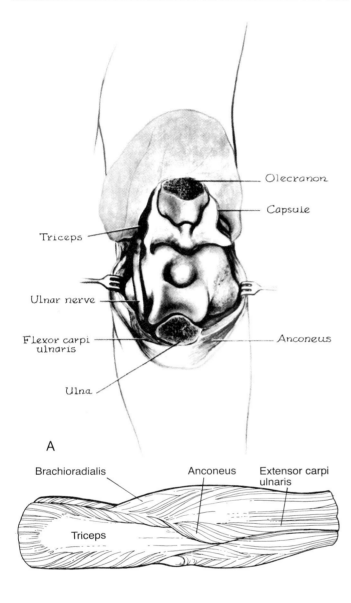

A

B

FIGURE 5–6. *A*, Posterior approach to the elbow. (From Kaplan EB. *Surgical Approaches to the Neck, Cervical Spine and Upper Extremity.* Philadelphia: WB Saunders, 1966, p 82.) *B*, Triceps-sparing posterior approach to the elbow.

by pain inhibition. Characterization of the endpoint as soft (usually caused by soft tissue) or hard (often the result of an osseous block) may also be important.
4. Strength Testing—Gross estimation of strength is possible in the clinical setting.

Flexion and extension strength is generally accomplished with the forearm in neutral rotation and the elbow flexed about 90°. Extension strength is normally 70% of flexion strength. Pronation and supination are also tested with the arm flexed, and supination is generally slightly more powerful than pronation.
5. Instability Testing—Straight varus and valgus instability is checked with the arm flexed about 25°, which unlocks the olecranon from its fossa. Varus instability is measured with the humerus internally rotated, and valgus instability with the humerus externally rotated (Fig. 5–12). A pivot shift test, similar to the examination for the knee, has been described. Insufficiency of the lateral collateral ligament of the elbow can lead to posterolateral instability. With the forearm fully supinated, the elbow is slowly extended while valgus, supination, and axial compressive forces are applied by the examiner (Fig. 5–13). Patients with posterolateral instability have subluxation of the radiohumeral joint posterolaterally from instability around the ulnohumeral joint.
6. Additional Testing—Additional examination should be directed by the findings from the initial history and physical examination. Radiologic evaluation, discussed in the next section, is an important part of the workup. An approach based on tissue type can be especially helpful for evaluating the problem elbow (Fig. 5–14).

III. Radiology of the Elbow
  A. Plain Radiographs—Plain films are still vital in the evaluation of elbow problems. Anteroposterior (AP) and lateral views are the minimal films required to investigate any elbow complaint. The standard AP view is taken with the forearm supinated. The epicondyles and radiocapitellar surfaces are easily seen, and the carrying angle can be measured. The lateral view is taken with the elbow flexed 90° with the forearm in neutral position. The distal humerus, coronoid, and radial head are well visualized on this view. The relationship between the radial head and capitellum should be constant on all views. The fats pads are well seen on the lateral views. Displacement of the fat pads, especially the posterior fat pad, is usually due to traumatic hemarthrosis. The supinator fat stripe, anterior to the radial head and overlying the supinator muscle, can also be affected by trauma (Fig. 5–15). Oblique views can also be helpful in cases of subtle pathology. The medial oblique view is taken with the forearm and arm internally rotated 45° and allows better evaluation of the trochlea, olecranon, and coronoid. The lateral

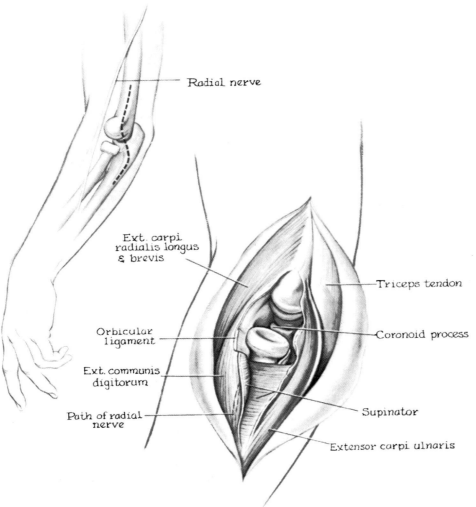

FIGURE 5–7. Lateral approach to the elbow. (From Kaplan EB. *Surgical Approaches to the Neck, Cervical Spine and Upper Extremity*. Philadelphia: WB Saunders, 1966, p 83.)

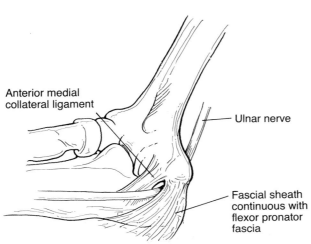

FIGURE 5–8. Cubital tunnel retinaculum.

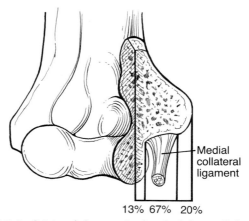

FIGURE 5–9. Origin of the anterior band of the medial collateral ligament. Note that only 20% of the medial epicondyle can be safely removed without jeopardizing this attachment. (Redrawn from O'Driscoll SW, Jalosynski R, Morrey BF, et al. Origin of the medial collateral ligament. J Hand Surg 17A:164–168, 1992.)

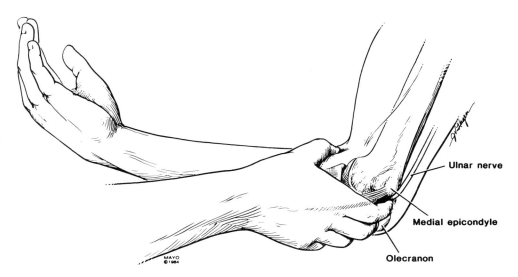

FIGURE 5–10. Palpation of the cubital tunnel. (From Regan WD, Morrey BF. The physical examination of the elbow. In Morrey BF [ed]. *The Elbow and Its Disorders*. 2nd ed. Philadelphia: WB Saunders, 1993, p 79.)

Ulnar nerve

Medial epicondyle

Olecranon

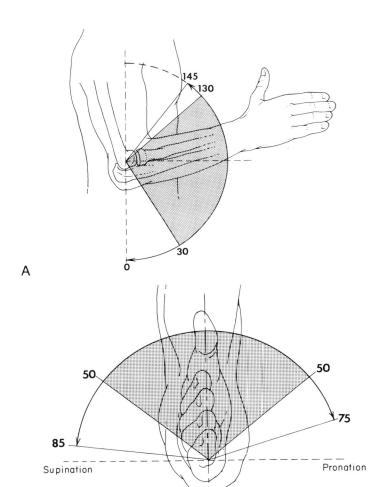

FIGURE 5–11. *A*, Normal flexion and extension of the elbow. The functional arc of motion is shaded. *B*, Normal pronation and supination. The functional arc of rotation is shaded. (From Regan WD, Morrey BF. The physical examination of the elbow. In Morrey BF [ed]. *The Elbow and Its Disorders*. 2nd ed. Philadelphia: WB Saunders, 1993, p 81.)

oblique view, taken in external rotation, allows good visualization of the radiocapitellar joint, medial epicondyle, radioulnar joint, and coronoid tubercle. The radial head view, a 45° caudal tilt lateral radiograph, can be helpful in cases of suspected radial head fractures.

B. Stress Radiography—Simple stress testing with varus/valgus force with AP radiographs can provide valuable information. An increase in the joint space of >2 mm is generally considered to be abnormal. The relationship of the ulna to the olecranon fossa is also altered with stress testing of unstable elbows. Gravity valgus stress testing can also be used to assess ulnar collateral ligament instability.

C. Other Studies—Tomography can be helpful in patients with complex fractures or in localization of loose bodies. Arthrography is also helpful, especially when combined with tomography. Magnetic resonance imaging has replaced many other imaging modalities because of its better ability to image soft tissues in multiple planes. It is especially helpful for detecting partial and complete collateral ligament injuries.

IV. Elbow Arthroscopy
A. Indications—Although elbow arthroscopy was originally proposed only for diagnostic purposes, the indications have expanded. The procedure is especially useful for synovectomy and removal of loose bodies (Fig. 5–16).
B. Operative Technique—A standard 4-mm 30° arthroscope is generally used. A smaller 2.7-mm scope is sometimes helpful for arthroscopy of the posterior elbow. Patients can be placed in a supine, prone, or lateral decubitus position with the arm placed over a padded bolster. Various positioning devices are commercially available. Precise portal placement

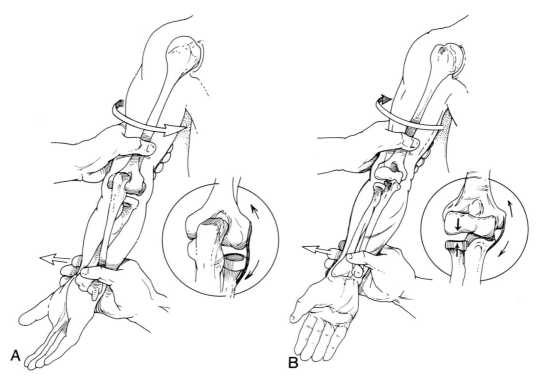

FIGURE 5–12. Assessment of varus (*A*) and valgus (*B*) instability. Note the rotation of the humerus during stress testing. (From Regan WD, Morrey BF. The physical examination of the elbow. In Morrey BF [ed]. *The Elbow and Its Disorders.* 2nd ed. Philadelphia: WB Saunders, 1993, p 83.)

is especially important because of the risk to the articular cartilage and neurovascular structures (Fig. 5–17). The course of the ulnar nerve is marked on the skin before arthroscopy. The anterolateral portal, located 1 cm distal and 1 cm anterior to the lateral epicondyle, is generally established first, after instilling fluid into the joint through the soft spot (midlateral portal). The anteromedial portal (2 cm distal and 2 cm anterior to the medial

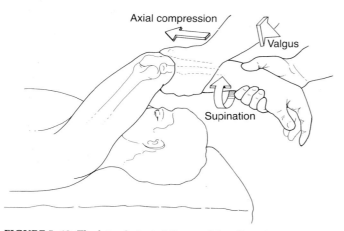

FIGURE 5–13. The lateral pivot shift test of the elbow for posterolateral rotatory instability. (Redrawn from O'Driscoll SW, Bell DF, Morrey BF. Posterolateral rotatory instability of the elbow. J Bone Joint Surg 73A:440–446, 1991.)

epicondyle) is usually established from inside out. A posterolateral portal is placed 1 to 3 cm proximal to the olecranon, immediately adjacent to the triceps tendon. An additional posterior portal can be established through the triceps tendon, but a posteromedial portal is generally not recommended because of undue risk to the ulnar nerve. Arthroscopy is carried out in a similar fashion as for other joints. The forearm can be pronated and supinated to confirm visualization of the radial head during initial orientation in the joint, and the ulnohumeral joint can be flexed and extended to view intra-articular structures more clearly.

C. Complications—The most significant complication of elbow arthroscopy is nerve injury. The incidence of nerve injury is unknown and probably underreported. The radial nerve and lateral antebrachial cutaneous nerves are at risk near the anterolateral portal. Placing this portal 3 cm distal to the epicondyle, as previously recommended, places the posterior interosseous nerve at risk for injury. The median nerve and medial antebrachial cutaneous nerves are at risk near the anteromedial portal. The ulnar nerve and posterior antebrachial cutaneous nerves are at risk with the posteromedial portal. The median nerve and brachial artery are at imminent risk with a posteromedial portal. To minimize these risks, only the

DIAGNOSTIC APPROACH:
THE PROBLEM ELBOW

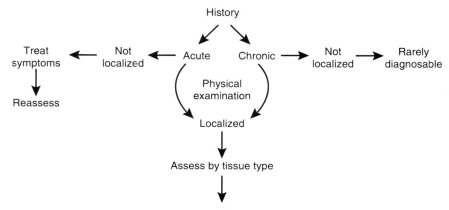

History

Treat symptoms ← Not localized ← Acute   Chronic → Not localized → Rarely diagnosable

Reassess

Physical examination

Localized

Assess by tissue type

Cartilage: Intra-articular injection, ^{99}Tc, arthroscopy
Bone: ^{99}Tc, tomogram
Ligament: Fluoroscopy stress, pivot shift, arthrogram, arthroscopy
Muscle: Objective strength measure, extra-articular injection, MRI (rare)
Nerve: Physical examination, injection, electromyography

FIGURE 5–14. Algorithm for the evaluation of the painful elbow. Note that final assessment is based on tissue type. (Adapted from Ferlic DC, Morrey BF. Evaluation of the painful elbow: the problem elbow. In Morrey BF [ed]. *The Elbow and Its Disorders.* 2nd ed. Philadelphia: WB Saunders, 1993, p 137.)

skin is incised with the knife blade, and a straight clamp is then used to spread to the capsule. Persistent drainage and a synovial fistula can occur, particularly with the anterolateral portal.

V. Compression Neuropathies
   A. Introduction—Many of the sites of upper extremity nerve entrapment syndromes are around the elbow (Fig. 5–18). Careful history taking and physical examination are essential in arriving at the correct diagnosis. Adding to the difficulty is the occasional simultaneous occurrence of other problems (e.g., lateral epicondylitis in combination with posterior inter-

osseous nerve compression) and the presence of more than one site of compression (the so-called double-crush syndrome). Electodiagnostic testing is an essential part of the evaluation.
   B. Cubital Tunnel Syndrome—This is the most common cause of nerve entrapment around the elbow and has a relatively high incidence among athletes. The anatomy of the cubital tunnel is illustrated in Fig. 5–8. Flexion of the elbow can narrow the cubital tunnel as the posterior fascial aponeurosis, the origin of the flexor carpi ulnaris, and the epicondylar olecranon ligament become taut. Hypermobility of the ulnar nerve, anomalous muscles, gan-

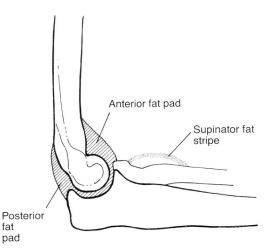

FIGURE 5–15. Location of the anterior and posterior fat pads and the supinator fat stripe.

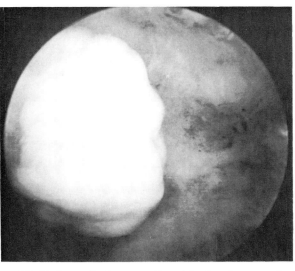

FIGURE 5–16. Loose body seen adjacent to the olecranon during arthroscopy.

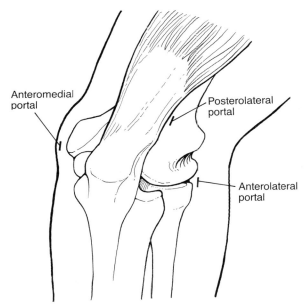

FIGURE 5–17. Portals for elbow arthroscopy.

Anteromedial portal

Posterolateral portal

Anterolateral portal

glia, osteophytes, and other lesions can also compress and injure the nerve in this area. A common symptom is paresthesia in the ring and small fingers, which is aggravated by elbow flexion and often awakens patients at night. Sensory loss in the dorsal and ulnar aspects of the hand usually precedes digital sensory loss. Clawing is a late finding. Pain with elbow hyperflexion and positive results of the Tinel test are common. Electrodiagnostic studies can confirm this diagnosis.

Treatment initially consists of extension splinting at night and avoidance of resting the elbow on a table during the day. Operative treatment options include transposition of the nerve either subcutaneously or submuscularly or a medial epicondylectomy. If an epicondylectomy is performed, care must be taken to remove only a small portion of the epicondyle, because excessive removal can cause iatrogenic valgus instability by injury to the anterior ulnar collateral ligament (see Fig. 5–9). Complete release of the nerve both proximally (including the arcade of Struthers) and distally is important to avoid further compression (Fig. 5–19). Although the techniques for transposition (subcutaneous, subfascial, submuscular, and others) have been reported to give equally good results, some concerns have been expressed about disruption of the vascular supply to the nerve with these techniques.

C. Pronator Syndrome—This is the most common of the compression neuropathies of the median nerve at the elbow in athletes. The median nerve can also be compressed by a supracondyloid process (ligament of Struthers), the lacertus fibrosus, the arch of the flexor digitorum superficialis, and various other lesions in this interval. Symptoms of median nerve compression often include a vague fatigue-like pain. This is usually brought on by repetitive strenuous activity. Numbness, which is often secondary, includes the radial three and one-half but may be only partial. Clinical findings may include pain, indentation, or induration of the flexor pronator musculature with prolonged resisted pronation. Resisted flexion of the middle finger proximal interphalangeal joint may also produce pain in some cases. Direct pressure on the pronator muscle mass 4 cm distal to its origin is consistent with the diagnosis of pronator syndrome. Unfortunately, electromyographic studies are often not specific in this condition. Therefore, the diagnosis is largely clinical. Nonoperative management includes activity modification and possibly occasional injections. Surgical release should include the lacertus fibrosus, the pronator origin, and the tendinous arch of the flexor digitorum superficialis (Fig. 5–20).

D. Posterior Interosseous Nerve Syndrome—The posterior interosseous nerve can be compressed at the proximal edge of the supinator at the arcade of Frohse (Fig. 5–21) or at a number of other less common locations. Complete loss of this nerve causes an inability to extend the metacarpophalangeal joints of the fingers and an inability to extend the thumb. Posterior interosseous nerve compression can occur in the setting of resistant tennis elbow. Pain or tenderness along the course of the nerve and pain in the elbow with resisted extension of the long finger with the elbow extended are common. Because this is purely a motor nerve, there are no associated sensory findings. Electromyographic studies are sometimes helpful. Surgical release of the proximal portion of the extensor carpi radialis brevis and the supinator muscle is usually successful.

E. Other Entrapments—The anterior interosseous nerve can be entrapped at its entrance into the pronator muscle near its origin. Patients with loss of this nerve have a characteristic pinch owing to loss of the flexor pollicis longus and flexor digitorum profundus to the index and middle fingers. Electromyographic findings of fibrillations are present in the affected muscles as well. Surgical release is occasionally required. The musculocutaneous nerve can be compressed at the lateral margin of the biceps aponeurosis at the level of the lateral epicondyle, and it also may occasionally require surgical release.

VI. Tendon Injuries
  A. Lateral Epicondylitis (Tennis Elbow)—Degenerative changes of the extensor muscle

Nerves involved in common entrapment syndromes:

Median—5, 9, 10, 13
Ulnar—4, 6, 11
Radial—3, 7, 8, 12
Other—1, 2

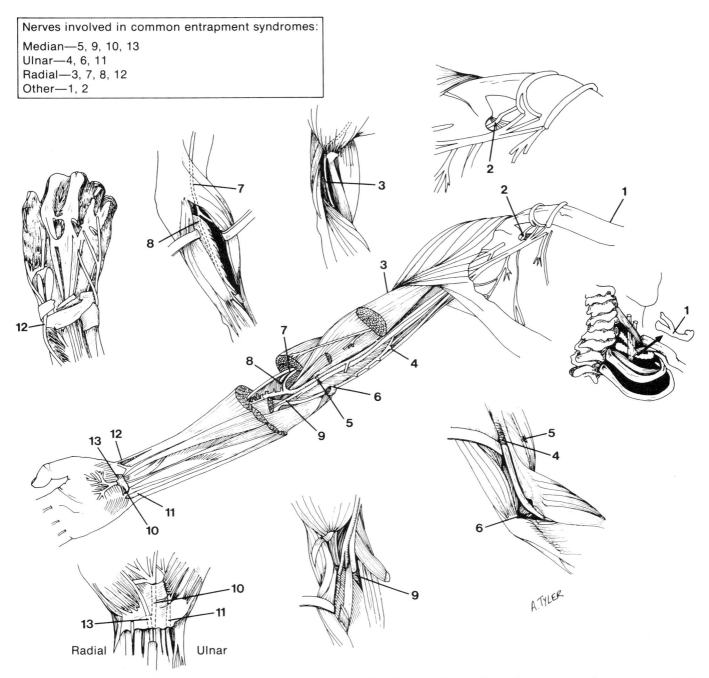

FIGURE 5–18. Composite of upper extremity sites of nerve entrapment. 1 = thoracic outlet syndrome; 2 = suprascapular nerve entrapment; 3 = high radial nerve entrapment; 4 = arcade of Struthers (ulnar nerve entrapment); 5 = ligament of Struthers (median nerve entrapment); 6 = cubital tunnel (ulnar nerve entrapment); 7 = radial tunnel; 8 = arcade of Frohse (posterior interosseous nerve entrapment); 9 = pronator (median nerve entrapment); 10 = carpal tunnel; 11 = Guyon's canal (ulnar nerve); 12 = Wartenberg syndrome (superficial radial nerve); 13 = flexor retinaculum (palmar cutaneous nerve). (From Miller MD. *Review of Orthopaedics.* Philadelphia: WB Saunders, 1992, p 123.)

group, primarily the tendon of the extensor carpi radialis brevis, is a common problem for middle-aged athletes. The condition is often caused by overuse or poor technique in racket sports and usually occurs during the back-hand stroke. The diagnosis is usually made by finding direct tenderness over the common extensor origin, just anterior to the lateral epicondyle, exacerbated by resisted extension.

Treatment in the early stages includes rest, anti-inflammatory measures, and activity modification. Physical therapy including ultrasound and high-voltage electrical stimulation can also be beneficial. Injection with a local anesthetic and steroid mixture in the paratendinous area can be helpful, but more than three injections should be avoided. Equipment modification including a more flexible

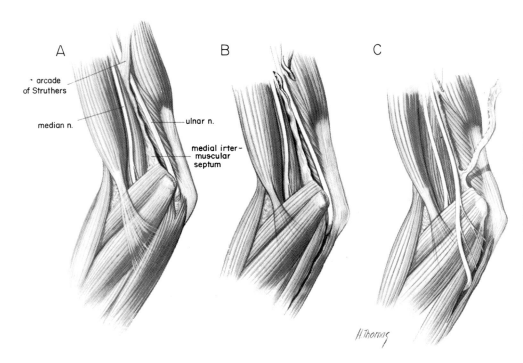

FIGURE 5–19. Anterior transposition of the ulnar nerve. Note intact arcade of Struthers (*A*), release of this structure (*B*), and release of the intermuscular septum and nerve transposition (*C*). (From Spinner M. *Injuries to the Major Branches of the Forearm.* 2nd ed. Philadelphia: WB Saunders, 1978.)

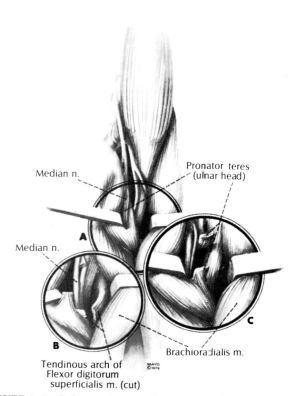

FIGURE 5–20. Release of the median nerve at the pronator origin (*A*), the flexor digitorum superficialis arch (*B*), and the ulnar head of the pronator teres (*C*). (From Morrey BF [ed]. *The Elbow and Its Disorders.* 2nd ed. Philadelphia: WB Saunders, 1993, p 828.)

racket frame, a larger racket head, looser string tension, and a larger grip may be helpful. Tennis elbow is now more common with the widespread use of stiffer wide-frame rackets. Correction of improper techniques can also be useful. A tennis elbow counterforce brace is also useful. Surgical options include release of the common extensor origin or simple debridement of pathologic tissue (extensor carpi radialis brevis origin) and vascular enhancement as described by Nirschl (Fig. 5–22). Histopathologic studies suggest that the process is a degenerative rather than an inflammatory condition, as originally believed.

B. Medial Epicondylitis (Medial Tennis Elbow or Golfer's Elbow)—This condition is less common than lateral epicondylitis and more difficult to treat. In tennis, symptoms occur with forehand shots in experienced players. The pathology appears to be at the interface between the pronator teres and flexor carpi radialis, but it is usually less discernible than lateral epicondylitis. Treatment is similar to that for tennis elbow. It is important to rule out other causes of medial elbow pain, including cubital tunnel syndrome and medial elbow instability, before considering surgical options. Multiple injections should be avoided.

C. Distal Biceps Avulsion—This is a relatively unusual injury that is related to a sudden force overload with the elbow near midflexion. The injury is more common in middle-aged male athletes and usually involves the dominant arm. Patients may note acute pain in the antecubital fossa associated with ecchymoses and

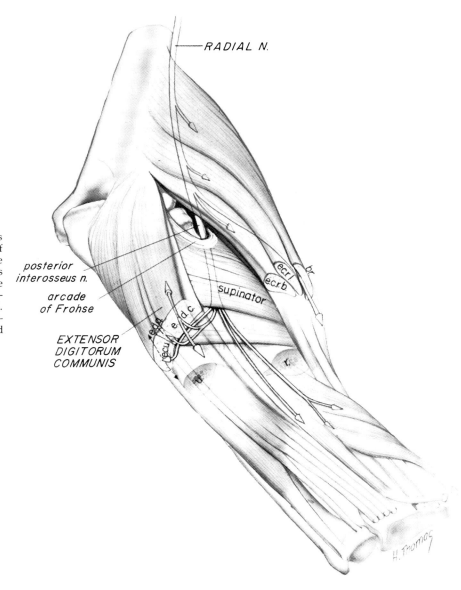

RADIAL N.

posterior
interosseus n.

arcade
of Frohse

EXTENSOR
DIGITORUM
COMMUNIS

ecr.l
ecr.b

br.

supinator

e.d.c

ecu.

FIGURE 5–21. The posterior interosseous nerve can be compressed at the arcade of Frohse after giving off its branches to the mobile wad (extensor carpi radialis brevis and longus [ecrb, ecrl]) and brachioradialis (br) and before its innervation of the extensor digitorum communis (edc) and extensor carpi ulnaris (ecu). (r = radial; u = ulnar.) (From Spinner M. *Injuries to the Major Branches of the Forearm.* 2nd ed. Philadelphia: WB Saunders, 1978.)

swelling as well as moderate weakness of elbow flexion and more marked weakness with supination. Surgical repair using a two-incision (Boyd-Anderson) technique is usually recommended (Fig. 5–23). Results of surgery are excellent.

  D. Distal Triceps Avulsion—This is an extremely rare injury usually caused by a decelerating counterforce during active elbow extension. Patients may present with sudden total loss of elbow extension and a palpable defect. Treatment is with direct repair, yielding generally good results.

VII. Elbow Instability
  A. Ulnar Collateral Ligament Injuries—Injuries to this ligament are usually a result of repetitive high valgus stress on the medial aspect of the elbow joint due to overhead throwing.

Excessive stresses during the acceleration phase of throwing can injure the anterior band of the ulnar collateral ligament. Associated ulnar nerve involvement is common. Patients typically are athletes who participate in throwing and present with localized medial elbow pain usually at the distal insertion of the ulnar collateral ligament. Patients may have valgus instability with endpoint laxity and commonly present with an elbow flexion contracture. Plain radiographs should be reviewed for loose bodies, ossification, or osteochondrotic lesions of the capitellum. Stress radiographs may demonstrate excessive medial joint opening. Magnetic resonance imaging can sometimes demonstrate loss of ligament integrity. Initial treatment includes rest, anti-inflammatory medication, and local modalities. Competitive athletes who wish to re-

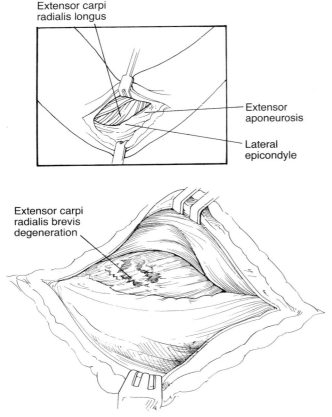

Extensor carpi radialis longus

Extensor aponeurosis

Lateral epicondyle

Extensor carpi radialis brevis degeneration

FIGURE 5–22. Operative exposure for lateral epicondylitis.

turn to throwing may ultimately require surgery. When primary repair is not possible, reconstruction using a tendon graft such as palmaris longus is recommended. This procedure involves passage of the autogenous graft through drill holes in a figure-eight fashion (Fig. 5–24).

B. Lateral Collateral Ligament Injuries—This condition has only recently been described. It is usually due to elbow dislocation or subluxation and less commonly results from varus stress. Patients may complain of recurrent clicking, snapping, or locking, usually while extending the elbow with the forearm in supination. Posterolateral rotatory subluxation can be demonstrated with the lateral pivot shift test of the elbow described by O'Driscoll and colleagues (see Fig. 5–13). This test usually produces apprehension in symptomatic patients. The actual subluxation and clunk from the reduction can usually be appreciated only with examination under anesthesia. Varus stress testing may be normal. The essential lesion with this instability appears to be in the lateral ulnar collateral ligament (see Fig. 5–3B). This ligament is one of the first structures disrupted with elbow subluxation or dislocation (Fig. 5–25). Patients with recurrent elbow subluxation may require surgery.

Reconstruction is similar to ulnar collateral ligament reconstruction (Fig. 5–26).

C. Dislocation—Elbow dislocation is not a common or unique injury in any specific sport. It is most commonly caused by elbow hyperextension from a fall on an outstretched hand and is more common in males. Posterior dislocations (named on the basis of the final position of the olecranon) are by far more common than anterior dislocations. Associated injuries include radial head, coronoid, epicondyle, and capitellar fractures. Ulnar nerve injury is also possible because the nerve is fixed in the cubital tunnel. Treatment includes reduction (traction-countertraction with manipulation of the olecranon distally and anteriorly to allow the coronoid to clear the trochlea) and immobilization for approximately 7 to 10 days. Shorter periods of immobilization are recommended for incomplete or perched dislocations (subluxations). The most common complication following elbow dislocations is loss of motion, particularly extension. Other problems include ectopic bone (more common with fracture-dislocations) and recurrent instability (discussed earlier).

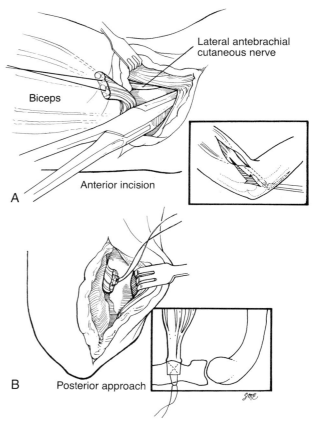

Lateral antebrachial cutaneous nerve

Biceps

Anterior incision

A

B Posterior approach

FIGURE 5–23. Repair of distal biceps rupture through a two-incision approach.

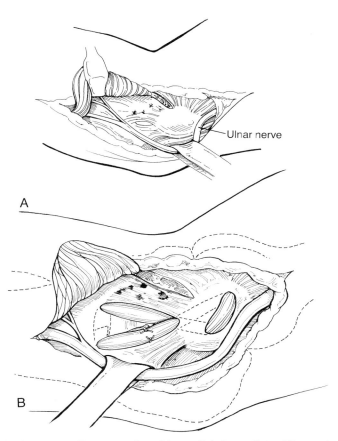

A

B

FIGURE 5–24. Reconstruction of the medial ulnar collateral ligament. *A*, Exposure and mobilization of the ulnar nerve. *B*, Reconstruction with a tendon graft.

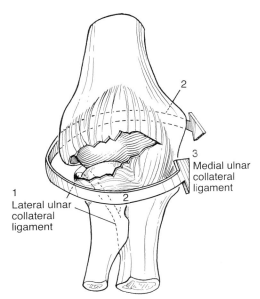

FIGURE 5–25. Elbow subluxation or dislocation disrupts the lateral ulnar collateral ligament first and not the medial ulnar collateral ligament. (Redrawn from O'Driscoll SW, Morrey BF, Korinek S, et al. Elbow subluxation and dislocation: a spectrum of instability. Clin Orthop 280:17–28, 1992.)

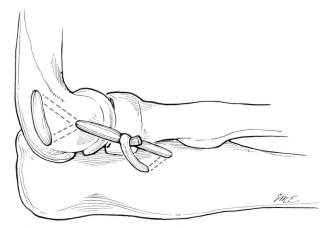

FIGURE 5–26. Reconstruction of the lateral ulnar collateral ligament. Note the similarity to reconstruction of the medial ulnar collateral ligament.

VIII. Articular Injuries
   A. Medial Epicondyle Fractures—Injuries to the medial epicondyle are relatively common in adolescents (Fig. 5–27). Repetitive valgus stresses in athletes who are throwers can result in a stress fracture of the medial epicondyle epiphysis. This condition, commonly referred to as *little league elbow*, is associated with point tenderness and an elbow flexion contracture. Fragmentation and widening of the epiphyseal lines may be seen. Rest and activity modification are usually successful, with return to throwing within 6 weeks. More significant stresses can sometimes result in a complete fracture. Surgical intervention may be required if the fragment displaces significantly with gravity (gravity stress test radiograph) or if it is entrapped into the joint.
   B. Osteochondritis Dissecans—Although its cause remains obscure, this condition is likely to be related to vascular insufficiency and repetitive microtrauma. Osteochondritis dissecans usually affects the capitellum but can also

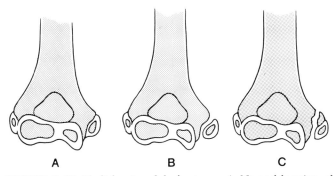

A   B   C

FIGURE 5–27. Medial epicondyle fractures. *A*, Normal location of the medial epicondyle. *B*, Salter-Harris I fracture of the medial epicondyle. *C*, Salter-Harris II fracture of the medial epicondyle. (From Morrey BF [ed]. *The Elbow.* Philadelphia: WB Saunders, 1993, p 258.)

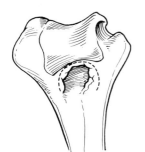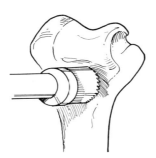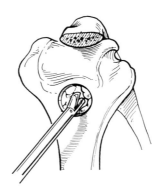

FIGURE 5–28. The Outerbridge-Kashiwagi arthroplasty, performed through a triceps-splitting approach, uses a Cloward drill to approach the coronoid fossa. The coronoid fossa can then be debrided of osteophytes. Note that the patient is supine with the elbow facing superiorly for this procedure.

involve the radial head. It most commonly occurs in young adolescent athletes who engage in throwing. Treatment is based on whether the fragment remains attached (rest) or if it is separated (arthroscopic removal and drilling). Avoidance of throwing is critical during the symptomatic stages of the disease.

C. Osteoarthritis—Patients with arthritis of the elbow usually complain of impingement pain in extension and may develop a flexion contracture. A history of significant overuse or repetitive trauma is characteristic. It is a common problem in football lineman, throwers, and racket sport athletes. Patients may have pain at the endpoint of forced extension or flexion. Radiographs are usually diagnostic. Operative treatment can include arthroscopic debridement, open decompression, distraction arthroplasty, and total elbow arthroplasty. The ulnohumeral (Outerbridge-Kashiwagi) arthroplasty allows decompression with minimal morbidity. A Cloward drill is used to remove a core of bone from the olecranon, allowing access to the anterior joint to remove the coronoid osteophytes (Fig. 5–28).

Selected References

Anatomy and Biomechanics

Bryan RS, Morrey BF. Extensive posterior exposure of the elbow. A triceps-sparing approach. Clin Orthop 116:188, 1982.
King GJW, Morrey BF, An KN. Stabilizers of the elbow. J Shoulder Elbow Surg 2:165–174, 1993.
London JT. Kinematics of the elbow. J Bone Joint Surg 63A:529–535, 1981.
Morrey BF. Anatomy and kinematics of the elbow. Instr Course Lect 40:10–16, 1991.
Morrey BF, An KN. Articular and ligamentous contributions to the stability of the elbow joint. Am J Sports Med 11:315, 1983.
Morrey BF, An KN, Stormont TJ. Force transmission through the radial head. J Bone Joint Surg 70A:250–256, 1988.
O'Driscoll SW, Horii E, Carmichael SW, et al. The cubital tunnel and ulnar neuropathy. J Bone Joint Surg 73B:613–617, 1991.
O'Driscoll SW, Jaloszynski R, Morrey BF, et al. Origin of the medial ulnar collateral ligament. J Hand Surg 17A:164–168, 1992.

Physical Examination

Jobe FW, Kvitne RS. Elbow instability in the athlete. Instr Course Lect 40:17–23, 1991.
Morrey BF, Askew LJ, An KN, Chao EY. A biomechanical study of normal functional elbow motion. J Bone Joint Surg 63A:872, 1981.
O'Driscoll SW, Bell DF, Morrey BF. Posterolateral rotatory instability of the elbow. J Bone Joint Surg 73A:440, 1991.
Regan WD, Morrey BF. The physical examination of the elbow. In Morrey BF (ed). *The Elbow and Its Disorders.* 2nd ed. Philadelphia: WB Saunders, 1993, pp 73–85.

Radiology

Berquist TH. MR imaging of the elbow and wrist. Magn Reson Imaging 1:15, 1989.
Berquist TH. Diagnostic radiographic techniques of the elbow. In Morrey BF (ed). *The Elbow and Its Disorders.* 2nd ed. Philadelphia: WB Saunders, 1993, pp 98–119.
Greenspan A, Norman A. The radial head, capitellar view. Useful technique in elbow trauma. Am J Roentgenol 138:1186, 1982.
Norell HG. Roentgenologic visualization of the extracapsular fat. Its importance in the diagnosis of traumatic injuries to the elbow. Acta Radiol 42:205, 1954.
Rogers SL, MacEwan DQ. Changes due to trauma in the fat plane overlying the supinator muscle: a radiographic sign. Radiology 92:954, 1969.

Arthroscopy

Andrews JR, Carson WG. Arthroscopy of the elbow. Arthroscopy 1:97, 1985.
Boe S. Arthroscopy of the elbow. Diagnosis and extraction of loose bodies. Acta Orthop Scand 57:52, 1986.
Carson W. Arthroscopy of the elbow. Instr Course Lect 37:195, 1988.
Guhl J. Arthroscopy and arthroscopic surgery of the elbow. Orthopedics 8:1290, 1985.
Lindenfeld TN. Medial approach in elbow arthroscopy. Am J Sports Med 18:413–417, 1990.
Lynch G, Meyers J, Whipple T, Caspari R. Neurovascular anatomy and elbow arthroscopy: inherent risks. Arthroscopy 2:191, 1986.
O'Driscoll SW, Morrey BF. Arthroscopy of the elbow: diagnostic and therapeutic benefits and hazards. J Bone Joint Surg 74A:84–94, 1992.

Compression Neuropathies

Craven PR Jr, Green DP. Cubital tunnel syndrome. J Bone Joint Surg 62A:986, 1980.
Eversman WW Jr. Entrapment and compression neuropathies. In Green DP (ed). Operative Hand Surgery. 2nd ed. New York: Churchill Livingstone, 1988, pp 1423–1478.
Farber JR, Bryan RS. The anterior interosseous nerve syndrome. J Bone Joint Surg 50A:521, 1968.
Glousman RE. Ulnar nerve problems in the athlete's elbow. Clin Sports Med 9:365, 1990.
Hartz CR, Linscheid RL, Gramse RR, Daube JR. Pronator teres syndrome: compressive neuropathy of the medial nerve. J Bone Joint Surg 63A:885, 1981.
Johnson RK, Spinner M, Shrewsbury MM. Median nerve entrapment syndrome in the proximal forearm. J Hand Surg 4:48, 1979.
Learmonth JR. Technique for transplanting the ulnar nerve. Surg Gynecol Obstet 75:792, 1942.
Lister GD, Belsole RB, Kleinert HE. The radial tunnel syndrome. J Hand Surg 4:52, 1979.
O'Driscoll SW, Horil E, Carmichael SW, Morrey BF. The cubital tunnel and ulnar neuropathy. J Bone Joint Surg 75B:613, 1991.
Roles NC, Maudsley RH. Radial tunnel syndrome. Resistant tennis elbow as a nerve entrapment. J Bone Joint Surg 54B:499, 1972.
Spinner M. The arcade of Frohse and its relationship to the posterior interosseous nerve paralysis. J Bone Joint Surg 50B:809, 1968.
Spinner M. The anterior interosseous nerve syndrome with special attention to its variations. J Bone Joint Surg 52A:84, 1970.
Spinner M, Linscheid RL. Nerve entrapment syndromes. In Morrey BF (ed). The Elbow and Its Disorders. 2nd ed. Philadelphia: WB Saunders, 1993, pp 813–832.
Wadsworth TG. The external compression syndrome of the ulnar nerve at the cubital tunnel. Clin Orthop 124:189, 1977.

Tendon Injuries

Boyd HB, Anderson LD. A method for reinsertion of the distal biceps brachii tendon. J Bone Joint Surg 43A:1041–1043, 1961.
Boyd HB, McLeod AC. Tennis elbow. J Bone Joint Surg 55A:1183, 1973.
Coonrad RW. Tennis elbow. Instr Course Lect 35:94–101, 1986.
D'Alessandro DF, Shields CL, Tibone JE, Chandler RW. Repair of distal biceps tendon ruptures in athletes. Am J Sports Med 21:114, 1993.
Farrar EL III, Lippert FG III. Avulsion of the triceps tendon. Clin Orthop 161:242–246, 1981.
Froimson AI. Treatment of tennis elbow with forearm support band. J Bone Joint Surg 53A:183, 1971.
Ilfeld FW. Can stroke modification relieve tennis elbow? Clin Orthop 276:182–185, 1992.
Morrey BF. Reoperation of failed surgical treatment of refractory lateral epicondylitis. J Shoulder Elbow Surg 1:47–55, 1992.
Nirschl RP. Sports—and oversue injuries to the elbow. In Morrey BF (ed). The Elbow and Its Disorders. 2nd ed. Philadelphia: WB Saunders, 1993, pp 537–552.
Nirschl RP, Pettrone F. Tennis elbow: the surgical treatment of lateral epicondylitis. J Bone Joint Surg 61A:832, 1979.
Regan W, Wold LE, Coonrad R, Morrey BF. Microscopic histopathology of chronic refractory lateral epicondylitis. Am J Sports Med 20:746–749, 1992.
Tarsney FF. Rupture and avulsion of the triceps. Clin Orthop 83:177–183, 1972.

Elbow Instability

Bennett JB, Green MS, Tullos HS. Surgical management of chronic medial elbow instability. Clin Orthop 278:62–68, 1992.
Conway JE, Jobe FW, Glousman RE, Pink M. Medial instability of the elbow in throwing athletes: surgical treatment by ulnar collateral ligament repair or reconstruction. J Bone Joint Surg 74A:67, 1992.
Habernek H, Ortner F. The influence of anatomic factors in elbow joint dislocation. Clin Orthop 274:226–230, 1992.
Jobe FW, Kvitne RS. Elbow instability in the athlete. Instr Course Lect 40:17, 1991.
Nestor BH, O'Driscoll SW, Morrey BF. Ligamentous reconstruction for posterolateral rotatory instability of the elbow. J Bone Joint Surg 74A:1235–1241, 1992.
O'Driscoll SW, Bell DF, Morrey BF. Posterolateral rotatory instability of the elbow. J Bone Joint Surg 73A:440, 1991.
O'Driscoll SW, Morrey BF, Korinek S, et al. Elbow subluxation and dislocation: a spectrum of instability. Clin Orthop 280:17–28, 1992.
Wilson FD, Andrews JR, Blackburn TA, McCluskey G. Valgus extension overload in the pitching elbow. Am J Sports Med 11:83, 1983.

Articular Injuries

Bauer M, Jonsson K, Josefsson PO, Linden B. Osteochondritis dissecans of the elbow: a long-term follow-up study. Clin Orthop 284:156–160, 1992.

Bennett JB. Articular Injuries in the athlete. In Morrey BF (ed). *The Elbow and Its Disorders*. 2nd ed. Philadelphia: WB Saunders, 1993, pp 581–595.

DeHaven KE, Evarts CM. Throwing injuries of the elbow in athletes. Orthop Clin North Am 1:801, 1973.

Morrey BF. Primary arthritis of the elbow treated by ulno-humeral arthroplasty. J Bone Joint Surg 74B:409, 1992.

Pappas AM. Elbow problems associated with baseball during childhood and adolescence. Clin Orthop 164:30, 1982.

Singer KM, Roy SP. Osteochondrosis of the humeral capitellum. Am J Sports Med 12:351–360, 1984.

Woodward AH, Bianco AJ. Osteochondritis dissecans of the elbow. Clin Orthop 110:35, 1975.

CHAPTER **6**

Wrist and Hand

I. Anatomy and Biomechanics
   A. Anatomy—The wrist joint consists primarily of the radiocarpal joint but also includes the ulnocarpal joint. The wrist comprises eight carpal bones, articulating proximally primarily with the radius and distally with the metacarpals.
      1. Radiocarpal Joint—This is an elipsoid joint that includes the distal radius and the scaphoid, lunate, and triquetrum. The volar radiocarpal ligaments provide stability to this joint.
      2. Ulnocarpal Joint—This joint is primarily composed of the triangular fibrocartilage complex (TFCC). This structure originates from the ulnar portion of the radius and extends to the ulnar styloid and base of the fifth metacarpal. The TFCC is attached to the ulnar margin of the lunate fossa of the radius and includes the ulnar collateral ligament, the dorsal and volar radioulnar ligaments, the articular disc (triangular fibrocartilage), the meniscal homologue, the extensor carpi ulnaris sheath, and the ulnolunate and ulnotriquetral ligaments (Fig. 6–1).
      3. Carpal Bones—The scaphoid, lunate, and triquetrum articulate with the radius and ulna at the wrist, and the trapezium, trapezoid, capitate, and hamate articulate with the metacarpals in the hand (Fig. 6–2). Several distinctive features of each bone bear special emphasis (Table 6–1).
      4. Hand—The hand comprises 5 metacarpals and 14 phalanges. Metacarpophalangeal (MP) joints and interphalangeal (IP) joints are supported by collateral ligaments, a capsule, a volar plate, and insertions of the intrinsic musculature (the extensor apparatus) (Fig. 6–3).
   B. Biomechanics
      1. Wrist—The wrist has been variously described as an intercalated link system, a column concept, and a ring design (Fig. 6–4). According to Gilford and colleagues, the links composing the wrist include the radius, the lunate, and the capitate, allowing less motion to be required at each link but at the expense of stability. The column concept, as described by Taleisnik, is based on a central (flexion-extension) column composed of the distal carpal row and the lunate, a lateral (mobile) column (scaphoid), and a medial (rotatory) column (triquetrum). In the ring concept, proposed by Lichtman and associates, the proximal and distal rows are semirigid posts stabilized by interosseous ligaments. The scaphotrapezial joint represents the radial link, and the triquetrohamate joint the ulnar link of the ring. Any break in the ring can produce carpal instability.
      2. Hand—The hand has been described as being composed of two transverse arches and five longitudinal arches. Stability is provided by the volar plate and collateral ligaments.

II. Diagnosis
   A. History—It is important to obtain information about the chronicity of symptoms, exacerbating factors, other joint involvement, and response to treatment. Systemic complaints may also be relevant.
   B. Physical Examination—An anatomic approach should be followed by careful inspection, palpation, evaluation of range of motion, neurovascular evaluation, and special tests. Tests for wrist instability are discussed in the appropriate sections.
   C. Radiographs—Routine views should include posteroanterior (PA), lateral, oblique, and scaphoid views. Special views may include a carpal tunnel view for carpal tunnel syndrome and possible hook of hamate fractures. Instability series include the anteroposterior (AP) clenched fist; PA in neutral, radial, and ulnar deviation; lateral in neutral, full flexion, and extension; and semipronated oblique and semisupinated oblique views. Other techniques can be helpful in cases of more subtle injuries. Radionuclide imaging done 2 to 3 days after injury can identify occult fractures. Bone scanning can identify an area of chronic arthrosis. Tomography can be helpful in identifying occult fractures, such as the hook of the hamate.

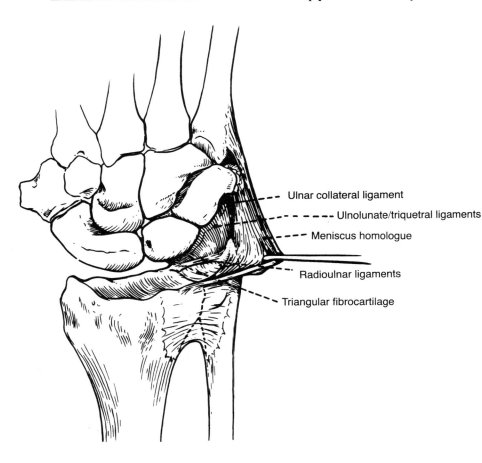

Ulnar collateral ligament

Ulnolunate/triquetral ligaments

Meniscus homologue

Radioulnar ligaments

Triangular fibrocartilage

FIGURE 6–1. Triangular fibrocartilage complex. (From Dell PC. Distal radioulnar joint dysfunction. Hand Clin 3:564, 1987.)

Cineradiography can identify abnormal carpal motion associated with instabilities. Arthrography can be useful in evaluating wrist injuries and tears of the triangular fibrocartilage complex. Magnetic resonance imaging (MRI)

arthrography has now been used with some encouraging results.

III. Wrist Arthroscopy
   A. Indications—Diagnostic arthroscopy may be indicated in patients with mechanical wrist pain (catching, popping, localized pain relieved by rest) that has not been diagnosed by other studies and is refractory to conservative management. Operative arthroscopy may be indicated for the treatment of certain ligament

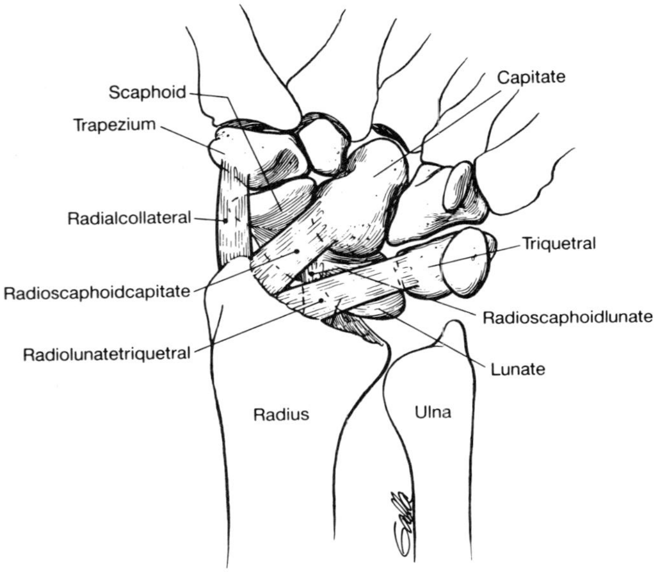

Scaphoid
Trapezium
Capitate
Radialcollateral
Triquetral
Radioscaphoidcapitate
Radioscaphoidlunate
Radiolunatetriquetral
Lunate
Radius
Ulna

FIGURE 6–2. Carpal bones and extrinsic ligaments of the wrist. (From Mooney JF, Siegel DB, Koman LA: Ligamentous injuries of the wrist in athletes. Clin Sports Med 11(1):129–139, 1992.)

TABLE 6–1. FEATURES OF THE CARPAL BONES

Bone	Important Features	Number of Articulations
Scaphoid	Tubercle (TCL, APB), distal vascular supply	5
Lunate	Lunar shape	5
Triquetrum	Pyramid shape	3
Pisiform	Spheroidal (TCL, FCR)	1
Trapezium	FCR groove, tubercle (opponens, APB, FPB, TCL)	4
Trapezoid	Wedge shape	4
Capitate	Largest bone, central location	7
Hamate	Hook (TCL)	5

TCL = transverse carpal ligament; APB = abductor pollicis brevis; FCR = flexor carpi radialis; FPB = flexor pollicis brevis.
(From Miller MD. *Review of Orthopaedics.* Philadelphia: WB Saunders, 1992, p 321.)

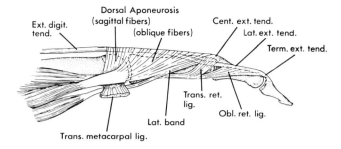

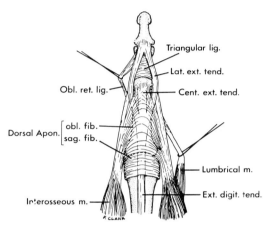

FIGURE 6–3. Dorsal extensor apparatus. (From Bora FW. *The Pediatric Upper Extremity.* Philadelphia: WB Saunders, 1986, p 93.)

tears, TFCC tears, articular cartilage injuries, and ulnar abutment syndrome, as well as for adjunctive treatment of some fractures.

B. Setup—Wrist arthroscopy is typically performed with the patient supine and using some type of traction apparatus. A 2.5- to

3.0-mm arthroscope with a 25° to 30° viewing angle is used. Some surgeons use a mechanical pump to balance inflow and outflow during the procedure. Various hand instruments such as a probe, basket forceps, suction baskets, and grasping forceps should be available. Small blades are attached to mechanical shavers for use in the wrist.

C. Portals—Three radiocarpal portals and three midcarpal portals are commonly used for wrist arthroscopy.

1. Radiocarpal Portals—Portals for wrist arthroscopy are designated on the basis of their relationship to the dorsal wrist compartments (Fig. 6–5). The *3–4 radiocarpal portal* is usually established first. A spinal needle is inserted between the tendons of the extensor pollicis longus and the extensor digitorum communis (EDC) tendons, and the wrist is distended with 5 to 10 mL of arthroscopic fluid. The portal is established with a number 11 blade, and the arthroscope is introduced into the joint. Through this portal, the scaphoid, scapholunate ligament, distal radius, and other ligaments can be easily visualized. The *4–5 radiocarpal portal* is created next to allow instrument insertion. This portal, located between the EDC and extensor digiti minimi (EDM) tendons, is about 1 cm ulnar to the 3–4 portal, and its position is best localized with a spinal needle before making a skin incision. Placing the arthroscope into this portal allows visualization of the ulnar side of the joint, including the TFCC and ulnocarpal ligaments. The *6R radiocarpal portal* is used for inflow (gravity system) or outflow (mechanical pump). It can also be used for visualization and instrumenta-

FIGURE 6–4. Three concepts of wrist kinematics. *A,* Link concept (Gilford). *B,* Column concept (Taleisnik). *C,* Ring concept (Lichtman).

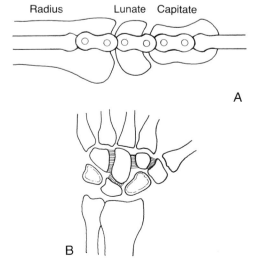

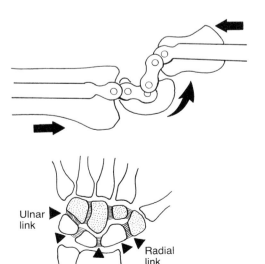

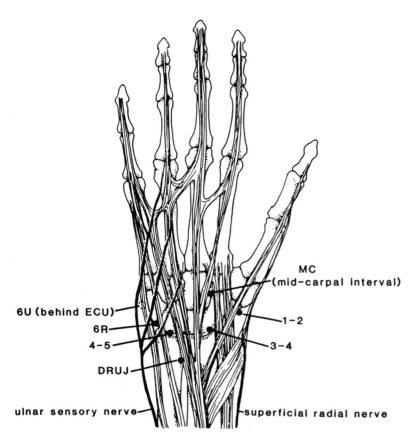

6U (behind ECU)

6R

4-5

DRUJ

ulnar sensory nerve

MC
(mid-carpal interval)

1-2

3-4

superficial radial nerve

FIGURE 6–5. Radiocarpal arthroscopic portals are designated based on their relationship to the dorsal wrist compartments. The midcarpal (MC) portal is located approximately 1 cm distal to radiocarpal portals. (ECU = extensor carpi ulnaris; DRUJ = distal radioulnar joint.)

tion. This portal is located radial to the extensor carpi ulnaris tendon (the portal could have been named 5–6 but is actually placed closer to the sixth compartment tendon, the extensor carpi ulnaris). Other portals that are occasionally used but are not routinely recommended because of risk to local structures include the 6U and the 1–2 radiocarpal portals.

2. Midcarpal Portals—Three midcarpal portals are in common use: the midcarpal radial (MCR), the midcarpal ulnar (MCU), and the scaphotrapezial-trapezoid (see Fig. 6–5). The midcarpal portals are necessary only when specifically indicated and are not required for routine wrist arthroscopy. The *MCR portal* is located 1 cm distal to the 3–4 radiocarpal portal along the axis of the radial border of the middle finger metacarpal. Located between the extensor carpi radialis brevis (ECRB) and EDC tendons, it allows visualization of the scapholunate, scaphocapitate, and scaphotrapezoid tendons. The *MCU portal* is located 1 cm distal to the 4–5 radiocarpal portal in line with the axis of the ring finger metacarpal. Located between the EDC and EDM tendons, it allows visualization of the lunocapitate, lunotriquetral, and triquetrohamate joints.

The *scaphotrapezial-trapezoid (STT) portal* is established between the extensor carpi radialis longus (ECRL) and ECRB tendons and is best located with traction on the thumb and index finger. This portal allows visualization of the scaphotrapezial and scaphotrapezoid joints.

D. Arthroscopic Technique—Routine diagnostic arthroscopy should be carried out in a systematic fashion. Debridement of stable partial tears of the radiocarpal or intercarpal ligaments and the TFCC has resulted in symptomatic relief in certain patients with wrist injuries. Diagnosis and treatment of articular cartilage lesions are also possible with the arthroscope. Adjunctive use of wrist arthroscopy in the treatment of distal radius fractures ensures restoration of articular congruity and documentation of the extent of ligamentous injury. Other uses for wrist arthroscopy may be on the horizon.

IV. Distal Radioulnar Joint Injuries
   A. TFCC Tears—Lesions of the TFCC are a common cause of ulnar wrist pain. Patients typically present with pain localized to the ulnocarpal joint and a history of a compression injury. Activities that load the wrist during pronation and supination (e.g., turning a key)

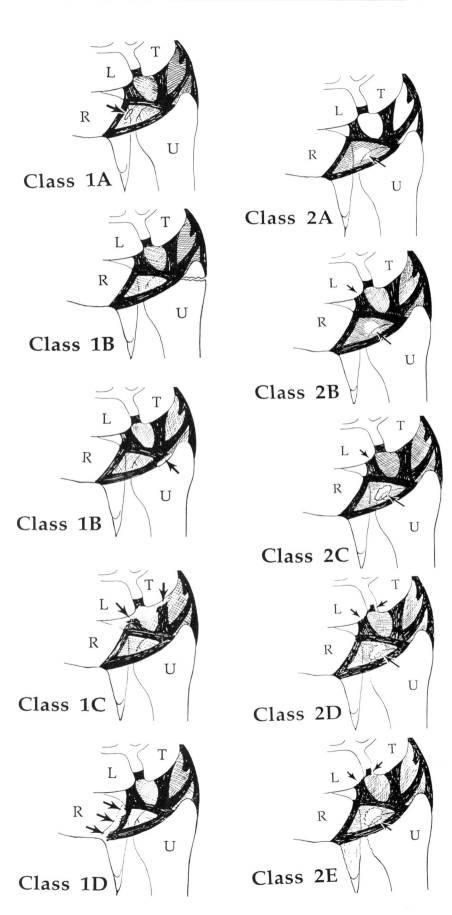

FIGURE 6–6. Palmer classification of TFCC injuries. (T = triquetrum; L = lunate; R = radius; U = ulna.) (From Palmer AK. Triangular fibrocartilage disorders: injury patterns and treatment. Arthroscopy 6:125–132, 1990.)

may exacerbate the symptoms. Arthrography has been helpful in establishing the diagnosis; however, many authorities have noted that arthroscopy is often more helpful for diagnostic and particularly for therapeutic purposes. The anatomy of the TFCC is detailed in Figure 6–1. Based on arthrography, arthroscopy, and dissection studies, Palmer and Werner classified injuries of the TFCC as shown in Figure 6–6 and Table 6–2. Much like the meniscus, central tears of the triangular fibrocartilage (disc) should be debrided, and peripheral tears repaired through arthroscopic or open techniques (Fig. 6–7).

B. Ulnocarpal Impaction Syndrome—Patients typically present with ulnar-sided wrist pain (especially with rotational or ulnar deviation loading), crepitus, and a length discrepancy of the ulna relative to the radius (ulnar positive variance) (Fig. 6–8). Cystic or sclerotic changes can also be seen in the lunate or ulnar head. The condition may be associated with premature closure of the radial epiphysis due to trauma (acquired Madelung deformity or other trauma), or it may be idiopathic. Treatment is individualized and includes supportive therapy, epiphyseal arrest (in children), or a shortening osteotomy. Feldon and colleagues described a wafer osteotomy in which 2 to 4 mm of cartilage and bone is removed from under the triangular fibrocartilage. In patients with posttraumatic arthritis, ulnar head resection (Darrach), arthrodesis with creation of a ulnar pseudarthrosis (Sauve-Kapandji), or a hemiresection-interposition arthroplasty (Bowers) (Fig. 6–9) may be appropriate.

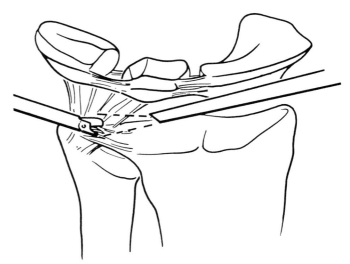

FIGURE 6–7. TFCC tear visualized through the 3–4 portal and resected through the 6R portal. (From McGinty JB. *Operative Arthroscopy*. New York: Raven Press, 1991, p 656.)

TABLE 6–2. CLASSIFICATION OF INJURIES OF THE TFCC

Class Description	Treatment
Traumatic Lesions (Type I)	
1A Horizontal tear adjacent to sigmoid notch*	Debridement
1B Avulsion from ulna +/− ulnar styloid fracture	Suture repair
1C Avulsion from carpus; exposes pisiform	Debridement
1D Avulsion from sigmoid notch	Debridement
Degenerative Lesions (Type 2)	
2A Thinning of TFCC without perforation†	
2B Thinning of disc with chondromalacia	
2C Perforation of disc with chondromalacia	
2D Perforation of disc, chondromalacia, partial tear of lunotriquetral ligament	
2E Perforation of disc, chondromalacia, complete tear of lunotriquetral ligament, ulnocarpal degenerative joint disease	

* Most common.
† Treatment for degenerative lesions includes debridement of loose degenerated discs, intra-articular resection of the ulnar head, and debridement of lunotriquetral ligament tears with percutaneous pinning of the lunotriquetral joint based on the pathology present.

V. Carpal Instabilities
 A. Scapholunate Instability—Although this is the most common type of carpal instability, diagnosis is often delayed. Patients may suffer a fall or direct blow to the wrist, with associated snuffbox tenderness. The Watson test (pain resulting from radial deviation of the hand while the scaphoid is stabilized with volar pressure) may be helpful, particularly with chronic injuries. Radiographs may demonstrate an increased scapholunate interval (>2 mm), a shortened appearance of the scaphoid, and a ring sign (cortical projection of the vertically displaced distal pole of the scaphoid) as seen on the AP view in supination. Lateral radiographs should be evaluated for an increased scapholunate angle (>70°) (Fig. 6–10).

Early treatment is controversial, although most authorities believe that casting alone is insufficient. Closed reduction and percutaneous pinning of the scapholunate joint and scaphocapitate joint for 8 to 10 weeks has been recommended by some surgeons. Others advocate open reduction and internal fixation (ORIF), usually through a dorsal approach with or without a combined dorsal and volar approach. Chronic instability (>3 months) can be a therapeutic challenge. Progressive arthritis and collapse are common. Most authorities recommend limited intercarpal arthrodesis or dorsal capsulodesis, although there remains considerable disagreement in this area.
 B. Ulnar Carpal Instability
  1. Triquetrohamate Instability—This is the most common form of ulnar instability. Patients may feel a painful clunk with ulnar

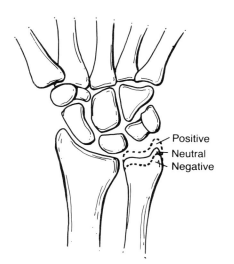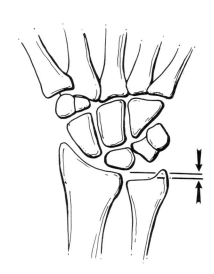

FIGURE 6–8. Ulnar variance. Ulnar positive variant is associated with ulnocarpal impaction syndrome. Ulnar minus (or negative) variant is associated with Kienbock disease. (From McCue FC, Bruce JF. The wrist. In DeLee JC, Drez D Jr [eds]. *Orthopaedic Sports Medicine.* Philadelphia: WB Saunders, 1994, p 929.)

and radial deviation from snapping of the triquetrum over the lunate articulation. Diagnosis is best confirmed with cineradiography. Conservative therapy including splinting and injections may be helpful. Surgical treatment includes limited intercarpal arthrodesis.

2. Triquetrolunate Instability—This instability is less common and may or may not be associated with a wrist click. The ballottement test (palmar and dorsal displacement of the triquetrum with one hand with simultaneous stabilization of the lunate with the opposite hand) may reproduce a patient's pain. Other tests and studies are less helpful. Treatment is similar and includes triquetrolunate arthrodesis for refractory symptoms (Fig. 6–11).

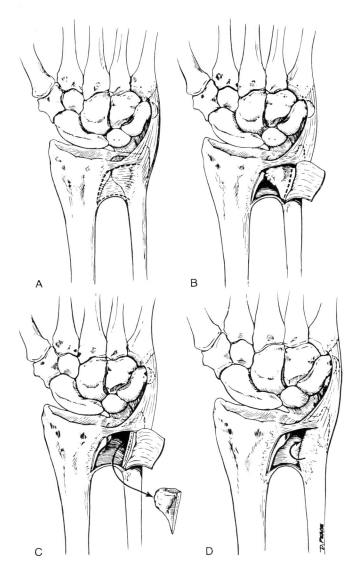

FIGURE 6–9. Hemiresection-interposition arthroplasty (Bowers). *A,* Ulnar-based capsular flap is planned. *B,* Flap is reflected, exposing the distal ulna. *C,* Oblique osteotomy. *D,* Interposition of the capsular flap. (From Dell PC. Distal radioulnar joint dysfunction. Hand Clin 3:575, 1987.)

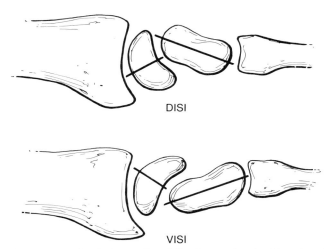

FIGURE 6–10. Scapholunate instability is associated with a dorsal intercalated segmental instability (DISI) pattern. (VISI = volar intercalated segmental instability.) Note the increased scapholunate angle (normal 30–60°). (From McCue FC, Bruce JF. The wrist. In DeLee JC, Drez D Jr [eds]. *Orthopaedic Sports Medicine.* Philadelphia: WB Saunders, 1994, p 918.)

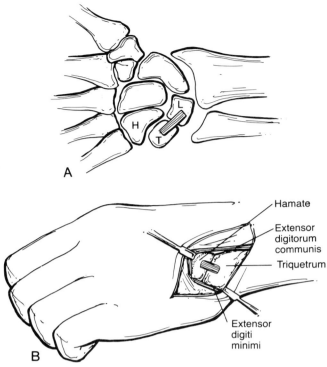

FIGURE 6–11. *A,* Triquetrolunate arthrodesis. (L = lunate; T = triquetrum; H = hamate.) *B,* Triquetrohamate arthrodesis. (From McCue FC, Bruce JF. The wrist. In DeLee JC, Drez D Jr [eds]. *Orthopaedic Sports Medicine.* Philadelphia: WB Saunders, 1994, p 925.)

VI. Fractures

A. Distal Radius Fractures—Although more common in the elderly population, these fractures can occur in athletes. Classification is based on the amount of articular involvement and comminution. Although still controversial, more aggressive treatment options may be necessary for displaced intra-articular fractures in the young, athletic population.

B. Scaphoid Fractures—These are the most common fractures involving the carpal bones and occur frequently in contact sports such as football. Because the vascular supply enters the scaphoid distally, proximal fractures have a high rate of nonunion and avascular necrosis (Fig. 6–12). Radiographs may be falsely negative early, and empirical treatment for snuffbox tenderness is often indicated. Bone scan 72 hours after injury can identify subtle fractures. For nondisplaced fractures, most authorities favor the use of a long arm thumb spica cast with the wrist in slight palmar flexion and radial deviation for 6 weeks, followed by the use of a short arm thumb spica cast until clinical and radiographic healing takes place. This treatment is controversial, however. Special padded or synthetic casts can be adapted to allow athletic participation in contact sports. ORIF may be necessary for displaced or severely angulated fractures.

Bone grafting and internal fixation is usually required if there is no evidence of healing after 6 months. For elite or professional athletes, ORIF allows earlier return to competition.

C. Hamate Fractures—These fractures most often involve the hook of the hamate in athletes, usually from a direct blow, either due to a fall or secondary to repeated trauma such as baseball batting or golf. Diagnosis is confirmed with a carpal tunnel view. Treatment may include excision of the hook through the fracture site. Fractures of the body of the hamate are less common and usually respond to 4 to 6 weeks of immobilization.

D. Fractures of Other Carpal Bones—Most nondisplaced fractures respond to 4 to 6 weeks of immobilization. Displaced fractures may require closed or open reduction and fixation (Fig. 6–13).

E. Fractures of the Metacarpals and Phalanges—Many of these fractures heal with closed reduction and immobilization if the fracture is stable after reduction. Closed reduction and percutaneous pinning can render an unstable fracture stable, allowing motion without open reduction. Techniques for percutaneous pinning include direct pinning for spiral phalangeal fractures (Fig. 6–14*A*), intramedullary fixation for transverse fractures (Fig. 6–14*B*, *C*), and fixation to an adjacent bone for meta-

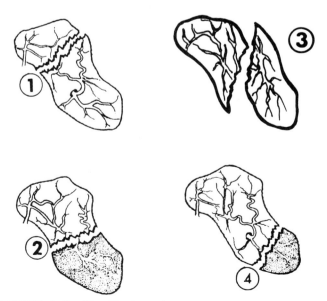

FIGURE 6–12. Classification of scaphoid fractures. (1 = neck; 2 = waist; 3 = body; 4 = proximal pole.) Note progressive risk of nonunion and avascular necrosis with proximal fractures. (From Wiesman BN, Sledge CB. *Orthopedic Radiology.* Philadelphia: WB Saunders, 1986, p 1060.)

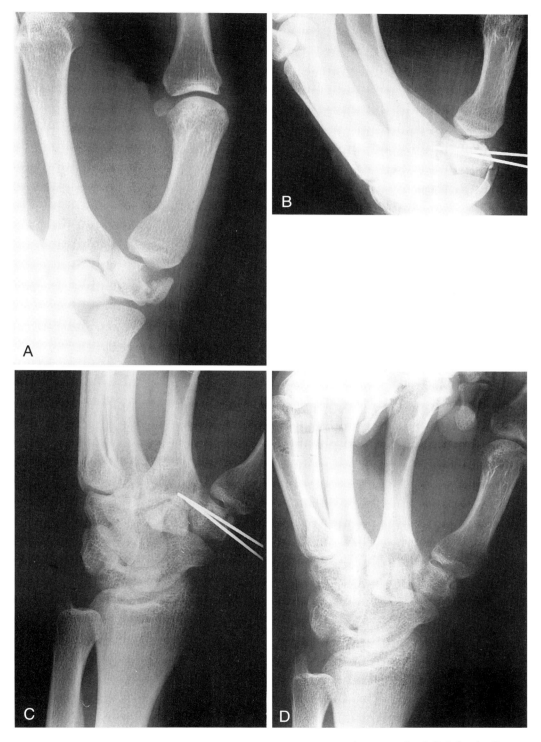

FIGURE 6–13. Displaced, longitudinal fracture-dislocation of the trapezial-1 metacarpal joint in a football defensive lineman. *A*, Radiographs following reduction (the joint was markedly unstable). *B*, Postoperative radiograph after open reduction and internal fixation. *C*, Radiographs taken 6 weeks postoperatively before pin removal. *D*, Radiographs taken 9 weeks postoperatively demonstrate healing of the fracture.

carpal shaft fractures (Fig. 6–14*D*). ORIF can be performed with various devices. This form of treatment is most commonly reserved for irreducible fractures or failure of other methods. Fractures most commonly requiring

ORIF include displaced intra-articular fractures and condylar fractures.

F. Bennett Fracture—Fracture of the base of the thumb metacarpal with radial displacement of the thumb requires reduction and stabiliza-

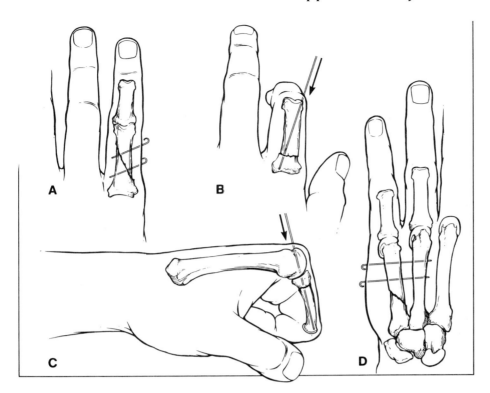

FIGURE 6–14. Methods of closed reduction and percutaneous pin fixation include direct pinning (*A*), intramedullary fixation (*B* and *C*), and fixation to an adjacent bone (*D*). (From Green DP, Strickland JW. The hand. In DeLee JC, Drez D Jr [eds]. *Orthopaedic Sports Medicine*. Philadelphia: WB Saunders, 1994, p 989.)

tion. Percutaneous stabilization to the adjacent metacarpal after reduction is usually adequate. ORIF may be more appropriate for competitive athletes, however, allowing more rapid return to play.

VII. Posttraumatic Problems of the Wrist
   A. Kienbock Disease—Avascular necrosis and collapse of the lunate is probably secondary to repetitive compressive forces causing microfractures of the cancellous bone. Mechanical factors, including ulnar negative variance, may predispose to this condition. Radiographs may demonstrate sclerosis, cysts, and carpal collapse, depending on the stage of the disease (Fig. 6–15). Treatment of the early stages of the disease includes relieving the compressive forces by ulnar lengthening or radial shortening. Limited intercarpal fusion with or without interpositional arthroplasty may be indicated for progressive stages of the disease.
   B. Osteochondrosis of the Capitate—This is an unusual disorder that appears to occur more commonly in gymnasts, probably as a result of repeated trauma. Partial excision of the capitate with or without limited intercarpal arthrodesis may be appropriate in some cases.
   C. Scaphoid Nonunion and Osteonecrosis—Untreated or persistent nonunion of the scaphoid is related to the development of late arthritis. Treatment of nonunions and avascular necrosis includes bone grafting and internal fixation. Salvage procedures include intercarpal

arthrodesis, proximal row carpectomy, and wrist fusion. Athletes may no longer be competitive if chronic symptoms necessitating these procedures develop.

VIII. Entrapment Neuropathies
   A. Introduction—Entrapment neuropathies were introduced in Chapter 5. The discussion in this chapter is limited to carpal tunnel syndrome and Guyon canal syndrome.
   B. Carpal Tunnel Syndrome—This common entrapment neuropathy is related to compression of the median nerve within the carpal tunnel (Fig. 6–16). This is a common problem among cyclists, throwers, and tennis players. Any condition that reduces the space within the confines of the carpal tunnel can cause symptoms (numbness or tingling in the radial three and one-half digits, clumsiness, and pain and paresthesias that may awaken a patient at night). Examination should include a complete neurologic examination and provocative testing (Phalen test, Tinel test, and median nerve compression test). Neurologic testing confirms the diagnosis. Splinting, injections, activity modification, and other conservative management are usually recommended. Surgical release of the transverse carpal ligament is recommended if symptoms persist. Arthroscopic release appears to offer some decrease in scar tenderness but also a higher risk of complications such as iatrogenic injury, especially when the procedure is per-

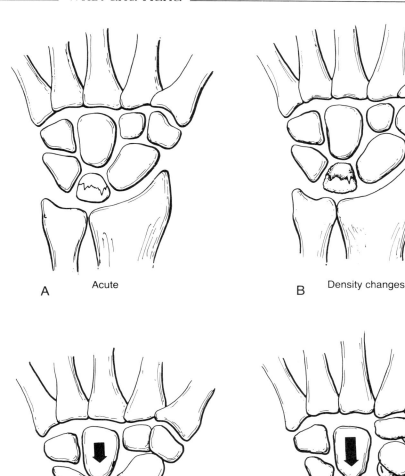

A   Acute

B   Density changes

C   Collapse of lunate

D   Pancarpal arthrosis

FIGURE 6–15. Stages of Kienbock disease. *A*, Stage I: normal or a radiolucent line. *B*, Stage II: lunate sclerosis. *C*, Stage III: lunate collapse. *D*, Stage IV: pancarpal arthrosis. (Redrawn from Lichtman DM, Alexander AHG, Mack GR, Gunther SF. Kienbock's disease—uptake on silicone replacement arthroplasty. J Hand Surg 7:343–347, 1982.)

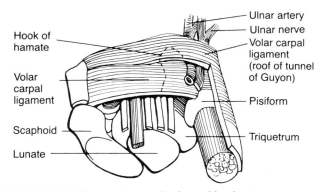

Hook of hamate

Volar carpal ligament

Scaphoid

Lunate

Ulnar artery

Ulnar nerve

Volar carpal ligament (roof of tunnel of Guyon)

Pisiform

Triquetrum

FIGURE 6–16. The carpal tunnel is formed by the transverse carpal tunnel, which is also the floor of the Guyon canal. (From McCue FC III, Bruce JF Jr. The wrist. In DeLee JC, Drez D Jr [eds]. *Orthopaedic Sports Medicine.* Philadelphia: WB Saunders, 1994, p 932.)

formed by surgeons less experienced with this technique.

C. Guyon Canal Syndrome (Handlebar Palsy)—This condition is unusual but appears to be more common in cyclists. Direct pressure over the Guyon canal, which transmits the ulnar nerve (Fig. 6–17), can result in pain and paresthesias in the ulnar one and one-half digits. Neurologic examination and testing usually confirm the diagnosis. Surgical release may be indicated if conservative measures fail. This syndrome commonly coexists with carpal tunnel syndrome.

IX. Tendinitis
   A. Introduction—Tendinitis of the wrist is one of the most common problems in sports. The cause is most often overuse, and athletes complain of localized pain exacerbated by activity.

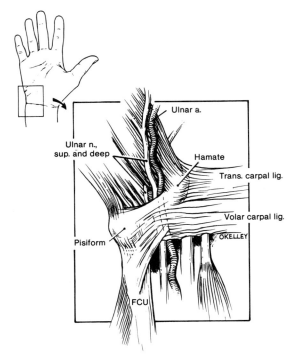

FIGURE 6–17. The ulnar nerve and artery pass beneath the pisohamate ligament into the Guyon canal, with the nerve lying ulnar to the artery. (FCU = flexor carpi ulnaris.) (From Green DP, Strickland JW. The hand. In DeLee JC, Drez D Jr [eds]. *Orthopaedic Sports Medicine.* Philadelphia: WB Saunders, 1994, p 1000.)

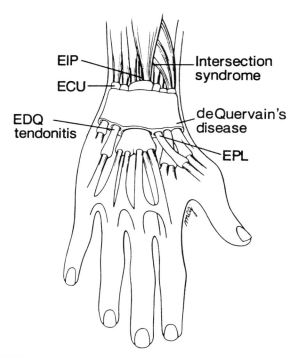

FIGURE 6–18. Location of common sites of tendinitis about the wrist. (EIP = extensor indicus proprius; ECU = extensor carpi ulnaris; EDQ = extensor diqiti quinti; EPL = extensor pollicis longus.) (From Kiefhaber TR, Stern PJ. Upper extremity tendinitis and overuse syndromes in the athlete. Clin Sports Med 11:43, 1992.)

Findings typically include local swelling and pain made worse with provocative testing. Tendinitis occurs most commonly in racket sports, rowing, volleyball, and gymnastics. A predictable series of events occurs after injury, consisting of inflammation, proliferation, maturation, and fibrosis. Progression to the final stage usually necessitates surgical intervention. Some of the more common sites of tendinitis about the wrist are shown in Figure 6–18.

B. De Quervain Disease—Stenosing tenosynovitis of the first compartment containing the abductor pollicis longus (APL) and extensor pollicis brevis (EPB) commonly occurs in golfers and in athletes who participate in racket sports. Patients present with localized pain and swelling. The Finkelstein test (ulnar deviation of the wrist with the thumb in the palm) reproduces the symptoms. Treatment includes rest and immobilization, local steroid injection, and rehabilitation. Refractory symptoms require surgical intervention. Release of the first compartment may require several incisions in the extensor retinaculum because the two tendons may be in separate compartments and the APL may have multiple slips (Fig. 6–19). Extreme care should be taken not to transect the dorsal sensory branch of the radial nerve.

C. Flexor Carpi Ulnaris and Radialis Tendinitis—Tendinitis of the wrist flexors is relatively common. Initial treatment consists of anti-inflammatory agents, activity modification, and possibly immobilization. Surgery, including tenolysis, is rarely necessary.

D. Extensor Carpi Ulnaris Subluxation—Athletes with this condition may present with painful snapping over the dorsoulnar aspect of the wrist during pronation and supination. Injury to the ulnar septum over the sixth dor-

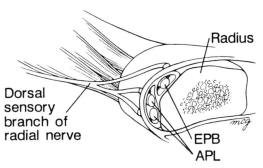

FIGURE 6–19. Surgical release of the first compartment for refractory de Quervain syndrome should include preservation of the dorsal sensory branch of the radial nerve and release of multiple compartments and slips. (EPB = extensor pollicis brevis; APB = abductor pollicis longus.) (From Kiefhaber TR, Stern PJ. Upper extremity tendinitis and overuse syndromes in the athlete. Clin Sports Med 11:44, 1992.)

sal compartment allows the extensor carpi ulnaris tendon to subluxate in supination and reduce in pronation. Care should be taken to distinguish this cause of ulnar wrist pain from TFCC injuries. Immobilization in a long arm cast with the wrist in pronation and slight dorsiflexion may allow healing. Failing this, fibro-osseous tunnel reconstruction with a flap of the extensor retinaculum may be successful (Fig. 6–20).

E. Intersection Syndrome—Inflammation at the intersection of the tendons of the first dorsal compartment (APL and EPB) and the second dorsal compartment (ECRL and ECRB) proximal to the dorsal extensor retinaculum can cause pain and swelling (Fig. 6–21). This condition is common in oarsmen and weight lifters, who have dubbed the audible crepitus associated with this condition "squeakers." Nonoperative treatment includes splinting, anti-inflammatory agents, and local injections. Surgical excision of inflamed tissue and decompression is rarely required, because this condition is usually self-limited.

F. Extensor Pollicis Longus Tenosynovitis—This condition can occur in racket players and is associated with pain aggravated by thumb motion. Local measures are usually effective, but rarely, surgical release is indicated.

X. Tendon Injuries in the Hand
A. Flexor Digitorum Profundus (FDP) Avulsion (Jersey Finger)—As the name suggests, avulsion of the FDP from its insertion on the distal phalanx occurs commonly in sports. The ring finger is most commonly injured. Leddy and

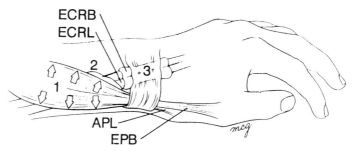

FIGURE 6–21. Intersection syndrome occurs at the crossing point of the first dorsal compartment muscles (APL and EPB) and those of the second dorsal compartment (ECRL and ECRB). (APL = abductor pollicis longus; EPB = extensor pollicis brevis; ECRL = extensor carpi radialis longus; ECRB = extensor carpi radialis brevis.) (From Kiefhaber TR, Stern PJ. Upper extremity tendinitis and overuse syndromes in the athlete. Clin Sports Med 11:45, 1992.)

Packer classified these injuries on the basis of the final position of the retracted tendon. Smith modified this classification to include a fourth type:

Type	FDP Final Position	Treatment Recommendation
I	Palm	Repair within 7 to 10 days
II	Flexor digitorum sublimis chiasm (PIP)	Repair within 3 months
III	A4 pulley	Repair within 3 months
IV	FDP avulsion and intra-articular fixation	Early repair and ORIF

Absence of FDP function, tested by stabilizing the proximal interphalangeal (PIP) joint while a patient actively flexes the distal interphalangeal (DIP) joint, is the hallmark of diagnosis. The location of the FDP stump can be localized on the basis of local tenderness, the position of the avulsed fragment of bone (if present), or MRI (Fig. 6–22). Although repair of some injuries can be postponed for 3 months, early repair is generally recommended once the injury is recognized. Repair is sometimes technically challenging because passing the tendon under the annular pulleys is difficult (A3, A4, and A5). These pulleys (especially the A4 pulley) must be preserved, and the tendon end may have to be trimmed for passage. Late treatment is difficult and may include observation, DIP arthrodesis, or tendon grafting, based on individual circumstances and the experience of the surgeon.

B. Mallet (Baseball) Finger—Avulsion of the terminal extensor tendon from the distal phalanx may or may not be associated with a bony avulsion (Fig. 6–23). The injury is caused by forcible flexion of the DIP while catching a ball

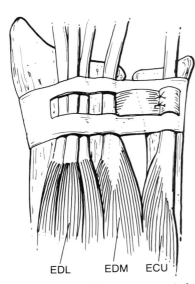

FIGURE 6–20. Stabilization of the extensor carpi ulnaris (ECU) with a flap of extensor retinaculum. Also shown are the extensor digitorum longus (EDL) and extensor digiti minimi (EDM) tendons. (Redrawn from Spinner M, Kaplan EB. Extensor carpi ulnaris. Clin Orthop 68:124–129, 1970.)

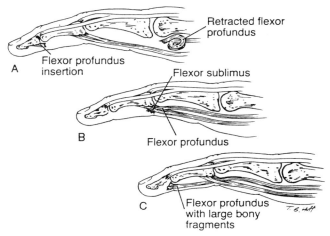

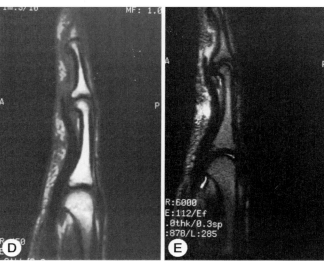

FIGURE 6–22. Leddy and Packer classification of FDP avulsions. *A,* Type I to palm. *B,* Type II to PIP. *C,* Type III to A4 pully. T1- *(D)* and T2-weighted *(E)* MRI of type II FDP avulsion. (*A–C* from Browner BD, Jupiter JB, Levine AM, Trafton PG. *Skeletal Trauma.* Philadelphia, WB Saunders 1992, p 1008.)

or hitting an object with the finger extended. Although treatment is still somewhat controversial, most authorities recommend continuous extension splinting to the DIP for 6 weeks, followed by nighttime splinting for an additional 6 weeks. It must be emphasized to patients that at no time during the initial 6 weeks of treatment should the DIP joint be allowed to fall into flexion, or an additional 6 weeks of continuous splinting is required thereafter. Late recognition of mallet fingers can result in deformities requiring surgical correction. Bony mallet fingers are treated similarly to soft tissue injuries unless volar fracture-subluxation of the distal phalanx is present, requiring ORIF.

C. Boutonniere Injury—Rupture of the central slip of the extensor apparatus near its insertion at the base of the middle phalanx can result in an established deformity if it is not recognized and treated early (Fig. 6–24). Acutely, patients have a swollen, painful PIP joint *with the point of maximum tenderness on the dorsum of the joint and inability to strongly extend the PIP joint.* Confirmation of the diagnosis can be accomplished by having patients flex the affected PIP joint 90° and actively extend the digit against resistance. If the central slip is intact, the DIP remains supple. If the central slip is ruptured, however, the lateral bands extend the PIP but also cause active DIP extension. Treatment involves splinting the PIP joint in full extension for a minimum of 6 weeks. It is important to leave the DIP joint free and to encourage passive flexion of this joint throughout the treatment period in order to maintain mobility of the lateral bands. Chronic injuries are difficult to treat. Surgical

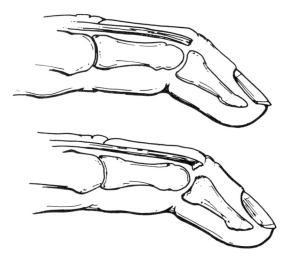

FIGURE 6–23. Mallet finger injuries can occur as soft tissue injuries only *(top)* or with an associated avulsion fracture *(bottom).* (From Green DP, Strickland JW. The hand. In DeLee JC, Drez D Jr [eds]. *Orthopaedic Sports Medicine.* Philadelphia: WB Saunders, 1994, p 951.)

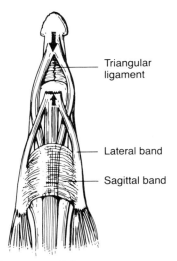

FIGURE 6–24. Boutonniere deformity can result from rupture of the central slip. If it is untreated, a flexion deformity of the PIP joint results from volar displacement of the lateral bands. (From Green DP, Strickland JW. The hand. In DeLee JC, Drez D Jr [eds]. *Orthopaedic Sports Medicine.* Philadelphia: WB Saunders, 1994, p 956.)

intervention, which is not always successful, may include tenolysis, transfer of the lateral bands, and repair of the extensor tendon.

XI. Ligamentous Injuries and Dislocations in the Hand
  A. Proximal Interphalangeal Joint
    1. Collateral Ligament Injury—The most common result of a jammed finger, these injuries occur frequently in athletes. Simple buddy taping for about 3 weeks is usually adequate for partial tears or sprains of the collateral ligaments. Most authorities also advocate buddy taping for a period of 6 weeks for complete tears, except for the radial collateral ligament of the index finger PIP, which requires surgical repair because of the need for stability of this joint. Such treatment is controversial, however.
    2. Volar Plate Injury (Dorsal PIP Dislocation)—Dorsal dislocations are much more common than volar dislocations at the PIP joint. Reduction of the joint is usually accomplished by the athlete, another player, or a trainer before presentation. After reduction, 3 to 6 weeks of buddy taping is usually adequate.
    3. Dorsal Fracture-Dislocation of the PIP—This injury can be disabling, particularly if recognized late. Initial treatment is with dorsal extension block splinting. The key is to ensure that the finger is flexed enough initially to reduce the joint and obtain articular congruity. The "V" sign of Light signifies an incomplete reduction (Fig. 6–25). Failure to achieve adequate reduction mandates open reduction or a volar plate arthroplasty. The dorsal extension splint is gradually straightened during the course of 4 to 6 weeks of treatment.
    4. Volar PIP Dislocation—These injuries are unusual. Because the central slip is necessarily injured with this dislocation, treatment includes immobilization of the PIP joint extension for 6 weeks, with active and passive DIP flexion.

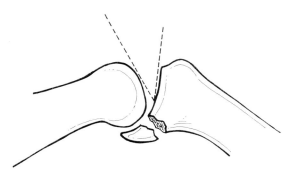

FIGURE 6–25. "V" sign as described by Light is consistent with an inadequately reduced joint after a bony volar plate injury.

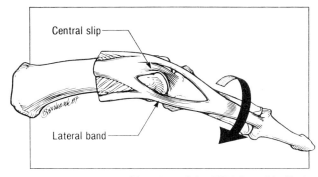

FIGURE 6–26. Rotatory subluxation of the PIP joint with displacement of a condyle of the proximal phalanx into the interval between the central slip and lateral band. (From Green DP, Strickland JW. The hand. In DeLee JC, Drez D Jr [eds]. *Orthopaedic Sports Medicine.* Philadelphia: WB Saunders, 1994, p 965.)

    5. Rotatory PIP Dislocation—Also unusual, this injury is usually a result of a twisting force. One condyle of the proximal phalanx buttonholes between the central slip and lateral band (Fig. 6–26). The lateral radiograph demonstrates a true lateral of one phalanx and an oblique of the adjacent phalanx. Closed reduction should be attempted by applying traction and a rotatory force on the digit with the MP and PIP joints flexed 90° and the wrist dorsiflexed. Simple buddy taping is all that is required after successful reduction. Open reduction is occasionally required if closed techniques are unsuccessful.
  B. Metacarpophalangeal Joint Injuries
    1. Collateral Ligament Injuries—These injuries are more common in athletes than in the general public and generally involve the radial collateral ligament. Localized tenderness and pain with lateral stress applied with the MP joint in flexion indicate the diagnosis. Treatment includes splinting with the MP joint in 50° flexion for 3 weeks.
    2. Dorsal Dislocation—These injuries should be reduced with hyperextension and volar displacement of the proximal phalanx with the wrist and IP joints flexed. After successful reduction, a short period of buddy taping is all that is required. Irreducible or complex dislocations are caused by buttonholing of the metacarpal head into the palm and interposition of the volar plate into the MP joint (Fig. 6–27). Three findings are usually present with these injuries: (1) parallelism of the proximal phalanx and metacarpal on lateral radiographs, (2) sesamoid located within a widened joint space, and (3) puckering of the volar skin. Open reduction is usually required, but one attempt at reduction using the technique described earlier may be reasonable.

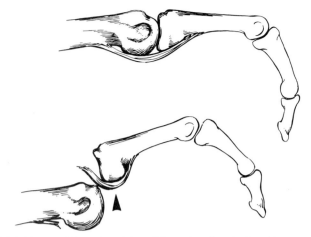

FIGURE 6–27. Normal position of the volar plate (*top*) and interposition of the volar plate between the base of the middle phalanx and the metacarpal head with a complex (irreducible) MP dislocation (*bottom*). (From Green DP, Strickland JW. The hand. In DeLee JC, Drez D Jr [eds]. *Orthopaedic Sports Medicine.* Philadelphia: WB Saunders, 1994, p 978.)

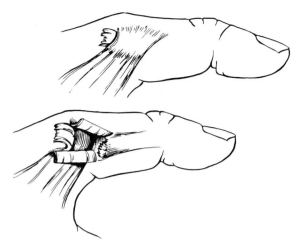

FIGURE 6–28. Stener lesion. Interposition of the adductor tendon between the two ends of the ulnar collateral ligament. (From Green DP, Strickland JW. The hand. In DeLee JC, Drez D Jr [eds]. *Orthopaedic Sports Medicine.* Philadelphia: WB Saunders, 1994, p 976.)

3. Volar Dislocation—This is an unusual injury. Reduction should be attempted by hyperflexing the MP joint and pushing the proximal phalanx back into position. Open reduction may be required.
C. Gamekeeper's (Skier's) Thumb—This injury is a result of a sudden valgus stress on the thumb MP joint. In complete injuries, the two ends of the ulnar collateral ligament are often left unopposed by interposition of the adductor tendon (Stener lesion) (Fig. 6–28). Stress radiographs, best performed under some form of anesthesia, allow differentiation between partial and complete injuries. Side-to-side differences of >10° to 15° or opening of >35° to 45° is consistent with a complete lesion. One study suggests that stress testing is necessary even with minimally displaced bony avulsion injuries. These bony injuries may actually represent fragmentation of the ulnar volar aspect of the proximal phalanx associated with complete disruption of the ulnar collateral ligament. Partial injuries are treated with immobilization, and most authorities recommend surgical repair of complete injuries.

Selected References

Anatomy and Biomechanics

Gilford WW, Bolton RH, Lambrinudi C. The mechanism of the wrist joint with special reference to fractures of the scaphoid. Guy's Hosp Rep 92:52–59, 1943.
Lichtman DM, Schneider JR, Swafford AR, et al. Ulnar midcarpal instability—Clinical and laboratory analysis. J Hand Surg 6A:515–523, 1981.
Palmer AK, Werner FW. Triangular fibrocartilage of the wrist: anatomy and function. J Hand Surg 6:153, 1981.
Taleisnik J. Post traumatic carpal instability. Clin Orthop 149:73, 1980.
Volz RG, Lieb M, Benjamin J. Biomechanics of the wrist. Clin Orthop 149:112, 1980.

Diagnosis

Green DP, Strickland JW. The hand. In DeLee JC, Drez D Jr (eds). *Orthopaedic Sports Medicine.* Philadelphia: WB Saunders, 1994, pp 945–1017.
Loeb PE, Mirabello SC, Andrews JR. The hand: field evaluation and treatment. Clin Sports Med 11:27–37, 1992.
McCue FC, Bruce JF. The wrist. In DeLee JC, Drez D Jr (eds). *Orthopaedic Sports Medicine.* Philadelphia: WB Saunders, 1994, pp 913–944.
Mirabello SC, Loeb PE, Andrews JR. The wrist: field evaluation and treatment. Clin Sports Med 11:1–25, 1992.

Arthroscopy

Cooney WP, Dobyns JH, Linscheid RL. Arthroscopy of the wrist: anatomy and classification of carpal instability. Arthroscopy 6:133–140, 1990.
North ER, Meyer S. Wrist injuries: correlation of clinical and arthroscopic findings. J Hand Surg 15A:915–920, 1990.
Osterman AL. Arthroscopic debridement of triangular fibrocartilage complex tears. Arthroscopy 6:120–124, 1990.
Poehling GG, Siegel DB, Koman LA, Chabon SJ. Arthroscopy of the wrist and elbow. In DeLee JC, Drez D Jr (eds). *Orthopaedic Sports Medicine.* Philadelphia: WB Saunders, 1994, pp 189–214.

Roth JH, Poehling GG, Whipple TL. Arthroscopic surgery of the wrist. Instr Course Lect 37:183–194, 1988.
Whipple TL. Diagnostic and surgical arthroscopy of the wrist. In Nichols JA, Hershman EB (eds). *The Upper Extremity in Sports Medicine.* St Louis: CV Mosby, 1990, pp 399–418.

Distal Radioulnar Joint Injuries

Aulicino PL, Siegel L. Acute injuries of the distal radioulnar joint. Hand Clin 7:283–293, 1991.
Bell MJ, Hill RJ, McMurtry RY. Ulnar impingement syndrome. J Bone Joint Surg 67B:126–129, 1985.
Bowers WH. The distal radioulnar joint. In Green DP (ed). *Operative Hand Surgery.* 3rd ed. New York: Churchill Livingstone, 1993, pp 973–1019.
Darrach W. Partial excision of lower shaft of ulna for deformity following Colles fracture. Ann Surg 57:764–765, 1913.
Dell PC. Traumatic disorders of the distal radioulnar joint. Clin Sports Med 11:141–159, 1991.
Feldon P, Belsky MR, Terrono AL. Partial ("wafer") distal ulna resection for triangular fibrocartilage tears and/or ulnar impaction syndrome. J Hand Surg 15A:826–827, 1990.
Friedman SL, Palmer AK. The ulnar impaction syndrome. Hand Clin 7:295–310, 1991.
Kapandji IA. The Kapandji-Sauve operation: its techniques and indications in non rheumatoid disease. Ann Chir Main 5:181–193, 1986.
Milch H. Dislocation of the end of the ulna—suggestion for a new operative procedure. Am J Surg 1:141–146, 1926.
Osterman AL. Arthroscopic debridement of triangular fibrocartilage complex tears. Arthroscopy 6:120–124, 1990.
Palmer AK. Triangular fibrocartilage disorders: injury patterns and treatment. Arthroscopy 6:125–132, 1990.
Taleisnik J. The Sauve-Kapandji procedure. Clin Orthop 275:110–123, 1992.

Carpal Instabilities

Alexander CE, Lichtman DM. Ulnar carpal instabilities. Orthop Clin North Am 15:307–320, 1984.
Blatt G. Capsulodesis in reconstructive hand surgery: dorsal capsulodesis for the unstable scaphoid and volar capsulodesis following excision of the distal ulna. Hand Clin 3:81–102, 1987.
Cooney WP III, Linscheid RL, Dobyns JH. Carpal instability: treatment of ligament injuries of the wrist. Instr Course Lect 41:33–44, 1992.
Linscheid RL. Scapholunate ligamentous instabilities (dissociations, subdislocations, dislocations). Ann Chir Main 3:323–330, 1984.
McCue FC, Bruce JF. The wrist. In DeLee JC, Drez D Jr (eds). *Orthopaedic Sports Medicine.* Philadelphia: WB Saunders, 1994, pp 913–944.
O'Brien ET. Acute fractures and dislocations of the carpus. Orthop Clin North Am 15:237–258, 1984.
Reagan DS, Linscheid RL, Dobyns JH. Lunotriquetral sprains. J Hand Surg 9A:502–514, 1984.
Watson HK, Ballet FL. The SLAC wrist: scapholunate advanced collapse pattern of degenerative arthritis. J Hand Surg 9A:358–365, 1984.
Watson HK, Hempton RF. Limited wrist arthrodesis I: the triscaphoid joint. J Hand Surg 5:320–327, 1980.

Fractures

Adler JB, Shafatan GW. Fractures of the capitate. J Bone Joint Surg 44A:1537–1547, 1962.
Cooney WP, Dobyns JH, Linscheid RL. Nonunion of the scaphoid. Analysis of the results from bone grafting. J Hand Surg 8:343–354, 1980.
Culver JE, Anderson TE. Fractures of the hand and wrist in the athlete. Clin Sports Med 11:101–128, 1992.
Gelberman RH, Menon J. The vascularity of the scaphoid bone. J Bone Joint Surg 62A:508–513, 1980.
Gellman H, Caputo RJ, Carter V, et al. A comparison of short and long thumb spica casts for nondisplaced fractures of the carpal scaphoid. J Bone Joint Surg 71A:354–357, 1989.
Green DP, Strickland JW. The hand. In DeLee JC, Drez D Jr (eds). *Orthopaedic Sports Medicine.* Philadelphia: WB Saunders, 1994, pp 945–1017.
Parker RD, Berkowitz MS, Brahms MA, Bohl WR. Hook of the hamate fractures in athletes. Am J Sports Med 14:517–523, 1986.
Polivy KD, Millender LH, Newberg A, et al. Fractures of the hook of the hamate: a failure of clinical diagnosis. J Hand Surg 9A:502–514, 1984.
Rand J, Linscheid RL, Dobyns JH. Capitate fractures. A long term follow-up. Clin Orthop 165:209–216, 1982.
Reister JN, Baker BE, Mosher JF, Lowe D. A review of scaphoid fracture healing in competitive athletes. Am J Sports Med 13:159–161, 1985.
Russe O. Fracture of the carpal navicular. J Bone Joint Surg 42A:759–768, 1960.
Stark HH, Jobe FW, Boyes JH, et al. Fracture of the hook of the hamate in athletes. J Bone Joint Surg 59A:575–582, 1977.
Zemel NP, Stark HH. Fractures and dislocations of the carpal bone. Clin Sports Med 5:709–724, 1986.

Posttraumatic Problems of the Wrist

Alexander AH, Turner MA, Alexander CE, et al. Lunate silicone replacement arthroplasty in Kienböck's disease: a long term follow-up. J Hand Surg 15A:401–407, 1990.
Almquist EE, Burns JF. Radial shortening for the treatment of Kienbock's disease—a 5 to 10 year follow-up. J Hand Surg 7:348–352, 1982.
Armstead RB, Linscheid RL, Dobyns JH, et al. Ulnar lengthening in the treatment of Kienbock's disease. J Bone Joint Surg 64A:170–178, 1982.
Chun S, Wicks BP, Meyerdierks E, et al. Two modifications for insertion of the Herbert screw in the fractured scaphoid. J Hand Surg 15A:669–671, 1990.
Gelberman RH, Salamon PB, Jurist JM, Posch JL. Ulnar variance in Kienbock's disease. J Bone Joint Surg 57A:674–676, 1975.
Lichtman DM, Mack GR, MacDonald RI, et al. Kienbock's disease: The role of silicone replacement arthroplasty. J Bone Joint Surg 59A:899–908, 1977.

Murakami S, Nakajima H. Aseptic necrosis of the capitate bone. Am J Sports Med 12:170–173, 1984.
Nalebuff EA, Poehling GG, Siegel DB, Koman LA. Wrist and hand: reconstruction. In Frymoyer JW (ed). *Orthopaedic Knowledge Update 4:* Home Study Syllabus. Rosemont, IL: American Academy of Orthopaedic Surgeons, 1993, pp 389–402.
Watson HK, Ryu J, DiBella. An approach to Kienbock's disease: triscaphe arthrodesis. J Hand Surg 10A:179–187, 1985.

Entrapment Neuropathies

Burke ER. Ulnar neuropathy in bicyclists. Physician Sportsmed 9:53–56, 1981.
Chow JCY. The Chow technique of endoscopic release of the carpal ligament for carpal tunnel syndrome: four years of clinical results. Arthroscopy 9:301–314, 1993.
Gelberman RH, Eaton R, Urbaniak JR. Peripheral nerve compression. J Bone Joint Surg 75A:1854–1878, 1993.
Katz RT: Nerve entrapments: an update. Orthopedics 12:1097–1107, 1989.
Paley D, McMurtry RY. Median nerve compression test in carpal tunnel syndrome diagnosis: reproduced signs and symptoms in the affected wrist. Orthop Rev 15:411–415, 1985.
Palmer DH. Endoscopic carpal tunnel release: a comparison of two techniques with open release. Arthroscopy 9:498–508, 1993.
Rowland EB, Kleinert JM. Endoscopic carpal tunnel release in cadavera. An investigation of the results of twelve surgeons with this training model. J Bone Joint Surg 76A:266–268, 1994.
Shea JD, McClain EJ. Ulnar nerve compression syndromes at and below the wrist. J Bone Joint Surg 51A:1095–1103, 1969.
Weinstein SM, Herring SA. Nerve problems and compartment syndromes in the hand, wrist, and forearm. Clin Sports Med 11:161–188, 1992.

Tendinitis

Burhkhart SS, Wood MB, Linscheid RL. Posttraumatic recurrent subluxation of the extensor carpi ulnaris tendon. J Hand Surg 7:1, 1982.
Dobyns JH, Sim FH, Linscheid RL. Sports stress syndromes of the hand and wrist. Am J Sports Med 6:236, 1978.
Finkelstein H. Stenosing tendovaginitis at the radial styloid process. J Bone Joint Surg 12A:509, 1930.
Kiefhaber TR, Stern PJ. Upper extremity tendinitis and overuse syndromes in the athlete. Clin Sports Med 11:39–55, 1992.
Wood MB, Dobyns JH. Sports-related extraarticular wrist syndromes. Clin Orthop 202:93–102, 1986.

Tendon Injuries

Green DP, Strickland JW. The hand. In DeLee JC, Drez D Jr (eds). *Orthopaedic Sports Medicine*. Philadelphia: WB Saunders, 1994, pp 945–1017.
Kaplan EB. Mallet or baseball finger. Surgery 7:784–791, 1940.
Lange RH, Engber WB. Hyperextension mallet finger. Orthopedics 6:1426–1431, 1983.
Leddy JP, Packer JW. Avulsion of the profundus tendon insertion in athletes. J Hand Surg 2:66–69, 1977.
Moss JG, Steingold RF. The long term results of mallet finger injury: a retrospective study of one hundred cases. Hand 15:151–154, 1983.
Rettig AC. Closed tendon injuries of the hand and wrist in the athlete. Clin Sports Med 11:77–99, 1992.
Smith JH. Avulsion of a profundus tendon with simultaneous intra-articular fracture of the distal phalanx. J Hand Surg 6:600–601, 1981.
Strickland JW. Management of acute flexor tendon injuries. Orthop Clin North Am 14:827–849, 1983.

Ligament Injuries

Betz RR, Browne EZ, Perry GB, Resnick EJ. The complex volar metacarpophalangeal-joint dislocation. J Bone Joint Surg 64A:1374–1375, 1982.
Campbell CS. Gamekeeper's thumb. J Bone Joint Surg 37B:148–149, 1955.
Eaton RG, Malerich MM. Volar plate arthroplasty of the proximal interphalangeal joint: a review of ten years' experience. J Hand Surg 5:260–268, 1980.
Green DP, Strickland JW. The hand. In DeLee JC, Drez D Jr (eds). *Orthopaedic Sports Medicine*. Philadelphia: WB Saunders, 1994, pp 945–1017.
Hinterman B, Holzach PJ, Schultz M, Matter P. Skier's thumb. The significance of bony injuries. Am J Sports Med 21:800–804, 1993.
Hubbard LF. Metacarpophalangeal dislocations. Hand Clin 4:39–44, 1988.
Isani A, Melone CP Jr. Ligamentous injuries of the hand in athletes. Clin Sports Med 5:757–772, 1986.
Kaplan EB. Dorsal dislocation of the metacarpophalangeal joint of the index finger. J Bone Joint Surg 39A:1081–1086, 1957.
Light TR. Buttress pinning techniques. Orthop Rev 10:49–55, 1981.
McElfresh EC, Dobyns JH, O'Brien ET. Management of fracture-dislocation of the proximal interphalangeal joints by extension-block splinting. J Bone Joint Surge 54A:1705–1711, 1972.
McLaughlin HL. Complex "locked" dislocation of the metacarpalphalangeal joints. J Trauma 5:683–688, 1965.
Palmer AK, Louis DS. Assessing ulnar instability of the metacarpophalangeal joint of the thumb. J Hand Surg 3:542–546, 1978.
Redler I, Williams JT. Rupture of a collateral ligament of the proximal interphalangeal joint of the fingers: analysis of eighteen cases. J Bone Joint Surg 49A:322–326, 1967.
Stener B. Displacement of the ruptured collateral ligament of the metacarpophalangeal joint of the thumb: a clinical and anatomical study. J Bone Joint Surg 44B:869–879, 1962.

III

Other Sports Medicine Problems

CHAPTER 7

Head and Spine

I. Head Injuries
   A. Introduction—Head injuries are relatively common in collision sports, and it is important for team physicians to understand at least the basics of injuries and guidelines for workup and return to play. Traumatic injuries of the brain can be considered in two categories, diffuse and focal. Each is discussed separately.
   B. Diffuse Brain Injury—Three types of diffuse brain injury are commonly recognized: (1) mild cerebral concussion, (2) classic cerebral concussion, and (3) diffuse axonal injury.
      1. Mild Cerebral Concussion—This entity is described as neurologic dysfunction without loss of consciousness. It commonly occurs in football and often is unreported. Mild concussions are further subclassified into three grades. Grade 1 is associated with confusion and disorientation without amnesia that clears within minutes. The player commonly notes that he had his "bell rung." If there are no associated symptoms (e.g., headache, dizziness, impaired orientation, photophobia), then the athlete may usually return to competition when the symptoms resolve. Grade 2 injuries are associated with retrograde amnesia that develops several minutes after the injury and lasts for a variable but usually brief period of time preceding the injury. Postconcussion syndrome, characterized by persistent headaches, irritability, and difficulty concentrating, is common after grade 2 injuries, and most authorities recommend that an athlete be kept out of competition for a week after the injury and for as long as any symptoms persist. Grade 3 injuries are less common but more severe. With these injuries, amnesia is present from the time of impact and usually has a posttraumatic component as well. Some authorities recommend restriction from competition for a minimum of a month for grade 3 injuries.
      2. Classic Cerebral Concussion—This occurs when a player is knocked out, usually for a brief period. As the athlete regains consciousness, the athlete passes through stages of stupor, confusion, and automatism before becoming fully alert. Proper consideration to airway and cervical spine control should be given to individuals with this injury. Players with loss of consciousness should not return to play that day. Overnight observation is appropriate for patients with prolonged loss of consciousness or deteriorating neurologic states. The duration of the loss of consciousness can be useful in determining when a player can return to participation. Players with loss of consciousness for >5 minutes should have computed tomography (CT) of the head and should not be allowed to return to competition for at least 1 week. The New York state boxing commission does not allow boxers with loss of consciousness to fight for 1 month. Other contact athletes who return and have a second episode of loss of consciousness should not be allowed to return to competition until the following season.
      3. Diffuse Axonal Injury—This occurs in individuals with loss of consciousness lasting more than 6 hours. Residual neurologic or personality deficits often occur. This can be a result of return to contact before resolution of concussion and postconcussion syndrome (second-impact syndrome).
   C. Focal Brain Syndromes—These are usually a result of traumatic intracranial hematomas including cerebral contusions, intracerebral hematomas, epidural hematomas, and subdural hematomas. The diagnosis is usually based on CT scan results (Fig. 7–1). A contusion usually demonstrates a hemorrhagic area with surrounding edema, an epidural hematoma is characterized by a biconvex/lentiform appearance, and a subdural hematoma has a concave/crecentric appearance on CT. Although epidural bleeding is classically described as being associated with loss of consciousness followed by a variable period of lucidity and then recurrence of a decreased level of consciousness, this cannot be relied on and is variable in a clinical setting. Subdural hematomas are associated with a high mortality rate, especially if associated with underlying cerebral contusion. Treatment of these injuries includes life support mea-

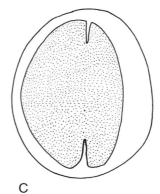

FIGURE 7–1. CT findings of contusion (A), epidural hematoma (B), and subdural hematoma (C).

sures and evacuation of the hematoma for larger intracranial hematomas.

II. Cervical Spine Injuries
   A. Introduction—Various cervical spine injuries can occur in athletes. Some of these injuries have minimal sequelae, and some are more serious, often with catastrophic outcomes. Most cervical spine injuries in sports are a result of axial loading of the spine with the neck flexed and the cervical spine straightened from its natural lordotic position. Changes in football rules prohibiting "spearing" have had a positive effect on the incidence of these injuries, but unfortunately, these devastating accidents still occur. Brachial plexus injuries, or "burners," were discussed in Chapter 4. Other injuries to the cervical spine are discussed next.
   B. Soft Tissue Injuries to the Cervical Spine— These injuries include subluxation of one vertebra on another and cervical disc rupture. In patients with subluxation, findings on static radiographs are normal. Flexion-extension films are required, and anterior translation of one vertebra on another in excess of 20% may be an indication for posterior fusion. Other criteria for instability include >3.5 mm of displacement and >11° angulation in relation to the adjacent vertebra (Fig. 7–2). After successful fusion of

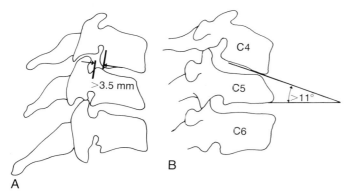

FIGURE 7–2. Both anterior displacement of >3.5 mm (A) and abnormal angulation of >11° (B) are associated with instability. (Modified from Shite AA, Johnson R, Panjabi MM, et al. Cervical instability following injury. Clin Orthop 109:85, 1975.)

one level with good residual motion and no remaining symptoms, selected athletes may return to contact sports. Cervical disc ruptures can result in transient quadriplegia and an anterior cord syndrome. With this syndrome, normal motor and sensory function is temporarily lost but position and vibration sense is preserved. Magnetic resonance imaging (MRI) has proved to be most valuable in the evaluation of this problem. Anterior diskectomy and fusion is infrequently required. Patients with healed anterior or lateral disc herniation treated conservatively or those patients who are treated operatively with a solid fusion and who have good motion and no neurologic deficits can return to contact sports. Contraindications to resumption of contact sports include central herniations and "hard" disc herniation with associated neurologic symptoms/findings.
   C. Cervical Spine Fractures and Dislocations—A complete discussion of acute cervical spine injuries is beyond the scope of this chapter; however, all team physicians should understand certain basic principles. Catastrophic cervical spine injuries in contact sports are most commonly caused by axial loading. Although these injuries are relatively rare in athletics, careful management of on-the-field injuries is paramount. Cervical spine immobilization, airway support, and safe transportation are essential. Fractures and facet dislocations causing cord impingement should be reduced by qualified physicians as soon as safely possible. Spinal shock is common after cervical spine injuries, and further recovery is possible until spinal shock has resolved. The end of spinal shock is heralded by return of the bulbocavernosus reflex. Acute management of cervical spine injuries should also include parenteral steroids. Methylprednisolone (30 mg/kg bolus followed by 5.4 mg/kg/hr) is recommended for the first 24 hours after injury. Fractures are generally considered unstable if they meet the criteria discussed earlier (>3.5 displacement or >20° angulation) or if they result in destruction of the anterior or posterior elements. Stable com-

pression fractures can usually be managed in a cervical collar, and athletes can return to competition after healing. Facet dislocations require reduction with or without stabilization. Unilateral facet dislocations result in displacement of approximately 25% of the vertebra, whereas bilateral dislocations result in >50% displacement. Unstable fractures and dislocations usually require a halo vest or operative treatment.

D. Cervical Stenosis—Narrowing of the anteroposterior (AP) diameter of the cervical spine can be congenital or developmental. The ratio of the spinal canal to the vertebral body, as described by Pavlov and associates, is a helpful method of evaluating lateral radiographs (Fig. 7–3). Cervical stenosis can be associated with neurapraxia and transient neurapraxia. This condition, although worrisome, is usually transient, and full recovery is normal. Recommendations for return to play for patients with cervical stenosis with transient symptoms are controversial. Some authorities suggest that there is no significant risk as long as patients have no associated cervical instability or degenerative changes. A high incidence of abnormal Pavlov ratios has been noted in collegiate and professional players who have no history of neck problems. The usefulness of this ratio is currently being challenged.

E. Upper Cervical Spine Abnormalities—Athletes with abnormalities of the upper two cervical vertebrae, including odontoid abnormalities,

atlanto-occipital fusion, Klippel-Feil deformities involving the dens or atlas, and other C1–C2 injuries, should be discouraged from participation in contact sports because of significant risk for further injury.

F. Spear Tackler's Spine—Football players who persistently use improper tackling techniques may develop this disorder, which includes developmental cervical stenosis (Pavlov ratio of <0.8 at one or more levels), loss of lordosis, and other preexisting spinal radiographic abnormalities. These individuals should not be allowed to return to contact sports because of a high risk of future significant injury. They may be allowed to return if their normal lordotic curve returns, if they show no evidence of disc disease or instability, and if they modify their tackling techniques.

III. Thoracic and Lumbar Spine Injuries

A. Soft Tissue Injuries—Sprains and strains of the back are common in athletics. Treatment includes anti-inflammatory medications, ice, and rehabilitation. Muscle spasms of the back can be controlled with appropriate medications. Supportive braces may also be helpful.

B. Fractures—Although unusual, several fractures of the thoracolumbar spine merit discussion.

1. Transverse Process Fractures of the Thoracic Spine—These injuries, which can also involve the bases of the ribs, are usually a result of a direct blow. Affected individuals have localized tenderness, and the fracture is usually identified on plain radiographs. Treatment is supportive. The use of a flak jacket may be appropriate for football players. Modalities, stretching, and other rehabilitation are often helpful. Formal bracing is not required.

2. Compression Fractures—These commonly involve the lower thoracic region and represent a failure of the anterior column. One must always be concerned about the possibility of a pathologic fracture, particularly in circumstances in which no significant trauma occurred and in upper thoracic spine injuries. A lateral radiograph is most helpful in judging the severity of the fracture. Most fractures involve compression of <25% of the anterior vertebral body height. Fractures with >50% compression or those involving the posterior elements should be evaluated with CT scanning to rule out posterior (burst) fractures. Bracing (6–12 weeks) in an extension orthosis and administration of analgesics are appropriate.

3. Fracture-Dislocation—These injuries are a result of high-energy impact and are highly associated with spinal cord injury. Early reduction and posterior fusion is indicated in most patients. Individuals with complete

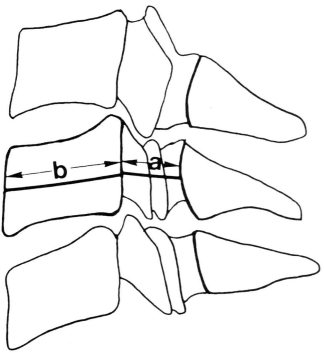

FIGURE 7–3. Pavlov ratio a : b. Ratios of <0.8 are consistent with stenosis. (From Pavlov H, Porter IS. Criteria for cervical instability and stenosis. Op Tech Sports Med 1:170, 1993.)

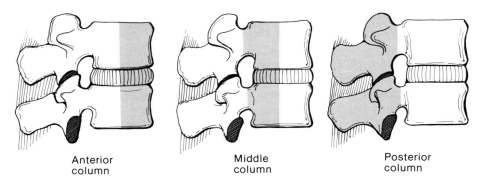

FIGURE 7–4. Three-column classification of spine injuries (Denis). (From Eismont FJ, Kitchel SH. Thoracolumbar spine. In DeLee JC, Drez D Jr [eds]. *Orthopaedic Sports Medicine*. Philadelphia: WB Saunders, 1994, p 1048.)

Anterior column

Middle column

Posterior column

neurologic deficits can be treated by bracing without surgery.

4. Lumbar Spine Fractures—These injuries are characterized on the basis of the columns involved (Denis) (Fig. 7–4). Isolated posterior column fractures (spinous process, transverse process) are treated nonoperatively. Unstable fractures (those involving two or more columns) are best treated by experienced spine surgeons and often require surgical stabilization, which necessarily restricts the athlete from returning to contact sports.

5. Vertebral Ring Apophysis Injury—Although these injuries are more common in athletes, particularly wrestlers and female gymnasts, their significance is unclear. In the thoracic spine, excavation of the anterior part of the vertebra is most common, but in the lumbar spine, persistent or enlarged apophysis is more common.

C. Disc Disease

1. Thoracic Disc Disease—Thoracic disc disease is unusual in athletes. Symptoms are vague and nonspecific radiating chest and upper back pain. MRI is the most useful

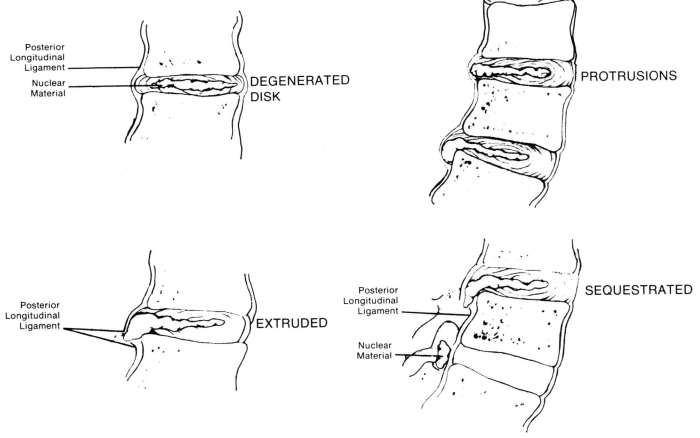

Posterior Longitudinal Ligament

Nuclear Material

DEGENERATED DISK

PROTRUSIONS

Posterior Longitudinal Ligament

EXTRUDED

Posterior Longitudinal Ligament

Nuclear Material

SEQUESTRATED

FIGURE 7–5. Nomenclature for disc pathology. (From Wiltse LL. Lumbosacral spine reconstruction. In *Orthopaedic Knowledge Update I.* Chicago: American Academy of Orthopaedic Surgeons, 1984, p 247.)

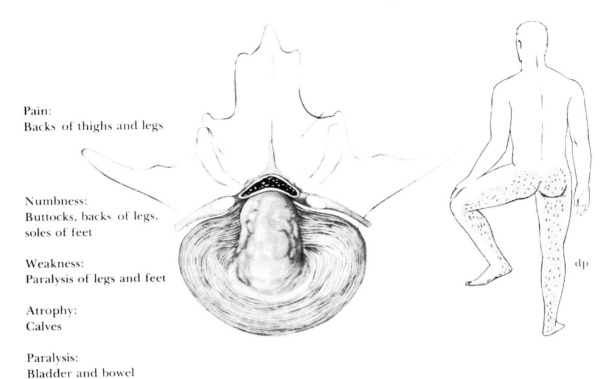

Pain:
Backs of thighs and legs

Numbness:
Buttocks, backs of legs,
soles of feet

Weakness:
Paralysis of legs and feet

Atrophy:
Calves

Paralysis:
Bladder and bowel

FIGURE 7–6. Cauda equina syndrome. (From DePalma AF, Rothman RH. *The Intervertebral Disc*. Philadelphia: WB Saunders, 1970, p 194.)

diagnostic test, but a high index of suspicion is required for ordering this evaluation. Treatment initially includes anti-inflammatory medications, physical therapy, bracing, or even injections. Surgery, usually through an anterior approach, may occasionally be required.

2. Lumbar Disc Disease—Lumbar disc disease is more common and can involve disc degeneration or herniation. Loss of water content in the disc typically occurs with age. Further degeneration can cause pain that is aggravated by activity. Weight lifting and other sports do not appear to increase the incidence of disc herniation. Treatment is supportive and includes exercise, modalities, and occasionally bracing. In addition to degenerating, discs can protrude, extrude, or become sequestered (Fig. 7–5). These last two categories involve herniation. Disc herniation is often associated with radicular leg pain. Careful neurologic testing is important

FIGURE 7–7. Spondylolysis. Note on the oblique radiograph (*A*) the disruption of the collar on the Scottie dog outline (*B*). (From Helms CA. *Fundamentals of Skeletal Radiology*. Philadelphia: WB Saunders, 1989, p 101.)

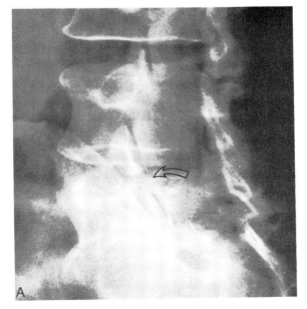

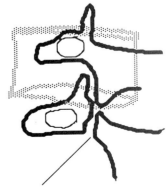

SPONDYLOLYSIS

A

B

TABLE 7–1. TYPES OF SPONDYLOLISTHESIS

Class	Type	Age	Pathology/Other
I	Congenital	Child	Congenital dysplasia of S1 superior facet
II	Isthmic*	5–50 years	Predisposition leading to elongation/fracture of pars (L5–S1)
III	Degenerative	Older	Facet arthrosis leading to subluxation (L4–L5)
IV	Traumatic	Young	Acute fracture/other than pars
V	Pathologic	Any	Incompetence of bony elements
VI	Postsurgical	Adult	Excessive resection of neural arches/facets

* Most common.

to determine nerve root involvement. Tension signs are sensitive indicators of nerve root compression. Bowel or bladder dysfunction (usually urinary retention), saddle anesthesia, and bilateral lower extremity symptoms may be associated with cauda equina syndrome (Fig. 7–6). This condition requires urgent surgery to avoid progressive or permanent neurologic loss. Treatment of other disc herniations usually involves a short period of rest, analgesics, therapy, and possibly epidural steroids. Various forms of

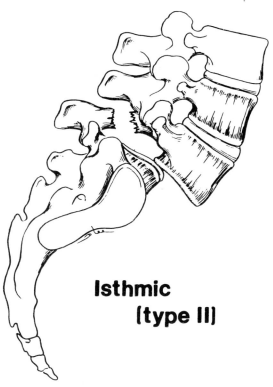

Isthmic (type II)

FIGURE 7–8. Isthmic (type II) spondylolisthesis is the most common form of spondylolisthesis. (From Rothman RH, Simeon FA. *The Spine*. Philadelphia: WB Saunders, 1982, p 264.)

surgical intervention have been proposed, including percutaneous, microsurgical, and even arthroscopically assisted techniques; however, the standard posterior partial laminectomy and discectomy still remains the gold standard.

D. Spondylolysis and Spondylolisthesis
  1. Spondylolysis—This condition is related to a defect (stress fracture) in the pars interarticularis of the spine. It is caused by a stress reaction of the pars, occurring most commonly in the lower lumbar levels. It may be caused by repetitive hyperextension of the lumbar spine, which explains its relatively high incidence among football interior linemen and gymnasts. Oblique radiographs are essential to the evaluation (Fig. 7–7). Bone scan (SPECT scan) and CT studies are helpful in the diagnosis and management of these injuries. Acute spondylolysis can be managed with rest and bracing in slight flexion. Reports of internal fixation of these defects are preliminary, and an athlete's ability to return to athletic activity after such a procedure is doubtful.
  2. Spondylolisthesis—This condition is related to the anterior displacement of one vertebral body over another. The severity of the slip is based on the percentage of the body that is displaced (I = 0–25%; II = 25–50%; III = 50–75%; IV = 75–100%; V (spondyloptosis) = >100%). Spondylolisthesis is also classified on the basis of its cause (Table 7–1; Fig. 7–8). Treatment of spondylolisthesis includes exercise and modalities. A very specific trunk stabilization rehabilitation program and postural training are useful in minimizing the symptoms in athletes with spondylolisthesis and foraminal stenosis. Lightweight orthotics may also be helpful. Higher-grade slippage (grade III and higher) may be associated with neurologic abnormalities and may require posterior fusion.

Selected References

Head Injuries

Bruno LA. Focal intracranial hematoma. In Torg JS (ed). *Athletic Injuries to the Head, Neck and Face.* 2nd ed. St Louis: Mosby-Year Book, 1991.

Cantu RC. Guidelines to return to sports after cerebral concussion. Physician Sportsmed 14:76, 1986.

Cantu RC. Criteria for return to competition after a closed head injury. In Torg JS (ed). *Athletic Injuries to the Head, Neck and Face.* 2nd ed. St Louis: Mosby-Year Book, 1991.

Gennarelli TA. Head injury mechanisms and cerebral concussion and diffuse brain injuries. In Torg JS (ed). *Athletic Injuries to the Head, Neck and Face.* 2nd ed. St Louis: Mosby-Year Book, 1991.

Jordan BD, Tsairis P, Warren RF. *Sports Neurology.* Rockville, MD: Aspen Press, 1989.

Lindsay KW, McLatchie G, Jennett B. Serious head injuries in sports. Br Med J 281:789–791, 1980.

Cervical Spine Injuries

Albright JP, Moses JM, Feldich HG, et al. Non-fatal cervical spine injuries in interscholastic football. JAMA 236:1243–1245, 1976.

Bracken MD, Shepard MJ, Collins WF, et al. A randomized, controlled trial of methylprednisolone or naloxone in the treatment of acute spinal cord injury. N Engl J Med 322:1405, 1990.

Pavlov H, Torg JS, Robie B, Jahre C. Cervical spinal stenosis: determination with vertebral body radio method. Radiology 164:771–775, 1987.

Schneider RC. The syndrome of acute anterior spinal cord injury. J Neurosurg 12:95–123, 1955.

Thompson RC. Current concepts in management of cervical spine fractures and dislocations. Am J Sports Med 3:159, 1975.

Torg JS, Gennarelli TA. Head and cervical spine injuries. In DeLee JC, Drez D Jr (ed). *Orthopaedic Sports Medicine: Principles and Practice.* Philadelphia: WB Saunders, 1994, pp 417–462.

Torg JS, Pavolv H, Genuario SE, et al. Neuropraxia of the cervical spinal cord with transient quadriplegia. J Bone Joint Surg 68A:1354–1370, 1986.

Torg JS, Sennett B, Vegso JJ, Pavlov H. Axial loading injuries to the middle cervical spine segment: an analysis and classification of twenty-five cases. Am J Sports Med 19:6–20, 1991.

Torg JS, Sennett B, Pavlov H, et al. Spear tacker's spine. An entity precluding participation in tackle football and collision activities that expose the cervical spine to axial energy inputs. Am J Sports Med 21:640–649, 1993.

Torg JS, Vegso JJ, O'Neill J, Sennett B. The epidemiologic, pathologic, biomechanical and cinematographic analysis of football-induced cervical spine trauma. Am J Sports Med 18:50–57, 1990.

White AA, Johnson RM, Panjabi MM. Biomechanical analysis of clinical stability in the cervical spine. Clin Orthop 109:85–93, 1975.

Thoracic and Lumbar Spine Injuries

Albrand OW, Corkill G. Thoracic disc herniation: treatment and prognosis. Spine 4:41–46, 1979.

Bradford DS, Boachie-Adjei O. Treatment of severe spondylolisthesis by anterior and posterior reduction and stabilization. A long-term follow-up study. J Bone Joint Surg 72A:1060, 1990.

Denis F. Spinal instability so defined by the three-column spine concept in acute spinal trauma. Clin Orthop 189:65, 1984.

Eismont FJ, Currier B. Surgical management of lumbar intervertebral disc disease. J Bone Joint Surg 71A:1266, 1989.

Eismont FJ, Kitchel SH. Thoracolumbar spine. In DeLee JC, Drez D Jr (eds). *Orthopaedic Sports Medicine.* Philadelphia: WB Saunders, 1994, pp 1018–1062.

Jackson D, Wiltse L, Dingeman R, Hayes M. Stress reactions involving the pars interarticularis in young athletes. Am J Sports Med 9:305, 1981.

Jacobs RR, Asher MA, Snider RK. Thoracolumbar spine injuries. Spine 5:463, 1986.

Keene JS, Albert MJ, Springer SL, et al. Back injuries in college athletes. J Spinal Disorders 2:190–195, 1989.

Mundt DJ, Kelsey JL, Golden AL, et al. An epidemiological study of sports and weightlifting as possible risk factors for herniated lumbar and cervical discs. Am J Sports Med 21:854–860, 1993.

Pedersen AK, Hagen R. Spondylolysis and spondylolisthesis. Treatment by internal fixation and bone grafting of the defect. J Bone Joint Surg 70A:15, 1988.

Smith MD, Bohlman HH. Spondylolisthesis treated by a single-stage operation combining decompression with in situ posterolateral and anterior fusion. J Bone Joint Surg 72A:415, 1990.

Sward L, Hellstrom M, Jacobsson B, Karlsson L. Vertebral ring apophysis injurty in athletes. Am J Sports Med 21:841–845, 1993.

Weber H. Lumbar disc herniation: a controlled prospective study with ten years of observation. Spine 8:131–140, 1983.

White AH, Derby R, Wynne A. Epidural injections for the diagnosis and treatment of low back pain. Spine 5:78, 1980.

CHAPTER 8

Medical Aspects of Sports Medicine

I. Introduction—It would be impossible to cover all medical aspects of sports medicine in this final chapter; nevertheless, several medical issues are receiving increasing attention from athletes and the media alike. Ergogenic drugs, sudden cardiac death, and problems particular to female athletes merit special emphasis.

II. Ergogenic Drugs
   A. Introduction—As athletic competition becomes more fierce and the financial rewards larger, today's athletes seek to obtain any competitive edge possible. Unfortunately, the side effects of these measures are often unknown or disregarded by athletes. The "drug du jour" changes as quickly as our abilities to detect substance abuse, and athletes may unwittingly become involved in progressively more dangerous drugs. As sports medicine physicians, it is our responsibility first to understand the magnitude and implications of the current problem and then to educate the athletes under our care.
   B. Anabolic Steroids—These drugs, which are synthetic derivatives of the hormone testosterone, are some of the most commonly abused agents. The effect of these drugs is an increase in muscle mass and strength. Adverse effects include alterations in liver function, changes in cholesterol levels, acne, cardiomyopathy, testicular atrophy, gynecomastia, alopecia, possible weakening of muscles and tendons, and psychologic changes. Objective measurement of psychologic changes was not possible in one study; however, subjective changes are common. Tighter controls and improved testing may reduce the incidence of the use of these drugs. Proper counseling of athletes is essential. The adverse side effects of the sometimes massive doses and "stacking" of compounds used by our athletes are not known. It is important for athletes to be aware of the risks involved.
   C. Human Growth Hormone—Human growth hormone is formed from recombinant deoxyribonucleic acid techniques using bacteria and is primarily administered to children with hormone deficiencies. Illegal use by athletes has become popular because athletes are not routinely tested for the drug (unlike steroids). Growth hormone has an enhancing effect on the size and weight of atrophied muscles and may increase lean body mass. Adverse effects include acromegaly, cardiomyopathy, coronary artery disease, hypertension, and giantism. These significant side effects are often misunderstood by the athlete-abuser.
   D. Amphetamines—These stimulants have an enhancing effect on athletic performance by masking fatigue and serving as anorectics for gymnasts, wrestlers, and divers. The adverse effects of these sympathomimetic drugs include central nervous system effects (tremulousness, anxiety, seizures), arrhythmias, nausea, and even death.
   E. Blood Doping—Induced erythrocythemia is accomplished by autologous reinfusion, heterologous blood infusion, or erythropoietin use. The idea is to increase the hemoglobin level of the athlete, thereby increasing, at least theoretically, an athlete's endurance. The adverse effects include transfusion reactions, transmission of hepatitis or acquired immunodeficiency syndrome, and increased blood viscosity, which may lead to congestive heart failure, hypertension, and cerebrovascular accidents.

III. Sudden Cardiac Death
   A. Sudden Death in Young Athletes—This is usually caused by a myocardial disorder, most commonly hypertrophic cardiomyopathy. This is an autosomal dominant disorder that affects the left ventricle. Hypertrophy of this chamber leads to a decrease in its volume and impedance of blood flow into the aorta. Most patients show no prodromal signs or symptoms. Other causes of sudden death in athletes younger than 30 years include anomalous coronary arteries, coronary artery disease, and conduction system abnormalities. Preparticipation history and physical examinations can sometimes identify patients at risk. The echocardiogram is the de-

finitive test but is not practical for screening purposes.

B. Sudden Cardiac Death in Older Athletes—This is usually related to preexisting coronary artery disease. Careful evaluation of risk factors and laboratory studies are important for older athletes. Stress electrocardiography can be a helpful screening tool.

IV. Exercise Physiology

A. Anaerobic Versus Aerobic Exercise—Anaerobic muscle action allows for a rapid source of energy from metabolism of glucose, resulting in the production of lactic acid. It is best suited for high-intensity, short-duration activities, and fatigue (from lactic acidosis) is usually the limiting factor. The aerobic system requires oxygen for metabolism and is better suited for endurance activities. Aerobic exercise uses mainly slow-twitch (red) type I muscle fibers. Anaerobic muscle fibers are fast twitch (white) or type II. The proportion of these fibers is genetically determined, and high-performance endurance athletes typically have a higher proportion of type I fibers. Sprinters, speed skaters, and other high-intensity, short-duration athletes usually have a higher proportion of type II fibers.

B. Muscle Contraction—Muscle contraction can be concentric or eccentric. Concentric muscle contraction results in muscle shortening; eccentric muscle action results in lengthening. Eccentric muscle action is important in dampening the forces across joints and is an essential part of preseason conditioning and training.

C. Strength Training—Although the distribution of type I and type II muscle fibers is predetermined, changes in training can alter the selective recruitment and can result in enlargement of specific muscle fiber types. Training for endurance sports consists of decreased tension and increased repetitions, which help increase the efficiency of type I fibers and increase the numbers of mitochondria, the capillary density, and the oxidative capacity. Training for strength/sprint sports consists of increasing tension and decreasing repetitions, leading to an increased number of myofibrils/fiber and selective hypertrophy of type II fibers. Either form of training slows the increase of lactate in response to exercise. Strength training includes isometric, isotonic, isokinetic, and functional exercises.

1. Isometric Exercise—Isometric exercise involves the development of tension within a muscle without a change in fiber length. Isometric contractions are usually performed against an immovable object. This form of training can result in muscle hypertrophy but not endurance. Strength gains are also specific to the joint angle at which the exercises are performed and do not improve motor performance.

2. Isotonic Exercise—This involves movement of weights at a constant resistance through an arc of motion. These exercises can be done concentrically or eccentrically, and resistance can be static (free weights) or variable (e.g., with Nautilus equipment). This type of training uses progressive resistance exercise. An amount of weight selected for training is based on the maximum amount that can be moved through a range of motion not to exceed 10 repetitions. The advantage of isotonic exercise is that it allows improved motor performance and feedback. However, it is difficult to load the muscle maximally through the entire arc of motion.

3. Isokinetic Exercise—This form of exercise is performed at a constant velocity with variable resistance throughout the range of motion. The muscle group is placed under uniform tension, and resistance occurs in proportion to the force applied throughout the entire range of motion. Advantages of isokinetic training include a lack of muscle soreness, great increases in strength throughout the entire arc of motion, enhanced motor performance, and decreased workout time. Disadvantages include the cost of equipment (e.g., Cybex), difficulty in assessing the effort made, and lack of positive feedback. Additionally, isotonic exercises are nonphysiologic and may cause patellofemoral pain.

4. Functional Exercises—These exercises restore strength and agility through dynamic movements and tend to be sport specific. Jump ropes, agility drills, and indoor sports can be used for rehabilitation. Closed-chain activities including Stairmaster, leg presses, and stationary cycling are an important part of this program. These exercises are easily performed and allow quick return to competition.

D. Stretching—Stretching has several effects, including increasing elasticity of connective tissue, motor nerve conduction velocity, range of motion, and flexibility. It also promotes better relaxation and improved fast isometric force development. It helps to prevent injury and improve performance, range of motion, and function. Types of stretching include ballistic, static, passive, and proprioceptive neuromuscular facilitation. Tension in muscle has active components (mediated by reflex activity) and passive components (connective tissue). The viscoelastic properties of the muscle-tendon unit are responsible for the increased length with stretching. When muscle is held at a higher tension, time-dependent stress-relaxation occurs to decrease the tension, as does an increase in length. With repetitive cyclic and static stretching, greater peak tensions and greater energy absorption occur at faster stretch rates. Recent studies have confirmed that more force is required to tear a muscle that is warm and stretched as compared to a cold, tight muscle-tendon unit.

V. Female Athletes
   A. Amenorrhea—Both primary amenorrhea (delay of menarche past the age of 16 years) and secondary amenorrhea (cessation of periods for more than 3 consecutive months) are common in female athletes. Some authorities suggest that amenorrhea is related to a body fat percentage falling below the threshold necessary for normal menstruation. Others suggest that it is stress related. Problems associated with amenorrhea include osteoporosis and stress fractures. Adequate calcium intake, alterations in training, and proper weight maintenance usually restore normal menstruation. Birth control pills are also useful in the treatment of selected female athletes with this problem.
   B. Orthopaedic Problems—Certain orthopaedic conditions appear to be more common in women. Patellofemoral syndrome, stress fractures, certain foot disorders, and anterior cruciate ligament injuries have an increased incidence in women. Patellofemoral problems in women may be related to a wider pelvis, greater valgus angles of the knees, increased femoral anteversion, and a less developed vastus medialis obliquus portion of the quadriceps. Stress fractures in women may be related to conditioning or to hormonal abnormalities. Foot disorders may be related to shoe wear or the stress of certain activities (e.g., ballet). The higher incidence of anterior cruciate ligament tears in women athletes may be related to ligamentous laxity, lack of sufficient strength of the dynamic restraints, or relative notch stenosis compared with their male counterparts.

Selected References

Ergogenic Drugs

Aronson V. Protein and miscellaneous ergogenic aids. Physician Sportsmed 14:209–212, 1986.

Bahrke MS, Wright JE, Strauss RH, Catlin DH. Psychological moods and subjectively perceived behavioral and somatic changes accompanying anabolic-androgenic steroid use. Am J Sports Med 20:717–724.

Brien AJ, Simon TL. The effects of red blood cell infusion on 10-km race time. JAMA 257:2761, 1987.

Cowart VS. Human growth hormone: the latest ergogenic aid? Physician Sportsmed 16:175, 1988.

Coyle EF. Ergogenic aids. Clin Sports Med 3:731–742, 1984.

Haupt HA. Anabolic steroids and growth hormone. Current concepts. Am J Sports Med 21:468–474, 1993.

Perlmutter G, Lowenthal DT. Use of anabolic steroids by athletes. Am Fam Physician 32:208, 1985.

Pope HG, Katz DL, Champoux R. Anabolic-androgenic steroid use among 1,010 college men. Physician Sportsmed 16:75, 1988.

Robinson JB. Ergogenic drugs in sports. In DeLee JC, Drez D Jr (eds). *Orthopaedic Sports Medicine.* Philadelphia: WB Saunders, 1994, pp 294–306.

Sawka MN. Erythrocyte reinfusion and maximal aerobic power: an examination of modifying factors. JAMA 257:1496, 1987.

Sudden Cardiac Death

Alpert SA. Athletic heart syndrome. Physician Sportsmed 12:103–107, 1989.

Braden DS, Strong WB. Preparticipation screening for sudden cardiac death in high school and college athletes. Physician Sportsmed 16:128–140, 1988.

Epstein SE, Maron BJ. Sudden death and the competitive athlete: perspectives on preparticipation screening studies. J Am Coll Cardiol 7:220–230, 1986.

Finney TP, D'Ambrosia RD. Sudden cardiac death in an athlete. In DeLee JC, Drez D Jr (eds). *Orthopaedic Sports Medicine.* Philadelphia: WB Saunders 1994, pp 404–416.

James TN, Froggatt P, Marshall TK. Sudden death in young athletes. Ann Intern Med 67:1013–1021, 1967.

Maron BJ, Epstein SE, Roberts WC. Causes of sudden death in competitive athletes. J Am Coll Cardiol 7:204–214, 1986.

Maron BJ, Roberts WC, McAllister HA, et al. Sudden death in young athletes. Circulation 62:218–219, 1980.

Van Camp SP. Exercise-related sudden deaths: risks and causes. Physician Sportsmed 16:97–112, 1988.

Exercise Physiology

Fleck SJ, Schutt RC. Types of strength training. Clin Sports Med 4:159–168, 1985.

Katch FI, Drumm SS. Effects of different modes of strength training on body compostion and arthropometry. Clin Sports Med 5:413–459, 1986.

Paulos LE, Grauer JD. Exercise. In Delee JC, Drez D Jr (eds). *Orthopaedic Sports Medicine: Principles and Practice.* Philadelphia: WB Saunders, 1994, pp 228–243.

Pipes TV. Isokinetic vs isotonic strength training in adult men. Med Sci Sports 7:262–274, 1975.

Taylor DC, Dalton JD, Seaber AV, et al. Viscoelastic properties of muscle-tendon units: the biomechanical effects of stretching. Am J Sports Med 18:300–309, 1990.

Yamamoto SK, Hartman CW, Feagin JA, Kimball G. Functional rehabilitation of the knee: a preliminary study. J Sports Med 3:228–291, 1976.

Female Athletes

Barrow G, Saha S. Menstrual irregularity and stress fractures in collegiate female distance runners. Am J Sports Med 16:209–215, 1988.

Clarke K, Buckley W. Women's injuries in collegiate sports. Am J Sports Med 8:187–191, 1980.

Cox J, Lenz H. Women in sports: the Naval Academy experience. Am J Sports Med 7:355–357, 1979.

Eisenberg T, Allen W. Injuries in a women's varsity athletic program. Physician Sportsmed 6:112–116, 1978.

Hunter L, Andrews J, Clancy W, Funk F. Common orthopaedic problems of the female athlete. Instr Course Lect 31:126–152, 1982.

Powers J. Characteristic features of injuries in the knee in women. Clin Orthop 143:120–124, 1979.

Protzman R. Physiologic performance of women compared to men. Observations of cadets at the United States Military Academy. Am J Sports Med 7:191–194, 1979.

Whiteside P. Men's and women's injuries in comparable sports. Physician Sportsmed 8:130–140, 1980.

Index